MEDICAL COLLEGE OF PENNSYLVANIA
AND HAHNEMANN UNIVERSITY
MOORE LIBRARY, EAST FALLS

DREXEL UNIVERSITY
HEALTH SCIENCES LIBRARIES
HAHNEMANN LIBRARY

Case Studies in Emergency Medicine and the Health of the Public

Edward Bernstein, MD, FACEP

Vice Chair for Academic Affairs, Department of Emergency Medicine and
Associate Professor of Emergency Medicine and Public Health
Boston University School of Medicine and School of Public Health
Attending Physician, Boston City Hospital and BU Medical Center

Judith Bernstein, RNC, PhD

National Policy and Resource Center on Women and Aging
Heller School, Brandeis University

D0140627

Jones and Bartlett Publishers
Sudbury, Massachusetts

Boston   London   Singapore

WB
105
C337
1996

Editorial, Sales, and Customer Service Offices

Jones and Bartlett Publishers
40 Tall Pine Drive
Sudbury, MA 01776
1-800-832-0034
1-508-443-5000

Jones and Bartlett International
Barb House, Barb Mews
London W6 7PA
UK

Library of Congress Cataloging-in-Publication Data

Case studies in emergency medicine and the health of the public /
  [edited by] Edward Bernstein, Judith Bernstein.
      p. cm.
    ISBN 0-7637-0029-0. — ISBN (invalid) 08672000290
    1. Emergency medical services—Case studies. I. Bernstein,
Edward, (date)
    [DNLM: 1. Emergencies—case studies. 2. Emergencies Medical
Services—United States. 3. Community Health Services—United
States. WB 105 C337 1996]
  RA645.5.C37 1996
  362.1'8'0973—dc20
  DNLM/DLC
  for Library of Congress   96-1930
                                                    CIP

Copyright © 1996 by Jones and Bartlett Publishers, Inc.

All rights reserved. No part of the material protected by this copyright notice may be
reproduced or utilized in any form, electronic or mechanical, including photocopying,
recording, or by any information storage and retrieval system, without written permission
from the copyright owner.

Acquisitions Editor: Jan Wall
Production Administrator: Anne S. Noonan
Senior Manufacturing Buyer: Dana L. Cerrito
Editorial Production Service: WordCrafters Editorial Services, Inc.
Typesetting: WordCrafters Editorial Services, Inc.
Cover Design: Marshall Henrichs
Printing and Binding: Braun-Brumfield
Cover Printing: John P. Pow Company

Printed in the United States of America

99 98 97 96   10 9 8 7 6 5 4 3 2 1

Contents

OCT 0 9 1996

Foreword

Never again will one person be able to encompass all knowledge. Specialization is necessary, important for practitioners, essential for the care of a patient, and crucial in the development of an area of knowledge or expertise. But with specialization comes new interdependence. The best specialists have broad vision. They see where their skills fit in; they retain an interest in the global view; and they benefit from exposure to other perspectives, problems, and talents.

Two decades ago the juxtaposition of emergency medicine and public health would have seemed unreasonable. Now it is an obvious match. From food poisoning to violence, to tobacco and mental health, or even environmental exposures and health promotion, *Case Studies in Emergency Medicine and the Health of the Public* clarifies what these fields have in common and, more important, how emergency physicians can have maximum impact on the health of the public. Attention to community health needs requires an involvement with the emergency department and, at the same time, responsibility for the health of the community. Therefore, both specialties will find value in the lessons presented in this book.

Grand rounds often start with the presenting complaint in the emergency department and proceed to the pathology involved. In too few cases, in prior decades, did grand rounds actually extend to the questions of how that visit could have been prevented. What were the community risk factors involved? What was the response from the hospital to the community as a result of this patient? And how did the emergency department's actions impact on public health? In this textbook, multiple case studies

provide that kind of comprehensive approach to the total picture of community and emergency department responsibilities.

It is currently the case that a substantial percentage of the population uses the emergency department as the source of routine care. As Lewis Goldfrank points out, awareness of a community outbreak of measles alerts emergency department personnel to the need for determining immunization status.[1] He notes the great discrepancy between what people judge to be the immunization protection level of their children and what the records show. Recent studies have shown that a major factor in suboptimal immunization in the United States is the belief by both parents and providers that children are already immunized when they are not. To have a tracking system for immunization coverage that links emergency departments, hospitals, clinics, and private offices and that could, with each admission, automatically show the patient's immunization experience, is just one example of how emergency departments could be better served by public health departments and, in turn, better serve the health of the public.

Likewise, as Kellermann points out, since emergency departments have continuous exposure to social problems as well as impressive credentials in detecting emerging trends in injuries, disease outbreaks, drug abuse, and access to care problems, it

---

1. Goldfrank LR, Emergency Medicine, *JAMA*, June 7, 1995, Vol. 273, No. 21.

becomes imperative for health departments to utilize this experience in ongoing surveillance activities.[2] In this day of electronic communication, there are few obstacles to this goal.

The time has come to enhance specialized attention to both emergency conditions and public health conditions. An improvement in both is possible through deliberate collaborative action. This textbook is an important step in recognizing this interdependence and suggesting areas for improvement.

William H. Foege, MD
Health Fellow, Carter Center
Atlanta, Georgia

---

2. Kellermann, AL. *What Is Clinical Emergency Medicine? The Role of Emergency Medicine in the Future of American Medical Care*, Josiah Macy, Jr. Foundation, New York, NY, 1995.

Introduction

This textbook is intended to expose health care practitioners to the public health aspects of acute medical illness and trauma, and to the challenging practice of emergency medicine. It also offers emergency medicine residents, nurses, EMTs, social workers, and physicians a more systematic and holistic approach with which to address patients' medical and personal problems. Public health students and researchers will find that the cases bring population-based epidemiological data to life and add personal meaning. For all groups, the book should generate ideas for collaboration.

Case Studies in Emergency Medicine and the Health of the Public is not a laundry list of problems, although the textbook identifies and analyzes the social reality and public nature of personal and medical problems seen in the emergency department. This textbook offers answers to the difficult problems facing emergency physicians and provides an array of useful public health approaches, clinical knowledge and skills, and models of protocols, preventive patient education, and public advocacy.

Fifty-eight contributors participated in the writing of these 32 chapters, representing the collaboration of diverse practitioners in our field: physicians, nurses, social workers, health educators and policy experts, MPHs and PhDs, women and minorities. Contributions represent both the public and private sector from around the country.

Each chapter is organized around one or more case studies from everyday practice. Several key questions are raised and discussed as each case progresses. The particular cases are followed by more general remarks addressing the public health aspects of the case and the specific role of emergency medicine. The scope of the teaching cases encompasses the needs of the diverse populations seen in the ED: infectious disease spread; alcohol, tobacco and other drugs of abuse; violence throughout the life cycle; and injury and environmental and occupational hazards. Changes are proposed for the ED medical encounter and interview, and examples are given for the emergency practitioner's role in public health, patient education, public policy, and health care delivery. Several model programs of ED-based preventive interventions are also presented as case studies.

Case Studies in Emergency Medicine and the Health of the Public is, at present, the only textbook of its kind, and fills a very real need. The cases come from everyday practice. The practicing physician on a busy shift sees many patients with public health problems: a group of wedding guests from out of state who ate Caesar salad dressing made from raw eggs 12 hours ago and now have severe abdominal cramps and diarrhea; a young male with a large scalp laceration who was hit over the head with baseball bat, has old scars on his chest from a previous stab wound, and talks of getting even while being sutured; an unrestrained intoxicated driver with head trauma and broken teeth; a patient with serious asthma who continues to smoke; and a woman with vaginal bleeding. In the midst of all these public health emergencies, the physician may also be called upon to console a rape victim and collect evidence properly. It is not difficult to imagine that these problems may be challenging and extremely frustrating to emergency physicians, who have limited time and counseling skill, yet know that a social worker is only available on weekdays between 9:00 A.M. and 5:00 P.M. Long patient waiting times, overcrowding, delays in admission, and a scarcity of resources and funding are not uncommon problems facing the emergency physician and threatening the basic health care support (the ED as safety net) that the public expects as a minimum from the health care system.

Emergency medicine is strategically placed for a public health role; it sits at the hub of the health care delivery system, connecting hospital and community, specialized inpatient and primary ambulatory services, and the prehospital and intensive care units. Approximately 25,000 physicians in 5,000 EDs see 100 million patients and interact with several hundred thousand health care providers. In addition, over 112 emergency medicine residency programs and 50 academic departments of EM are involved in teaching tens of thousands of medical students and residents who rotate through the department from other services, as well as emergency medicine residents. At this critical juncture in the health care "revolution," there is a public need to understand the place of emergency medicine in providing quality health care to the entire population.

The failure to develop a comprehensive national health plan has switched focus to the states, where rapid changes in health care financing and delivery are taking place. The U.S. has become a vast laboratory for testing a myriad of plans and options. Much of this momentum is positive, but there is potential for reforms driven by market forces to overlook the needs of a variety of population groups. In the decade to come, millions of people will lack insurance altogether, and millions more may find their access to prompt and user-friendly medical attention restricted. Managed care organizations may initially take the short-term view that ED care is costly and may not perceive the long-term cost-saving and humanitarian benefits of the safety net that emergency medicine provides. Reimbursement may be cut, but ED census and complexity of diagnostic problems and patient mix will most likely increase. We will be taking care of sicker patients for longer,

as observation units are integrated into our practice. Clinicians, administrators, and policy makers must be convinced of the need to assure adequate resources, funding, reimbursement, training, and support for health care provided in the ED.

Emergency medicine is in flux. It has traveled a long road from its historical roots as a trauma specialty, developed in the 1960s in response to public concern that soldiers wounded on the battlefield in Vietnam had a better chance of survival than did the injured on our nation's highways. Along with EMS system funding came support and recognition for emergency medicine as an acute care specialty. Over the course of the last 25 years, a recognized speciality has evolved and broadened its base of activities. Organized emergency medicine began to respond to public health issues in the mid 1980s when chapters of the American College of Emergency Medicine lobbied their state legislatures and participated in public education campaigns to change attitudes toward use of seatbelts and toward drinking and driving and to enact legislation to change behavior. More recently, many chapters have programs to reduce societal violence and improve the care of victims. As a result of this growing movement, the Society of Academic Emergency Medicine established a Public Health and Education Committee in 1991 with the charge to develop a position paper entitled *A Public Health Approach to Emergency Medicine: Preparing for the Twenty-First Century*. The position paper and its recommendations (reprinted as Chapter 1), with an original draft of more than 60 pages, is the foundation for the present textbook. Today, public health issues are well represented in our journals and national meetings, and even that part of our discipline that is crisis-oriented—advanced trauma life support and advanced cardiac life support—includes prevention as an important link in the survival chain.

This book is a beginning, a first step in preparing ourselves for health care in the twenty-first century. Attention to the public health context will bring benefits to both practitioners and patients. There is no natural barrier between personal troubles, social problems, and medical illnesses. *Case Studies in Emergency Medicine and the Health of the Public* makes clear how medical and personal problems have their origin in public health and societal problems; and, conversely, how the ill health of individuals can affect the larger population. Our patients come from communities and return to those communities. Emergency physicians, in a real sense, have their fingers on the pulse of their patients and the pulse of the community. Breaking down artificial barriers will improve outcomes, lower the long-run costs of health care, and make the practice of medicine more compassionate and satisfying.

Edward Bernstein, MD
Judith Bernstein, PhD

List of Contributors

Deirdre Anglin, MD
Assistant Professor of Emergency Medicine
Los Angeles County University of Southern
    California Medicine Center
Los Angeles, California

L. Kristian Arnold, MD, FACEP
Assistant Clinical Professor of Emergency
    Medicine
Boston University School of Medicine
Boston, Massachusetts

Renate Austin, MD
Former Assistant Residency Director and Assistant
    Clinical Professor of Emergency Medicine,
    Boston University Medical School
Attending Boston City Hospital and Boston
    University Medical Center
Boston, Massachusetts

Diane Barry, Program Manager
CSAT Demonstration Grant: Project ASSERT
Department of Emergency Medicine
Boston City Hopsital
Boston, Massachusetts

Jay M. Baruch, MD
Emergency Medical Services
Department of Emergency Medicine
Bellevue Hospital Center
New York, New York

Edward Bernstein, MD, FACEP
Associate Professor of Emergency Medicine and
    Public Health
Boston University Medical School and School of
    Public Health
Attending Physician, Boston City Hospital and BU
    Medical Center and Vice-Chair for Academic
    Affairs, BUSM
Boston, Massachusetts

Erica D. Bernstein
Certified HIV Testing Counselor
MD/PhD Student, Medical College of
    Pennsylvania and Hahnemann University
Philadelphia, Pennsylvania

Judith Bernstein, RNC, PhD
National Policy and Resource Center on Women &
    Aging
Heller School, Brandeis University
Waltham, Massachusetts

Jeffrey Brubacher, MD, MSc
Fellow in Medical Toxicology
Bellevue Hospital Center
New York, New York

Geraldine Burton, Health Promotion Advocate
CSAT Demonstration Grant: Project ASSERT
Department of Emergency Medicine
Boston City Hopsital
Boston, Massachusetts

E. Martin Caravati, MD, MPH
Associate Professor
Division of Emergency Medicine
University of Utah Health Sciences Center
Salt Lake City, Utah

Miriam Cotler, PhD
Professor, Health Sciences
California State University
Northridge, California

Mark Davis
President, Live Save Medical, Inc.
Boston, Massachusetts

Gail D'Onofrio, MD
Residency Director and Assistant Professor
Department of Emergency Medicine, Boston
    University Medical School
Attending Physician, Boston City Hospital and BU
    Medical Center
Boston, Massachusetts

Lily Dow, BS, MPA
Executive Director
Adolescent Social Action Program
Department of Family and Community
    Medicine
University of New Mexico School of Medicine
Albuquerque, New Mexico

Judith Dyson-Mounds, Supervisor
CSAT Demonstration Grant, Project ASSERT
Department of Emergency Medicine
Boston City Hospital
Boston, Massachusetts

Carlos R. Flores, MD, FACEP
Asssitant Director
Emergency Medicine Services
New York University Hospital
New York, New York

Eric S. Freedland MD, FACEP
CEO, Live Save Medical, Inc.
Assistant Clinical Professor
Department of Emergency Medicine
Boston University Medical School
Boston, Massachusetts

Richard M. Goldberg, MD, FACEP
Associate Professor of Emergency Medicine
Research Coordinator
Department of Emergency Medicine
Los Angeles County–University of Southern
    California
School of Medicine
Los Angeles, California

Lewis R. Goldfrank, MD, FACP, FACEP, ABMT
Director of Emergency Medical Services
Bellevue Hospital Center and New York
    University Medical Center
Associate Professor of Clinical Medicine
New York University School of Medicine
New York, New York

Robert M. Gougelet, MD
Assistant Professor
Department of Emergency Medicine
University of New Mexico School of Medicine
Albuquerque, New Mexico

Stephen W. Hargarten, MD, MPH, FACEP
Associate Professor and Interim Chairman
Department of Emergency Medicine
Medical College of Wisconsin
Madison, Wisconsin

Barbara Herbert, MD
Attending Physician
Department of Emergency Medicine
Boston City Hospital
Boston, Massachusetts

Rick Hayne, RN, PhD
Emergency Department
St. Joseph Medical Center
Burbank, California

Kathleen Higgins, RN
Emergency Department
Boston University Medical Center
Boston, Massachusetts

Elizabeth Holliger, MD
Center for Injury Control
Rollins School of Public Health and the Division of
    Emergency Medicine, Department of Surgery
Emory University School of Medicine
Atlanta, Georgia

Anita L. Hurtig, PhD
Director, Psychosocial Clinic and Clinical Associate
    Professor
Division of General and Emergency Pediatrics
University of Illinois
Chicago, Illinois

Jeffrey S. Jones, MD, FACEP
Associate Professor of Medicine
Michigan State University College of Human
    Medicine
Research Director, Department of Emergency
    Medicine
Butterworth Hospital
Grand Rapids, Michigan

Norman D. Kalbfleisch, MD, FACEP
Assistant Professor of Emergency Medicine
Oregon Health Sciences University
Portland, Oregon

Laura E. Kaufman, MA
Executive Director, Boston Women's Fund
Boston, Massachusetts

Arthur L. Kellermann, MD, MPH, FACEP
Associate Professor and Director Center for Injury
    Control
Rollins School of Public Health and the Division
    of Emergency Medicine, Department of
    Surgery
Emory University School of Medicine
Atlanta, Georgia

Thomas D. Kirsch, MD, MPH, FACEP
Assistant Professor, Emergency Medicine
Johns Hopkins University School of Medicine
Baltimore, Maryland

Alison Lane-Reticker, MD, FACEP
Director of Emergency Medicine
St. Francis Hospital and Medical Center
Hartford, Connecticut

David L. Levine, MD
Chief Resident Department of Emergency
    Medicine
Boston City Hospital and Boston University
    Medical Center
Boston, Massachusetts

Judith A. Linden, MD
Attending Physician
Boston City Hospital and Boston University
    Medical Center Department of Emergency
    Medicine
Boston University Medical School
Boston, Massachusetts

John F. Marcinak, MD
Associate Professor
Dept. of General and Emergency Pediatrics and
    Infectious Diseases
University of Illinois at Chicago
Chicago, Illinois

Richard M. McDowell, MD, FACEP
Chairman, Department of Emergency Medicine
Crozer Chester Medical Center
Philadelphia, Pennsylvania

Don Wesley Mounds
Director, Project Directions
Department of Emergency Medicine
Boston City Hospital
Boston, Massachusetts

Peter H. Moyer, MD, FACEP
Chairman, Department of Emergency Medicine
Associate Professor of Emergency Medicine
Boston University Medical School
Boston, Massachusetts

Susan Payne, PhD, Program Evaluator
CSAT Demonstration Grant: Project ASSERT,
    formerly
Associate Professor, Health Services Department
Boston University Medical School, School of Public
    Health
Boston, Massachusetts

Mark D. Pearlmutter, MD, FACEP
Assistant Professor of Medicine
Tufts University School of Medicine
Chief Department of Emergency Medicine
St. Elizabeth's Hospital
Boston, Massachusetts

Kyran P. Quinlan, MD
Assistant Professor of Pediatrics
Division of Pediatrics
University of Chicago
Chicago, Illinois

Niels K. Rathlev, MD, FACEP
Director, Emergency Department
Carney Hospital
Associate Professor of Emergency Medicine
Boston University School of Medicine
Boston, Massachusetts

Stephen Rollnick, PhD
Principal Clinical Psychologist
Department of Clinical Psychology
Whitchurch Hospital
Cardiff, Wales

Steven Rosenzweig, MD
Clinical Assistant Professor
Division of Emergency Medicine
Department of Surgery
Jefferson Medical College
Philadelphia, Pennsylvannia

Elaine W. Rousseau, PhD
Director of Research
Arizona Center on Aging
University of Arizona Health Sciences Center
Tucson, Arizona

Arthur B. Sanders MD, FACEP, FACP
Professor of Emergency Medicine
University of Arizona College of Medicine
Attending Physician
University of Arizona Health Sciences Center
Tucson, Arizona

Kenneth Savage
Live Save Medical, Inc.
Boston, Massachusetts

Carol Jack Scott, MD, MSEd.
Principal and Consultant, The Medical Education
    Group, Inc.
Clinical Assistant Professor
Department of Emergency Medicine
University of Maryland Medical Center
Baltimore, Maryland

Kim Seawright
CSAT Demonstration Grant, Project ASSERT
Department of Emergency Medicine
Boston City Hospital
Boston, Massachusetts

Todd Stanley, BS
CSAT Demonstration Grant, Project ASSERT
Department of Emergency Medicine
Boston City Hospital
Boston, Massachusetts

Brent Stevenson, Health Promotion Advocate
CSAT Demonstration Grant, Project ASSERT
Department of Emergency Medicine
Boston City Hospital
Boston, Massachusetts

Donna Sue, MD
Resident, Emergency Medicine
Johns Hopkins University School of Medicine
Baltimore, Maryland

Michael Tarmey, RN, MS
Director of Nursing
Heritage Hospital
Somerville, Massachusetts

Roosevelt Travnitz, MSW, LCSW
Emergency Department
St. Joseph Medical Center
Burbank, California

Nina B. Wallerstein, PhD
Associate Professor of Family and Community
    Medicine
University of New Mexico School of
    Medicine
Albuquerque New Mexico

Stephen P. Waxman, MD, FACEP
Clinical Assistant Professor of Medicine
New York University Medical School
New York , New York

Jocelyn C. White, MD
Assistant Clinical Professor
Oregon Health Sciences University
Legacy Good Samaritan Hospital
Portland, Oregon

Unit I

Emergency Medicine and Public Health

1

Introduction to "A Public Health Approach to Emergency Medicine"

THOMAS KIRSCH

WHY CONSIDER A PUBLIC HEALTH APPROACH TO EMERGENCY MEDICINE?

Public health has been defined as

> One of the efforts organized by society to protect, promote and restore the people's health. It is . . . directed to the maintenance and improvement of health of all the people through collective or social action. The programs, services and institutions involved emphasize the prevention of disease and the health needs of the population as a whole. The goals are . . . to reduce the amount of disease, premature death and disease-produced discomfort and disability in the population.[1]

Superficially, there are few similarities between the perceived excitement and action of emergency medicine and the more bureaucratic measures of public health. Emergency medicine (EM) deals with the individual patient; public health (PH) with whole populations. EM is curative; public health preventive. In reality, there are many related areas because of EM's unique position in the medical world. EM acts as the interface between the community and the health care system and between specialized inpatient care and primary care. EM has also become the safety net for persons without insurance or other means of access to medical care, and this situation has resulted in emergency department overcrowding and delayed care, especially in poor urban areas.[2] Because EDs are often the source of primary care for socioeconomically depressed populations, emergency care physicians have become more aware of the health problems of vulnerable populations and, consequently, many have become more interested in prevention. Substance abuse, infectious diseases, environmental health, and even issues such as immunizations have become the concerns of EPs.

A Brief History of Public Health

Both public health and emergency medicine have historic links to the military. Early sanitation efforts started in army camps, because until World War I the majority of deaths in wartime occurred as a result of disease, not fighting.[3] Advances in field care during the Korean and Vietnam wars provided opportunities for the development of the emergency and trauma care system in the U.S. President Johnson noted that more people were dying on the highways from motor vehicle trauma each year than in Vietnam.

Since antiquity and until relatively recently, public health measures were the only successful health interventions. It was not until the development of vaccines and antibiotics in the twentieth century that curative medical practices began to have any significant impact on diseases.[4] Ancient history has many references to public health practice. Restrictions from eating certain foods and laws governing food preparation in the Old Testament were a response to the problems of food-borne infections. Even some epidemiologic methods were described in the Old

3

Testament and by Hippocrates.[5] Early public health efforts focused mostly on sanitation. The Romans built massive aqueducts and sewer systems to provide clean water and handle wastes. Efforts were also made to prevent or control epidemics through the use of quarantine and proper disposal of the dead.

Few real public or curative health advances were made during the Middle Ages. In the late seventeenth and early eighteenth centuries, the theoretical and mathematic basis for public health and epidemiology was developed. However, the great blossoming of both curative and public health didn't begin until about 150 years ago with the proof and widespread acceptance of the germ theory. For the first time, medicine was based on scientific studies rather than on theory and personal observation. At the same time, with the proof of disease transmission by microorganism, public health had a specific target for intervention and both specialties had a common enemy: the pathologic microorganism.

During the same time period, improved sanitation and personal hygiene began having a major impact on infectious diseases in the industrializing countries. Epidemiology also developed into a practical, and not just theoretical, field. Perhaps the most famous public health practitioner was John Snow of Great Britain, who used epidemiologic reasoning to identify the source of a cholera outbreak in London in 1854. His intervention to prevent access to the contaminated water and effectively end transmission was a resounding proof of the success of public health efforts. John Snow mapped out the neighborhoods where there were cholera deaths and observed the cluster of deaths around London's Broad Street Pump. He simply turned the handle off the pump to literally end the epidemic. By the late 1890s, medicine was also making a difference in health, primarily through its contributions to public hygiene.[3]

With the laissez-faire attitude of the United States government at the time, public health was initially seen as a function of private physicians. Gradually, near the end of the nineteenth century, the field of professional public health began on the East Coast with the establishment of municipal public health agencies in Providence, Rhode Island, Boston, and New York City. This led to the establishment of state public health agencies and, finally, to the creation of the Department of Health and Human Services in the early 1900s.

Issues Common to Public Health and Emergency Medicine

The issues that EM and public health share in common are numerous and varied. The most obvious area of mutual interest is in injury control, because it is in emergency departments that injuries are primarily treated. As a result, collaboration between EPs and PH practitioners in the prevention of injuries and interpersonal violence has gradually developed. EDs are also a common site for the treatment of infectious diseases, particularly sexually transmitted diseases, AIDs, and respiratory and gastrointestinal infections. More recently, the resurgence of tuberculosis has led to great concern about the potential of disease transmission in EDs.[6] Substance abuse, including abuse of alcohol, drugs, and cigarettes, is a common primary or secondary reason for ED visits. In treating an acute COPD exacerbation, caring for an intoxicated trauma patient or intubating a patient apneic from narcotic use, substance abuse accounts for a large percent of ED visits. Health for underserved populations and minority health are obvious concerns of EM, since it is these populations which turn to the ED for their primary care. Toxicology is commonly considered a subspecialty of emergency medicine, but is also a branch of the public health field of environmental health. This specialty includes not only poisoning, but also health problems related to heat and cold and to industrial toxins. The ED is also an excellent potential site for the surveillance of infectious diseases and injuries because of the large populations it serves. Finally, because some EPs are, by default, primary care physicians there has been discussion in the literature of the benefits of providing immunizations and other preventive services in the ED.[7,8] It is often to the ED that patients turn when what was once a preventable health problem requires curative care.[9-11] Obviously, EM cannot solve all of the health problems of the U.S. However, with a concerted effort targeting a specific problem, the specialty can have a greater impact on the health of our society than by only providing curative care.[12]

Constraints

The extent to which EM can support the public health system and provide preventive services is limited by both how the specialty of emergency medicine defines its mission and by the financial and resource constraints placed on it by society. EDs can be an expensive source of care. Their high patient volume and the diverse problems that patients present also limit the time available for additional interventions. Probably the greatest constraint is purely financial: EPs are not reimbursed for the preventive services that they may want to provide. With the increasing influence of HMOs and the ongoing potential for health care reform at the state level, it is unclear whether managed care will create incentives for preventive services. What EPs can accomplish in filling in the gaps in the public health system must be either within the context of their current clinical mandate or additional funding and resources must be provided by the health care system for new services.

The Society of Academic Emergency Medicine (SAEM) position paper, *A Public Health Approach to Emergency Medicine*, was adopted in 1994. It represents an important milestone in that it attempts to broaden the scope and paradigm that currently influences the practice of emergency medicine. It provides background materials, recommendations, and a vision for the emergency physician's role in primary and secondary prevention, professional education, research, and ED-based surveillance. It is also the foundation and impetus for this book, *Case Studies in Emergency Medicine and the Health of the Public.*[13]

NOTES

1. Last JM, *A dictionary of epidemiology*, 2nd ed. New York: Oxford University Press, 1988, p. 107.

2. United States General Accounting Office. *Emergency departments: Unevenly affected by growth and change in patient use.* Washington, DC: Government Printing Office, 1993.

3. Dolan JP, Adams-Smith WN. *Health and society: A documentary history of medicine.* New York: Seabury Press, 1978.

4. Starr P. *The social transformation of American medicine.* New York: Basic Books, Inc., 1982, p. 138.

5. Lilienfeld AM, Lilienfeld DE. *Foundations of epidemiology*, 2nd ed. New York: Oxford Univ. Press, 1980.

6. Barnes, PF, Bloch AB, Davidson PT, Snider DE Jr. Tuberculosis in patients with human immunodeficiency virus infection. *N Eng J Med* 1991; 324: 1644–1650.

7. Polis MA, Davey VT, Collins ED, et al. The emergency department as part of a successful strategy for increasing immunization. *Ann Emerg Med* 1988; 17: 1016–18.

8. Rodenwald LE, Szilagyi PG, Humistan SG, et al. Is the emergency department visit a marker for undervaccination? *Pediatrics* 1993; 91:605–11.

9. Center for Disease Control. Tuberculosis morbidity, 1992. *MMWR* 1993; 42:363.

10. Centers for Disease Control. Measles, United States, 1992. *MMWR* 1993; 42:378–81.

11. Centers for Disease Control. Measles vacccination levels among selected groups of pre-school-aged children, United States, 1990. *MMWR* 1991; 40:36–9.

12. Institute of Medicine. *The future of public health.* Washington, DC: National Academy Press, 1988.

13. Bernstein E, Goldfrank LR, Kellerman AL, et al. A public health approach to emergency medicine: Preparing for the 21st century. *Acad Emerg Med* 1994: 1(3):277–86.

A PUBLIC HEALTH APPROACH
TO EMERGENCY MEDICINE:
Preparing For The Twenty-first Century

Position Paper of the Society for Academic Emergency Medicine

ABSTRACT

This [chapter] focuses on the implications of an inadequate public health/preventive health care system for Emergency Medicine (EM), the role that EM providers can play in remedying critical health problems, and the benefits gained from a public health approach to EM. A broad definition of public health is adopted, suggesting shared goals of both public health and EM. Critical problems posed for EM include alcohol, tobacco, and other drug abuse; injury; violence; sexually transmitted diseases and the human immunodeficiency virus (HIV) infection; occupational and environmental exposures; and the unmet health needs of minorities and women. A blueprint for future merging of public health issues with EM is presented which includes the application of public health principles to (1) clinical practice, (2) public education, community involvement, and public policy advocacy, (3) development of medical school and residency public health/prevention curricula and teaching methods, and (4) research opportunities and surveillance. Finally, recommendations are proposed that require restructuring the present health care system to provide resources, incentives, and organizational changes that promote an integration of public health and preventive services in the practice of EM.

Bernstein, Edward, M.D.; Goldfrank, Lewis R, M.D.; Kellermann, Arthur L, M.D., M.P.H.; Hargarten, Stephen W, M.D., M.P.H.; Jui, Jonathon, M.D.; Fish, Susan S, Pharm. D., M.P.H.; Herbert, Barbara H, M.D.; Flores, Carlos, M.D.; Caravati, Martin E, M.D., M.P.H.; Krishel, Scott, M.D.; Stevens, Carl D, M.D., M.P.H.; Kirsch, Thomas D, M.D., M.P.H.; Lowe, Robert A, M.D., M.P.H.; Lowenstein, SR, M.D., M.P.H.; Baraff, Larry J, M.D.; and Orsay, Elizabeth J Mueller, M.D.; Ling, Louis J, M.D., Sklar, David P, M.D., for the SAEM Public Health and Education Committee. Reprinted with permission of the Society of Academic Emergency Medicine. Published by Hanley & Belfius, Inc., Philadelphia, and as an article, Bernstein E et al. *Acad Emerg Med* 1994; 1, 277–286.

INTRODUCTION

Emergency medicine (EM) links hospital and community, specialized inpatient care and primary care, pre-hospital and intensive care. From their unique vantage point, emergency physicians can recognize and analyze many serious health and social problems that result in premature death and disability. This analysis can be shared with the communities in which we work in order to initiate action in partnership with them.

The 1988 Institute of Medicine report, "The Future of Public Health," asserts that the present public health system is underfunded, fragmented, poorly integrated with clinical services, and deficient in governmental, medical provider, and public support. As a result, the public health system is unable to fill its vital role as the early-warning system and safeguard for society.[1] These deficits in public health measures, preventive services, and primary care access have resulted in overcrowded emergency departments (EDs) and limited access for those with real emergencies.[2]

COMMON CONCERNS AND GOALS

Emergency medicine and public health share many concerns and goals that form a basis for mutual collaboration. They also share a range of problems. Failure of the public health system has forced possibly preventable conditions, such as chronic and communicable diseases, poisoning, injury, the results of violence, addiction, untreated mental illness, and malnutrition, to surface in the ED. Although economic incentives in the current health care system reward treatment rather than prevention, constant exposure to tragedy is a strong motivation for emergency physicians to find alternatives to treatment in EDs. Such alternatives require an understanding of public health concepts and a commitment to extend practice out of the ED and into the community.

IMPACT OF PUBLIC HEALTH ADVANCES ON EM

Public health advances have had a dramatic impact on societal well-being and safety. Initially, public health made its greatest advances in the area of communicable disease control through improved sanitation, better living conditions, and immunization. More recently, a public health model based on the interaction among host, agent, and physical and socio-economic environment has been adapted to address such diverse problems as cancer, cardiovascular disease, injury, violence, and alcohol, tobacco, and other drug abuse.

Over the last two decades, a number of successes have been documented: an increase in public commitment to diet and exercise, a demand for environmental protection of air and water, legislation for safer workplaces, a decline in smoking, a reduction in alcohol-related traffic fatalities, and an increase in the use of seat belts.

Reductions in traffic-related injuries provide a striking example of a successful public health and policy intervention. Fatal motor vehicle crashes declined 42% in the past decade, from 2.95 per 100 million vehicle miles traveled in 1980 to 1.7 in 1991. Nighttime motor vehicle crashes, which involve more young drivers and alcohol, declined 30%, and pedestrian deaths were down 28% during the same period.[3] Drivers 15 to 24 years old had a 32% decline in alcohol-related fatalities from 1982 to 1989.[4]

Critical factors accounting for these gains include citizen activism, the social influence of groups such as Mothers against Drunk Driving (MADD) and Students against Driving Drunk (SADD), media coverage, school and community education programs, and a governmental response that led to 700 legislative acts and public mandates for enforcement.[5,6] Recent national, state, and community efforts have attempted to decrease alcohol availability and consumption, increase excise taxes, restrict alcohol advertising, decrease reckless driving, promote safety belt use, and advocate air bags, safer cars, and safer roads.[6,7] The National Highway Traffic Safety Administration estimated that in 1990, among front-seat passengers older than 4 years of age, seat belt use prevented 4,800 deaths and 125,000 moderate-to-critical injuries.[8] As of July 1993, 45 states and Washington, D.C., had enacted seat belt laws, and utilization rates had climbed to 59%.[9] EM providers and their organizations have assisted in these gains by working to improve the pre-hospital and trauma system, researching injury and other health care issues, testifying before state legislatures and Congress, and participating in public education campaigns for safety restraint usage and the deterrence of drunk driving.[10,11]

CRITICAL PUBLIC HEALTH-EM PROBLEMS

An in-depth analysis of the critical problems of substance abuse, injury and violence, infectious diseases [including sexually transmitted diseases (STDs) and human immunodeficiency virus (HIV) infection], occupational and environmental exposures, and minority and women's health needs demonstrates the relationship between public health issues and ED function. These problems require serious study, for they are at the root of ED overcrowding and have strained and reshaped the practice of EM.

Substance Abuse

Drugs. Annual illegal drug sales are estimated at $30 to $100 billion. The economic cost of drug abuse to society is over $58 billion. From 1958 to 1990, cocaine-related emergencies doubled. Emergency physicians treat the myriad effects of drug abuse, including seizures, sudden death, infections, respiratory arrests, delirium, disorientation, and hallucinations, as well as drug-related injuries, suicides, and homicides. Many urban areas have become war zones controlled by drug dealers selling crack cocaine. Punishment has been the principal strategy used in this war, but the cost of treatment is one-tenth the cost of incarceration, and every $1 invested returns $4 in savings. According to the National Institute of Drug Abuse, 107,000 persons are currently awaiting treatment for drug abuse treatment.[12]

Tobacco. Emergency physicians care for the acute complications of smoking including myocardial infarctions, strokes, cancer, chronic obstructive pulmonary diseases, and asthma exacerbations. Smoking rates are probably higher among ED patients because young patients, minorities, the less educated, and the poor have higher rates of smoking and less access to health care (unpublished report, S. Lowenstein). The estimated health care cost for cigarette smoking is over $65 billion annually. Each year over 430,000 Americans die (one-sixth of all U.S. deaths) of smoking-related diseases.[13,14] Although smoking has declined in recent years, 28% of adults continue to smoke.[13] The tobacco industry plays a major role in the continued use of tobacco, spending $3.3 billion per year on advertising and promotion. An example of this influence is the negative correlation between the amount of cigarette advertising and the coverage of the hazards of smoking in magazines.[15]

Alcohol. ED personnel regularly see firsthand the devastation caused by alcohol in patients, their families, and their communities. Proportions of ED patients who have recently consumed alcohol range from 10% to 46%.[16] Five to ten percent of adults in this country are considered dependent on alcohol, and 20% are problem drinkers. By 1995, medical and societal costs of alcohol abuse are predicted to reach $150 billion.[17] Injury is the most common cause of death for Americans between the ages of 1 and 44 years, and alcohol use is implicated in 25% of fatalities caused by falls and fire, 30% of suicides, 35% of drownings, and 50% of motor vehicle crashes and homicides.[18]

Intentional and Unintentional Injury

Patients who are injured, whether intentionally or unintentionally, account for over 25% of ED visits.[19] Intentional and unintentional injuries accounted for 150,000 deaths and 57 million injuries in 1989.[20] The societal cost in 1992 was estimated at $200 billion.[21] Every year almost 1% of the population (over 1.9 million people) is hospitalized with an **unintentional injury**.[20] Unintentional injuries cause 100,000 deaths each year. Motor vehicle crashes are the leading cause of fatal unintentional injuries, followed by falls, poisonings, fires and burns, and drownings. Three percent of Americans will be disabled at some point in their lifetimes and 1.4% will die as a result of motor vehicle crashes.[20]

Falls, which primarily affect children and the elderly, are the second most costly cause of injury in the United States, with a one-year cost of $47.3 billion in 1991. The elderly have ten times greater risk of hospitalization than children and eight times the risk of dying from a fall, at three times the cost.[21]

Each year, approximately one-third of injury-related deaths are **intentional** injuries in the form of suicides or homicides. Suicide is the eighth leading cause of death. Homes with firearms are almost five times more likely to be the scenes of suicides than are comparable homes without firearms.[22] Adolescents, elderly men, and those with mental illness, chronic illness, and substance abuse are at special risk and represent an important segment of ED patients. Although suicides have long been considered a "mental health" problem and violent deaths and injuries a "law enforcement" problem, both are obviously primary concerns for public health and EM.

Homicide is the leading cause of death among black men aged 15 to 34 years.[23] Homicides conform to a preventable pattern that disproportionately affects high-risk populations and have a predictable chain of events involving weapons, alcohol and/or drugs, and arguments between relatives or acquaintances.[24-26] Firearm violence accounts for more deaths among black male teenagers than all natural causes combined.[27] Although handguns comprise no more than 30% of all firearms in private hands, they are involved in the deaths of more than twice as many citizens each year as shotguns and rifles combined.[28] Domestic violence is reaching epidemic proportions and has become a major focus of organized medicine, with the American Medical Association reporting that "the rate of injury to women from battering surpasses that of car accidents and muggings combined."[29]

Infectious Diseases

Emergency physicians are often the only source of care for patients with acute infectious diseases and for patients at risk but not yet infected, and these patients constitute a large part of EM practice.

STDs. Recent data suggest that increasing vigilance and effort are needed to combat new or resurgent outbreaks of communicable STDs. There were 620,478 cases of gonococcal disease and 128,569 cases of syphilis reported to the Centers for Disease Control (CDC) in 1991,[30] but the actual number of cases may be more than double these amounts.[31] Untreated syphilis, especially, leads to neurologic and cardiac complications, and the chancres [associated with syphillis] are a known risk factor for the transmission of acquired immunodeficiency syndrome (AIDS).[32]

Hepatitis B and C. There are approximately 300,000 new cases of hepatitis, with 4,000 to 5,000 deaths from hepatitis B each year, at an annual cost of $500 million.[33] The high-risk groups for hepatitis are similar to those for other STDs. Emergency physicians play a critical role in treatment, case identification, preventive services (vaccines and immune gammaglobulin), patient education, and other public health interventions for these diseases.

Tuberculosis. There were 26,673 cases of tuberculosis (TB) reported to the CDC in 1992.[34] This is a 1.5% increase over 1991 and continues the upward trend of the past five years. The recent emergence of multi-drug-resistant TB among immunosuppressed patients poses a difficult challenge to the emergency physician. The high-risk populations for TB include minorities, the urban poor, immigrants, intravenous drug users, and immunocompromised patients. Emergency physicians are often the source of care for these high-risk groups and must work in conjunction with public health officials to screen the high-risk groups, initiate treatment, and arrange for follow-up and long-term care. Emergency physicians must also ensure that our EDs are not a source of transmission of TB to our patients, other health care workers, and ourselves.

Other infectious diseases. Other infectious diseases such as diarrhea, respiratory diseases, and those infections preventable by vaccination (measles, mumps, pertussis, pneumococcal pneumonia, and influenza) are commonly treated in the ED. Recent studies have shown that up to 50% of children less than age 5 years old have been inadequately immunized,[35] which led to the measles epidemic of 1989-1991 (more than 55,000 cases and 132 deaths).[36] During this epidemic, the majority of cases occurred among the urban poor. Recent studies have shown that the ED can play a critical role in the identification and immunization of the unvaccinated.[37,38]

HIV Exposure

The spread of HIV infection has reached epidemic proportions. By September 1992, a total of 242,146 cases of AIDS had been reported in the United States, and 64% of these persons had died.[39] Ten years ago there were only 1,000 new cases; however, in 1992, 47,106 new cases were diagnosed in the United States.[40] Approximately one million people in the United States are infected with HIV.[41] There is an overrepresentation of minorities, but public health policy has not yet reflected these issues [nor does] the distribution of resources. Many studies have been conducted in the ED to assess the prevalence of HIV infection in the emergency patient population.[42-46] These studies demonstrate that 0.4% to 8.9% of all patients are HIV-positive, with the lower rates occurring in suburban hospitals and the highest in the poor, inner-city areas. These studies point out that 1) health care workers in the ED are often exposed to HIV-infected patients, 2) patients from the inner city with HIV infections commonly use the ED for routine health care, and 3) education about safer sex and the risk of intravenous drug use continues to be an ED responsibility.

Ethical dilemmas concerning discrimination and infringement on the freedom of individuals have emerged regarding issues such as educating adolescents about safer sex and acknowledging differences in sexual orientations.[47,48] Questions remain about confidentiality, mandatory testing, the special responsibilities of health care providers who are HIV-infected, advance directives, euthanasia, and abortions for HIV-infected women.

The cost of caring for a patient with AIDS from the time of diagnosis to death is estimated to be $50,000 to $150,000.[49] The cost of one year's supply of zidovudine (AZT) to treat AIDS is approximately $5,000,[50] and many life insurance and health insurance companies are reluctant or unwilling to provide coverage to AIDS patients. Legislation is lacking to provide for broad program development, especially funding for mental health, drug rehabilitation, and preventive programs for populations at risk.

Despite these barriers, there have been successes that provide encouragement for public health programs that will have a positive impact on the ED. Early detection of HIV infection is now possible with new techniques such as polymerase chain reaction, and some progress is being made in the search for a therapeutic vaccine. Clinicians have improved their knowledge of the treatment of HIV-infected persons, and HIV teaching modules are now part of nursing and medical school curricula. Epidemiologic surveillance techniques have improved, permitting more effective allocation of resources and expertise in targeting high-risk populations.

Innovative campaigns have been developed among populations at risk; the best of these use extensive community educational and support efforts. Information about safer sex and condoms has become available in many high schools. The whole spectrum of AIDS activists, from hemophiliacs to Act-Up members, has demonstrated the power of consumers to have a voice in what health professionals do, and state and local communities have passed legislation prohibiting discrimination against HIV-infected individuals.

Nevertheless, it is difficult to provide quality care for persons with HIV infection and AIDS who depend solely on the ED for education, detection, and treatment. EM by itself cannot compensate for widespread deficiencies in response to this epidemic.

Occupational and Environmental Exposures

Work-related injury is a significant public health concern and a preventable cause of disability and death. Each year, approximately 2 million injuries result in disability, 75 million days of work are lost, and 7,000 to 11,000 workers die. The annual cost of work-related injuries is greater than $48 billion.[51] Common problems seen in the ED are injuries from assaults, crashes, falls, and burns, hand trauma from repetitive motion, skin disorders, asthma, toxic inhalations, pesticide and lead exposure.

Environmental exposures are equally serious. For example, more than 5,000 lung cancers are attributed to exposure to radon.[52] Lead poisoning remains an important problem in children,[53] who may report to the ED with hyperactivity, headache, behavioral changes, or anemia. The American Lung Association estimates that the cost of exposure to outdoor air pollutants is from $50 to $60 billion, with approximately 50,000 to 120,000 premature deaths annually.[53] Serious health problems may result from exposure to hazardous waste site, radioactive materials, and transportation-related chemical spills. Community emergency planning and preparedness for disasters remain inadequate in most regions.

Minority Health

The public health issues of minorities are varied and complex. Minorities face increased morbidity and mortality as a result of social, economic, and political barriers to health care.[54,55] Our present health care system has failed this segment of our society, as evidenced by the inability to gather basic health care data for some groups[56] and the inability to address the health care needs of all minorities.

Health care issues vary among the different racial and ethnic minority groups. Each group has its own cultural, social, economic, and political characteristics that define its public health needs. The Hispanic population, for example, is composed of many diverse ethnic groups with diverse problems.[57,58] Blacks have the highest overall cancer incidence and mortality rate of any minority group, with higher death rates for lung cancer[59] and cervical cancer[60] than those of whites. Their five-year survival rate for all cancer is approximately 38% compared with 52% of whites.[59] The death rates for heart disease, hypertension, and diabetes are higher for blacks than for whites, and the life expectancy for blacks is six years shorter.[61] Factors that have been implicated in these differences include smoking, environmental and occupational exposure to carcinogens, diagnosis at a late stage of illness, treatment difference, and socioeconomic disadvantage.[62-64] Treatment difference is illustrated by a lack of access to high-technology procedures. Compared with white males, black males are half as likely to have coronary angiography, one-third as likely to undergo coronary artery bypass surgery, and two-thirds as likely to receive renal transplantation.[61,65]

Only 61% of pregnant black women receive first-trimester prenatal care, and the black infant mortality rate is 2.3 times the white infant mortality rate.[60] Excluding Cuban Americans, only 60% of Hispanics initiate prenatal care in the first trimester, compared with 80% of whites. The neonatal mortality rate is higher for Puerto Ricans (whether continental or Caribbean) than for Cuban Americans.[66]

Hispanics face difficulties in access to health care as a result of their socioeconomic status and language barriers; many of these individuals have employers who do not provide health insurance.[67,68] The incidence of type II diabetes for Mexican Americans and Puerto Ricans is two to three times the rate for the non-Hispanic population,[67,68] and the incidence of diabetes-related end-stage renal disease is six times that for whites.[57] There also appears to be a higher incidence of cancer of the cervix among Hispanic women. It has been suggested that this is due to the inadequate access to preventive services.[67,68]

Native Americans have an unintentional injury death rate that is 2.5 times higher than that for the overall U.S. population and other minorities. They have higher rates for motor vehicle crashes, residential fires, and drownings. In some areas, Native Americans have pedestrian death rates that are 100 times the average rate.[69,70]

The American Medical Association Council on Ethical and Judicial Affairs published a report in *JAMA* in 1990 entitled, "Black-White Disparities in Health Care," and stated that "whether the disparities in treatment decisions are caused by differences in income and education, socio-cultural factors, or failure by the medical profession, they are unjustifiable and must be eliminated."[61] The complexity of a public health approach to minority health care is evident. We are faced with a growing minority population with varying needs that is underserved and overrepresented in our EDs.

Women's Health

Care of women in the ED is complicated by knowledge deficits resulting from long-standing societal attitudes toward women (e.g., scientific ignorance about as basic a physiologic experience as menopause). Medicalization of pregnancy into a disease state results in transformation of a normal delivery in the ED into a medical emergency. Ideologic battles concerning safe contraception and reproductive rights also affect both information and care rendered to women in the ED.[71] Because medical research has failed to include women or has included them only peripherally, emergency physicians have an inadequate research basis for prevention and treatment of many diseases.[72,73] For example, car crash-worthiness and safety restraint have been tested over the last 25 years on anthropomorphic dummies designed for the 90th percentile male body size, and injuries resulting from safety restraints worn by women have not been studied.[74] Similarly, emergency physicians may not optimally treat cardiac events in 35-year-old women complaining of symptoms similar to those of indigestion.[73]

Pelvic inflammatory disease (PID) is a major cause of infertility and ectopic pregnancy in women,[75] and is the second leading cause of maternal death in the United States.[76] The incidence of newly acquired HIV infections in women has risen steadily. Women now represent 11% of all reported cases and are the fastest-growing population of infected people. Between 1988 and 1989, the number of cases in women rose by 29%, while the number of cases in men rose by 18%.[77] Diseases specific to women have only recently been included in AIDS-defining diagnoses. Inclusion of women in new drug trials continues to be debated.[78]

It has been estimated that the population of the United States contains more rape victims (3,750,000) than combat veterans (2,480,544).[79] Although one in three U.S. women experience childhood or adult physical or sexual violence during their lifetimes, there is no organized system of care for female victims of violence.[80,81] Following battering, women are 16 times more likely to develop a serious drinking problem, and one in ten attempts suicide. A battering relationship often leads to homelessness for women and children.[82] Barriers exist for women seeking substance abuse treatment; they are rarely able to keep children with them at treatment facilities. Although few treatment options are available for pregnant women, paradoxically, in some settings, only pregnant women qualify for treatment.[83]

THE EM ROLE IN ADDRESSING CRITICAL PUBLIC HEALTH PROBLEMS

A public health approach to EM means applying the principles of public health in 1) clinical practice (secondary prevention); 2) public education campaigns, community involvement, and public policy advocacy (primary prevention); 3) medical student/resident training; and 4) research and surveillance.

Clinical Practice (Secondary Prevention)

Questions must be added to the conventional history to identify patients who abuse alcohol and drugs and those who are victims of child, spouse, or elder abuse. Problems with immunization status, lack of contraception information or access, or failure to obtain regular Pap smears will not be recognized without a specific effort to obtain such information. Occupational or home-related injuries such as falls need treatment, but so do the conditions that made the injuries possible. A brief ED case-finding survey questionnaire may be helpful. The CAGE questionnaire and the simple question, "Have you ever had a drinking problem?" plus evidence of alcohol consumption in the previous 24 hours are examples of brief screening questions currently being researched in a number of EDs. These questions have a combined sensitivity of 90% and specificity of 85% for detecting alcoholism compared with the "gold stand-

ard," the Michigan Alcohol Screening Test (MAST).[84,85] Thousands of ED patients with substance abuse-related problems are evaluated every day by emergency physicians, yet few are referred for evaluation and treatment[86,87] despite evidence that treatment works.[88] Both brief interventions by physicians and referral for alcohol or drug treatment programs have the potential for positive impacts on future behavior and health.

Emergency physicians have an especially important role to play in the detection of injuries caused by violence. Many patients are reluctant to divulge the true causes of their injuries. One study has shown that without a formal screening protocol, emergency physicians routinely fail to identify three of every four battered women. Although ED protocols require establishing a link to social support groups, shelter, and the legal system, many EDs do not have an organized system of care and protection for women who are victims of violence. Often, wounds are treated, while the offender/victim relationships and circumstances of the injury are neglected. The battered woman is released without activation of the criminal justice system, without family intervention, and without a plan for the safety of the woman and her children. Unfortunately, battering thrives in secrecy and escalates over time.[81,82] Emergency providers can play a significant role in protecting women from the risk of repetitive and escalating violence.

One study has suggested that violent trauma has a five-year recurrence rate of 44% and a five-year mortality rate of 20%. Alcohol and other drug abuse and unemployment were identified as risk factors.[89] The first encounter with a victim of assault needs to be an opportunity for intervention. Emergency physicians need to be better prepared to interview, counsel, and release victims of violence after establishing a plan for safety.

The ED can be an ideal environment for the detection, brief intervention, and referral of preventable conditions. Patients previously resistant to educational messages about smoking or blood pressure control may be more receptive to counseling when they understand the implications of end-organ failure represented by a trip to the ED with asthma, shortness of breath, or chest pain. The power of physician-generated advice and motivational interviewing has been demonstrated in other clinical settings.[90-92] Yet, many emergency providers do not initiate smoking cessation counseling and referral in the ED, despite the proven success in other settings of brief advice to quit.[93] In the often-emotionally-charged environment of the ED, the impact of teaching by physicians, nurses, social workers, and counselors may be even greater. Preventive patient education must be specific to age, gender, culture, site, and complaint, and should be incorporated into practice guidelines.[94-96] The ED is often the only health care site for some people who seek care during crises; it also may be the only site where the most disenfranchised persons can be reached.

In addition to these screening and educational efforts, emergency physicians can provide preventive services. Immunization of young and old,[37] treatment of STD contacts, screening for hypertension and breast cancer,[97] referral for smoking cessation,[98] and Pap smears[99] can all be provided without greatly extending the length of the ED visit. Referral to primary care services is appropriate and essential to provide follow-up for an acute condition or continuity of care for a chronic condition. Patients must be assisted in making the transition to a primary care setting by ED team members who provide education, follow-up and linkage with a clinic or private physician. Preventive services must be a shared responsibility among physicians, nurses, social workers, discharge planners, and other health professionals. Hospital administrators, as well as physicians, must support systems of emergency care that encourage prevention through screening, risk factor identification, counseling, and referral. Reimbursement for such services is essential.

Public Education Campaigns, Community Involvement, and Public Policy Advocacy (Primary Prevention)

Through work within communities, professional organizations, and the media, emergency physicians can become credible and influential advocates for public health. Emergency physicians witness the tragic consequences of firearm use, violence, alcohol and other drug abuse, smoking, and noncompliance with car seat belts, motorcycle helmet, and bicycle helmet laws. Members of the ED staff are often approached by news media to comment on a variety of health issues, which can be used as vehicles to advance a number of public health concerns.

Emergency physicians can also influence public policy through personal lobbying and scheduled testimony before local, state, or federal officials. Emergency physicians advocating public health in general and lobbying for public policy to enhance health promotions, disease prevention, and injury control specifically reinforce the public's view of emergency physicians as patient and community advocates and essential members of our nation's health care system.[11,100,101]

Medical Student and Resident Physician Training

Academic emergency physicians can broaden their interaction with medical students and support the validity of primary prevention as an effective strategy for illness and injury control by including public health issues in the medical school curriculum. Emergency physicians often present case studies related to alcohol abuse, drug abuse, tobacco, violence, and injury control and prevention to pharmacology, pathology, and introduction to clinical medicine courses. During Advanced Cardiac Life Support courses, emergency physicians bring out the role of the community and prevention as vital links in the chain of survival.

In a number of training programs, medical students and residents are receiving instruction in basic epidemiology and public health measures. They function as part of a multidisciplinary team to work within communities to identify and link patients to community resources. Exposure to health issues affected by cultural variables can be taught effectively if experientially based in community projects, and EM should provide leadership in designing such innovative curricula.[102]

Research and Surveillance

During the past decade, two major advances have placed EM in a position to make important contributions to research in injury and disease prevention. First, a framework has been developed that utilizes the concept of victim-host interaction with the environment, permitting systematic exploration of strategies to disrupt the chain of events leading to preventable illness and injury and to reduce diseases frequently encountered in the ED.[7]

Second, there has been an improvement in our knowledge of the impacts of diseases. There is now a body of descriptive literature that documents incidences in defined populations as well as demographic and geographic factors that place patients at risk. There are several types of research that can be employed to enrich the knowledge base for a public health approach to EM. Population-based incidence studies are necessary to clarify diseases. Case-control studies provide insight into risk factors. Intervention and program evaluation research describes the efficacy, effectiveness, safety, and economic, ethical, social, and legal impacts of prevention measures.[103] Obstacles to such research include inadequate funding, lack of databases (especially for nonfatal injuries), inadequate professional training, societal inertia, and fatalistic attitudes. Overcoming these barriers may bring large benefits in improved patient care and decreased mortality and morbidity.[104]

Effective efforts to prevent injury and illness require the evaluation of population, community, and societal needs. Pilot projects must show that specific interventions reduce the risks of targeted diseases in defined populations. The initial success of a program can be measured by observing increased rates of lower-risk behaviors (e.g., not driving while intoxicated) or risk-protective behaviors (e.g., using safety belts).

Once pilot interventions have been proven effective, they can be implemented on a larger scale to produce demonstrable changes in disease rates, which will be detectable in population-based studies. To conduct these large projects, EM researchers should collaborate in multi-center studies and participate in public health coalitions. Emergency physicians must work closely with government agencies active in the political arena because most health initiatives that affect disease at the population level demand some legislative or regulatory action and community-based implementation.

Emergency physicians are uniquely positioned to make major contributions to public health research, particularly in the fields of injury control, violence, substance abuse, disease prevention, women's health, and minority health. High priority should be given to the development of ED information systems that facilitate injury and disease surveillance, ED quality improvement, and evaluation of community health programs. Bench researchers in EM should expand their present scope of laboratory

investigation to include studies of the biomechanics of trauma and the pathophysiology of acute neural injury. Analysis of national injury data sets and collaborative projects with public safety agencies (e.g., the police) also hold great promise. ED surveillance provides the necessary database for prevention and financing, access, and evaluation of acute care.

Surveillance is defined as the "ongoing systematic collection, analysis, and interpretation of health data essential to the planning, implementation and evaluation of public health practice, closely integrated with the timely dissemination of these data to those who need to know. The final link in surveillance is the application of these data to prevention and control. . . ."[105]

Examples of ED-based surveillance systems are the Drug Abuse Warning Network (DAWN), the National Electronic Injury Surveillance System (NEISS), which is operated by the Consumer Product Safety Commission, and the Sentinel Injury Surveillance System for Gunshot and Stab Wounds (SISS), a CDC-funded program. Emergency physicians can play a key role in developing ED injury databases with consistent coding (e.g., E-codes or mechanism-of-injury modifiers of the ICD9 codes), which provide public health agencies, researchers, and other interested individuals and organizations with accurate information about injured ED patients.

The ED is an excellent site for injury and disease surveillance because of its high volume. The population that uses EDs is at high risk and the geographic areas/census tracks provide the denominator for rate-based population data. CDC reporting of notifiable diseases and collaboration with local public health agencies in case reporting and intervention are critical. In order to develop accurate surveillance, a uniform data set, including standards for case definitions and accurate population based-information is needed.

THE ROLE OF ORGANIZED EM IN IMPLEMENTING PUBLIC HEALTH POLICY

Emergency medicine's role in public health and its place in national health care reform can be strengthened by emergency medicine's providing leadership in the following areas:

1. Work with other primary care providers to include preventive education and services into the description of reimbursable services.

2. Develop a compendium of ED patient education resources.

3. Include patient education and counseling in the mission. Important areas to address include STDs, HIV infection, smoking, nutrition, hypertension, warning signs of myocardial infarction, early detection of cancer, asthma, injury, violence, substance abuse, and use of helmets and safety restraints and other safety devices. Priorities must be set and the most effective intervention for the most serious problems developed and evaluated.

4. Incorporate public health concerns into curriculum materials and into certification and in-house training examinations.

5. Develop practice guidelines, standards, and protocols for the treatment of persons presenting to the ED, including patients with alcohol, tobacco, and other drug abuse, STDs, and HIV infection, and those who have been victims of violence. These protocols would encompass case finding, documentation, patient education, and discharge planning that includes a plan for safety and referral as well as linkage to a primary care site or provider.

6. Pursue advanced training and research in public health, epidemiology, and public policy with particular attention to the critical problem areas.

7. Collaborate with the CDC to develop a national uniform data set for ED injury and disease surveillance and with state and local health departments to improve disease surveillance, case finding, and follow-up.

8. Advocate for public health concerns and for the health care debate to include preventive services and public health measures. Collaborate with patient and community groups to form coalitions for change.

CONCLUSIONS

The current debate about health care reform must address solutions to critical public health and emergency medicine problems as well as the impacts of race, gender, sexual orientation, physical condition, and age on health. To improve the quality of life and provide for a truly healthy population, we must ensure that resources will be available for the nation's social, educational, and environmental needs as well as for public health measures and preventive and comprehensive medical services.

Emergency medicine has a unique opportunity to contribute to health care reform by instituting a comprehensive and collaborative public health approach to Emergency medicine.

REFERENCES

1. Institute of Medicine. The Future of Public Health. Washington, DC: National Academy Press, 1988.
2. U.S. General Accounting Office. Emergency Departments: Unevenly Affected by Growth and Change in Patient Use. Washington, DC: U.S. Printing Office, 1993.
3. National Highway Traffic Safety Administration. Fatal Accident Reporting System 1991: A Review of Traffic Crashes in the U.S. Washington, DC: U.S. Department of Transportation, 1992.
4. Centers for Disease Control. Update: Surveillance of alcohol related fatalities among youth and young adults-U.S., 1982-1989. MMWR. 1991; 40:178–87.
5. Centers for Disease Control. Alcohol related traffic fatalities-US, 1982-1989. MMWR. 1990; 39:890–1.
6. Hingson R, Howland J, Schiavone T, Damiata M. The Massachusetts saving lives program: six cities-widening the focus from drunk driving to speeding, reckless driving and failure to wear safety belts. J Traffic Med. 1990; 18:123–30.
7. National Committee for Injury Prevention and Control. Injury prevention: meeting the challenge. Am J Prev Med. 1989; 5:192–270.
8. Centers for Disease Control. Safety belt use and motor vehicle related injuries: The Navajo nation, 1988-1991. MMWR. 1992; 41:705–8.
9. Insurance Institute for Highway Safety (IIHS). Child restraints and belt laws. State Law Facts, 1993.
10. Bernstein E, Lowe R. Survey of public health and health policy issues addressed in emergency medicine training programs. Acad Emerg Med. 1990; 2:7–10.
11. Bernstein E, Roth P, Yeh C, Lefkowits DJ. The emergency physician's role in prevention. Pediatr Emerg Care. 1988; 4:207–11.
12. NIDA. Drug Abuse Treatment: An Economical Approach to Addressing the Drug Problem in America. Washington, DC: ADAMHA, 1991.
13. Bauman KE. On the future of applied smoking research: is it up in smoke? Am J Pub Health. 1992; 82:14–6.

14. Amler RW, Dull HB. Closing the Gap: The Burden of Unnecessary Illness. Oxford: Oxford University Press, 1987.

15. Warner KE, Goldenhar LM, McLaughlin CG. Cigarette advertising and magazine coverage of the hazards of smoking. N Engl J Med. 1992; 326:305–9.

16. Cherpital, CJS. Breath analysis and self-report as measures of alcohol-related emergency room admissions. J Stud Alcohol. 1989; 50:155–61.

17. U.S. Department of Health and Human Services. 7th Special Report to the U.S. Congress: Alcohol and Health. Washington, DC. 1990, pp 1–42.

18. National Committee for Injury Prevention and Control. Injury prevention: meeting the challenge. Am J Prev Med. 1989; 5:6.

19. Committee on Trauma Research, Institute of Medicine. Injury in America: A Continuing Public Health Problem. Washington, DC: National Academy Press, 1985.

20. Rice DP, McKenzie EJ. Cost of Injury in the United States: A Report to Congress. San Francisco, CA: Institute for Health and Aging, 1989.

21. Runge JW. The cost of injury. Emerg Med Clin North Am. 1993; 11:241–53.

22. Kellermann AL, Rivara FP, Somes G. Suicide in the home in relation to gun ownership. N Engl J Med. 1992; 327:467–72.

23. Centers for Disease Control. Homicide surveillance, 1979-1988. MMWR. 1992; 41:1–34.

24. Earl F, Slaby RG, Spirito A. Prevention of violence and injury due to violence. In CDC: Setting the National Agenda for Injury Control in the 1990s: Position Papers from Third National Injury Control Conference. Atlanta: Centers for Disease Control, 1992, pp 160–294.

25. Prothrow-Stith D, Spivak, H. Homicide and violence: contemporary health problems for America's black community. In Braithwaite RL, Taylor SE (eds). Health Issues in the Black Community. San Francisco: Jossey-Bass Publishers, 1992, pp 132–43.

26. Rosenberg ML, Mercy JA. Violence. In Last JM, Wallace RB (eds). Public Health & Preventive Medicine, 13th ed. Norwalk, CT: Appleton & Lange, 1992, pp 1035–9.

27. Wintemute G, Hanock M, Loftin C, McGuire A, Pertschuk M, Teret S. Policy options on firearm violence. In Samuel SE, Smith MD (eds). Improving the Health of the Poor. Menlo Park, CA: Henry Kaiser Foundation, 1992.

28. Kellermann AL, Lee RK, Jercy JM, Banton J. The epidemiologic basis for the prevention of firearm injuries. Annu Rev Public Health. 1991; 12:17–40.

29. Council on Ethical and Judicial Affairs of the AMA. Physicians and domestic violence. JAMA. 1992; 267:3190–3.

30. Centers for Disease Control. Summary of notifiable diseases, United States, 1991. MMWR. 1992; 40:1–55.

31. Thacker SB, Berkelman RL. Public health surveillance in the United States. Epidemiol Rev. 1988; 10:164–90.

32. Simonsen JN, Cameron WC, Gakinya MN, et al. Human immunodeficiency virus infection among men with sexually transmitted diseases-experience from a center in Africa. N Engl J Med. 1988; 319:274–8.

33. Centers for Disease Control. Hepatitis Surveillance Report no. 52. Atlanta: U.S. Department of Health and Human Services, Public Health Service, 1989.

34. Centers for Disease Control. Tuberculosis morbidity, 1992. MMWR. 1993; 42:363.

35. Centers for Disease Control. Measles vaccination levels among selected groups of pre-school aged children, United States, 1990. MMWR. 1991; 40:36–9.

36. Centers for Disease Control. Measles, United States, 1992. MMWR. 1993; 42:378–81.

37. Polis MA, Davey VT, Collins ED, Smith JP, Rosenthal RE, Kaslow RA. The emergency department as part of a successful strategy for increasing immunization. Ann Emerg Med. 1988; 17:1016–18.

38. Rodewald LE, Szilagyi PG, Humiston SG, et al. Is an emergency department visit a marker for undervaccination. Pediatrics. 1993; 91:605–11.

39. Centers for Disease Control. AIDS Clearinghouse. Atlanta: Centers for Disease Control, 1993.

40. Haverkos HW. Reported cases of AIDS: an update. N Engl J Med. 1993; 329:511.

41. Centers for Disease Control. The HIV/AIDS epidemic: the first 10 years. MMWR. 1991; 40:357–63.

42. Centers for Disease Control. Update: human immunodeficiency virus infections in health-care workers exposed to blood of infected patients. MMWR. 1987; 36:285.

43. Baker JL, Kelen GD, Sivertson KT, Quinn TC. Unsuspected human immunodeficiency virus in critically ill emergency patients. JAMA. 1987; 257:2609.

44. Kelen GD, Fritz S, Qaqish B, et al. Unrecognized human immunodeficiency virus infection in emergency department patients. N Engl J Med. 1988; 318:1645.

45. Kelen GD, DiGiovanna T, Bisson L, Kalainov D, Sivertson KT, Quinn TC. Human immunodeficiency virus infection in emergency patients: epidemiology, clinical presentations, and risk of health care workers. The Johns Hopkins experience. JAMA. 1989; 262:516.

46. Strum JT. HIV prevalence in a midwestern emergency department. Ann Emerg Med. 1991; 20:272.

47. Connor SS. AIDS: Social, legal and ethical issues of the "third epidemic." Bull. Pan American Health Organ. 1989; 23:95–107.

48. Knopp R, Adams J, Derse A, et al. The HIV-infected emergency health care professional. Ann Emerg Med. 1991; 20:1036–40.

49. Hellinger FJ. Forecasting the personal medical care costs of AIDS from 1988 through 1991. Public Health Rep. 1990; 105:1–12.

50. Solomon DJ, Hogan AJ, Bouknight RR, Solomon CT. Analysis of Michigan medicaid costs to treat HIV infection. Public Health Rep. 1989; 104:416–24.

51. Baker SP, Conroy C. Occupational injury prevention. In CDC: Setting the National Agenda for Injury Control in the 1990s: Position Papers from Third National Injury Control Conference, Atlanta: Centers for Disease Control, 1992, pp 327–74.

52. Dvorak V. Ionizing radiation. In Last JM, Wallace RB (eds). Public Health & Preventive Medicine, 13th ed. Norwalk, CT: Appleton & Lange, 1992, pp 503–12.

53. U.S. Public Health Service. Year 2000 Objectives, Healthy People 2000: National Health Promotion and Disease Protection Objectives. Washington, DC: USPHS, 1991, pp 313–21.

54. Pappas G, Queen S, Hadden W, Fisher G. The increasing disparity in mortality between socioeconomic groups in the United States, 1960 and 1986. N Engl J Med. 1993; 329:103–9.

55. Becker LB, Han BH, Meyer PM, et al. Racial difference in the incidence of cardiac arrest and subsequent survival. N Engl J Med. 1993; 329:600–6.

56. Amaro H. In the Midst of Plenty: Reflections on the Economic and Health Status of Hispanic Families. Presented at the American Psychological Association Convention, August 1992.

57. Council on Scientific Affairs. Hispanic health in the United States. JAMA. 1991; 265:248–52.

58. Poma P. The Hispanic health challenge. J Natl Med Assoc. 1988; 80:1275–7.

59. Baquet C, Gibbs T. Cancer and Black Americans. In Braithwaite RL, Taylor SE (eds). Health Issues in the Black Community. San Francisco: Jossey-Bass Publishers, 1992, pp 106–20.

60. Avery B. Health Status of Black Women. In Braithwaite RL, Taylor SE (eds). Health Issues in the Black Community. San Francisco: Jossey-Bass Publishers, 1992, pp 35–51.

61. Council on Ethical and Judicial Affairs. Black-white disparities in health care. JAMA. 1992; 263:2344–6.

62. Nickens H. Report on the Secretary's Task Force on Black and Minority Health: A summary and a presentation of health data with regard to blacks. J Natl Med Assoc. 1986; 78:577–80.

63. Centers for Disease Control. Report of the Secretary's Task Force on Black and Minority Health. MMWR. 1986; 35:109–12.

64. Centers for Disease Control. Years of potential life lost before age 65, by race, hispanic origin and sex-United States, 1986-88. MMWR. 1992; 41:13–23.

65. Whittle J, Congliano J, Good CB, Lofren RP. Racial differences in the use of cardiovascular procedures in the internal medicine department of the VA Medical System. N Engl J Med. 1993; 329:621–7.

66. Becerra J, Hogue C, Atrash H, Perez N. Infant mortality among Hispanics: a portrait of heterogeneity. JAMA. 1991; 265:217-21.

67. Munoz E. Care for the Hispanic poor: A growing segment of American society. JAMA. 1988; 260:2711–2.

68. Ginzberg E. Access to health care for Hispanics. JAMA. 1991; 265:238–41.

69. U.S. Public Health Service. Year 2000 Objectives, Healthy People 2000: National Health Promotion and Disease Protection Objectives. Boston: Jones and Bartlett, 1992, pp 602–4.

70. Gallaher MM, Fleming DW, Berger LR, Sewell M. Pedestrian and hypothermia deaths among Native Americans in New Mexico between bar and home. JAMA. 1992; 267:1345–8.

71. The Boston Women's Health Collective. Our Bodies, Ourselves. New York: Simon and Schuster, 1992.

72. Bennett JC for the Board of Health Science Policy, Institute of Medicine, National Academy of Science. Inclusion of women in clinical trials-policies for population subgroups. N Engl J Med. 1993; 329:288–92.

73. Wenger NK, Speroff L, Packard B. Cardiovascular health and disease in women. N Engl J Med. 1993; 329:247–56.

74. NHTSA. Federal Motor Vehicle Safety Standard 208. Washington, DC. NHTSA, 1968.

75. Chow WH, Daling JR, Cates W, Greenburg RS. Epidemiology of ectopic pregnancy. Epidemiol Rev. 1987; 9:70–94.

76. Koonin MN, Atrash HK, Lawson HW, Smith JC. Maternal mortality surveillance, United States, 1979-1986. In: CDC Surveillance Summaries 1991. MMWR. 1991; 40:1–55.

77. Centers for Disease Control. AIDS in women-United States. MMWR. 1990; 47:845–6.

78. Corea G. The Invisible Epidemic: The Story of Women and AIDS. New York: Harper & Collins, 1992.

79. Rosenberg ML, et al. Violence in America: A Public Health Approach. Oxford: Oxford University Press, 1991.

80. Faludi S. Backlash. New York: Crown Publishers, 1991.

81. McLeer SV, Anwar R. Education is not enough: a systems failure in protecting battered women. Ann Emerg Med. 1989; 18:651–3.

82. Stark E, Flitcraft AH. Spouse abuse. In Last JM, Wallace RB (eds). Public Health and Preventive Medicine, 13th ed. Norwalk, CT: Appleton & Lange, 1992, pp 1040–3.

83. Amaro H. Testimony on women's health research before Senate Committee Labor & Human Resources field hearing at Boston University Medical School, January 1993 (unpublished).

84. Cyr MG, Wartman SA. The effectiveness of routine screening questions in the detection of alcoholism. JAMA. 1988; 59:41–4.

85. Adams WL, Magruder-Habib K, Trued S, Broome HL. Alcohol abuse in elderly emergency department patients. J Am Geriatr Soc. 1992; 40:1236–40.

86. Bernstein E. National conference to link primary care, HIV, alcohol and drug abuse treatment. Acad Emerg Med. 1992; 4:8–10.

87. Lowenstein SR, Weissberg M, Terry D. Alcohol intoxication, injuries and dangerous behaviors and the revolving emergency department door. J Trauma. 1990; 30:1252–8.

88. Miller W. The effectiveness of treatment for substance abuse: Reasons for optimism. J Subst Abuse Treat. 1992; 9:93–102.

89. Sims DW, Buins BA, Farouck NO, et al. Urban trauma: a chronic recurrent disease. J Trauma. 1989; 29:940–947.

90. Miller WR, Rollnick S. Motivational Interviewing: Preparing People to Change Addictive Behavior. New York: Guilford Press, 1991.

91. Rollnick S, Heather N, Bell A. Negotiating behavior change in the medical setting: the development of brief motivational interviewing. J Ment Health. 1992; 1:25-37.

92. Walsh D, Hingson RW, Merrigan DM, et al. The impact of a physician's warning on recovery after alcoholism treatment. JAMA. 1992; 267:663–7.

93. Schwartz TL. Review and Evaluation of Smoking Cessation Methods, the U.S. and Canada. Washington, DC: U.S. DHHS, 1987, (NIH publications no. 87–7940).

94. Vogt T. Paradigm and prevention. Am J Public Health. 1993; 83:795–6.

95. U.S. Preventive Service Task Force. Guide to Clinical Preventive Services: An Assessment of the Effectiveness of 169 Interventions. Baltimore: Williams and Wilkin, 1989.

96. Collins TR, Goldenberg K, Ring A, Nelson K, Konen J. The Association of Teachers of Preventive Medicine's recommendations for postgraduate education in prevention. Acad Med. 1991; 66:317–20.

97. Goldman JM, Fegler R, Stinhagen A, Shofer FS. Is there a need for preventive care in emergency medicine [abstract]. Ann Emerg Med. 1990; 19:487.

98. Fiore MC. The new vital sign: assessing and documenting smoking status. JAMA. 1991; 266:3183–4.

99. Hogness CG, Engelstad LP, Linck LM, Schorr KA. Cervical cancer screening in an urban emergency department. Ann Emerg Med. 1992; 21:933–9.

100. Hargarten S. Injury control. Emerg Clin North Am. 1993; 11:255–61.

101. Jernigan DH, Mosher T. Public action and awareness to reduce alcohol-related problems: a plan of action. J Public Health Policy. 1988; 9:17–41.

102. Sklar D, Hall H. Community oriented learning for emergency medicine residents. Acad Emerg Med. 1990; 2:8–9.

103. Centers for Disease Control. A framework for assessing the effectiveness of disease and injury prevention. MMWR. 1992; 41:1–11.

104 Martinez R. Opportunity knocks. What will we do? Ann Emerg Med. 1992; 21:169–171.

105. Centers for Disease Control. Comprehensive Plan for Epidemiologic Surveillance. Atlanta: Centers for Disease Control, 1986.

Unit II

Critical Problems, Unmet Needs

2

Tuberculosis and Homelessness

STEPHEN P. WAXMAN

CONTENTS

- Epidemiology
- Rapid diagnosis
- Isolation
- Direct observed therapy
- PPD immunology
- Tuberculosis and HIV
- Infection control
- Public health issues
- The role of the ED practitioner

CHAPTER SUMMARY

Tuberculosis is an ancient disease that infects one-third of mankind. Annually, 8 million new cases and 3 million deaths are reported. Poverty, malnutrition, overcrowding, and social neglect have always been critical to the survival and success of this organism.

A decline in the incidence of tuberculosis actually began in industrialized countries *before* the introduction of antituberculosis antibiotics. Improved standards of living and recognition of the benefit of isolating active cases in sanatoria contributed to a decline in active disease of 6% per year in the United States from 1953 to 1985.[1]

After 1985, however, there was a resurgence of TB. From 1985 through 1992, the number of reported cases rose by 20%. Reasons cited include an increase in immigration from countries in Asia and Central and South America that have high rates of tuberculosis; an increase in pockets of poverty and overcrowding in our own urban centers; an increase in the prevalence of substance abuse; an increase in the number of persons living in congregate settings such as nursing homes, prisons, and homeless shelters; and the HIV epidemic.[2] Over the same time period, funding for public health programs that could have anticipated and controlled this resurgence was slashed. From 1980 to 1990, the incidence of reported tuberculosis increased 132 percent in New York City.[3]

In 1989, the Centers for Disease Control (CDC) announced the goal of eliminating TB by the year 2010.[4] This goal was an expression of confidence in (1) the capacity of our medical and scientific institutions to diagnose, treat and cure the disease; (2) the capacity of our social and political institutions to eliminate the circumstances that promote disease; (3) the willingness of the American public to expand access to care for those who are infected; and (4) the availability of funds and service providers to educate and protect those who are at risk. A major commitment to public health is an absolute prerequisite to progress.

The homeless patient with tuberculosis crystallizes the interconnections between the medical care system, the political system, and the economic system. With a high prevalence of substance abuse, malnutrition, AIDS, psychiatric disease, poor medical compliance, and close congregate living, the homeless in our urban centers tax our medical and social care capabilities. Tuberculosis, especially multidrug resistant tuberculosis, is a major threat to patients, to their caregivers, and to the society at large.

Case #1

WB is a 59-year-old black male who works for a messenger service in New York City. He complains of a cough for one month and progressive fatigue, weakness, weight loss, and night sweats. He has had intermittent low-grade fevers.

WB now lives in a room in a boarding house, but prior to this he lived in a shelter for 6 months. He has smoked cigarettes for 40 years and spends every evening with his friends sharing bottles of wine or hard liquor. He was last hospitalized 5 years ago for a fractured ankle sustained while intoxicated. He does not recall ever having a skin test for tuberculosis.

On physical examination, WB is tall, thin, and coughs frequently. Vital signs are WNL except for a temperature of 101°F. Chest exam reveals rhonchi in the right upper thorax chest anteriorly. Abnormal labs include a Hematocrit of 29% and a white cell count of 12,300/mm³ (73 neutrophils, 6 bands, 16 lymphocytes, and 4 monocytes). Chest radiograph shows RUL and RML infiltrates.

Q: Should this man be isolated from other patients and staff?

Despite technologic advances in isolating the infectious material of patients with respiratory diseases, the most critical element in limiting the spread of tuberculosis is early suspicion, physical isolation, and rapid initiation of antimycobacterial antibiotics. All clinicians, especially those at the earliest point of encounter, should think of tuberculosis and isolate suspicious cases long before definitive diagnosis.

WB was sick with a cough and constitutional symptoms for over 4 weeks. This chronicity of symptoms implies a process like a malignancy or an atypical pneumonia. His history of substance abuse, physical neglect, and episodic living in homeless shelters should heighten suspicion of mycobacterium tuberculosis. Early isolation in specially designed rooms that produce at least 6 fresh-air

exchanges per hour, that are negatively pressurized relative to hallways or adjoining rooms, and that are exhausted to the outside (away from nearby intake vents) are critical measures for limiting the spread of infection. Staff should be alerted to wear personal respirators when treating these patients.

Emergency departments and outpatient clinics are areas that are particularly vulnerable to nosocomial spread of tuberculosis. Patients in these areas often lack specific diagnoses, spend long amounts of time in close proximity to other patients and staff, and rarely exercise caution when they cough or sneeze. Suspicion, early isolation, and the liberal use of UV lamps in all patient areas will help to limit the spread of disease.

Q: How did this patient acquire tuberculosis?

On further interview, WB said he grew up with his grandparents in Brooklyn, New York. Both grandparents at different times in his childhood had to be hospitalized for prolonged amounts of time for pulmonary tuberculosis. In all likelihood, WB was exposed to mycobacterium tuberculosis in his childhood, and his present disease is due to reactivation of dormant organisms.

Mycobacterium tuberculosis is carried in airborne particles known as droplet nuclei, produced when a person with infectious TB coughs, sneezes, or speaks. These particles are so small that normal air currents keep them suspended in air for long periods of time. Although infection can be established after inhalation of even one tubercle bacillus, the risk of becoming infected increases as the amount of time spent with infectious patients increases.[5] In addition, patients who harbor large numbers of TB organisms, as in cavitary disease, or who cough excessively without covering their mouths, pose an enhanced risk. According to the National Institute of Allergy and Infectious Diseases, there is a 50% chance of infection after being exposed to someone with active tuberculosis for 8 hours a day over 6 months.

Once infected, approximately 5% of people will develop clinical symptoms of active disease within the first 3 months. If latent infection is established, as manifested by a positive tuberculin skin test, there is a 5 to 10% life time risk of developing active tuberculosis in the future. Groups known to have a high risk of developing reactivation tuberculosis include the elderly, individuals on steroids or chemotherapy, diabetics, individuals who are malnourished, chronic alcohol and IV drug users, and, of course, individuals who are infected with HIV.[6]

Q: How rapidly can we make a diagnosis of tuberculosis in this patient?

All patients suspected of having tuberculosis should have a chest radiograph, a tuberculin skin test, sputum testing for acid-fast staining and culture, and blood cultures for mycobacteria. Up to 80% of HIV-negative patients whose sputum cultures ultimately grow M. tuberculosis will have positive acid-fast smears.[7] The specificity of acid-fast smears for tuberculosis is 90%.[8]

Case Continuation

WB had a chest radiograph that was classic for reactivation tuberculosis: bilateral upper lobe infiltrates with a suggestion of early cavitation and hilar adenopathy. He had three positive AFB (acid-fast bacilli) smears on the day of admission and sputum cultures were positive for mycobacteria about 12 days later. He was immediately begun on a four-drug regimen.

Rapid diagnosis and initiation of treatment is critical to stopping the spread of tuberculosis. Classic methods for laboratory diagnosis of tuberculosis are time consuming. Sputum cultures take 4 to 6 weeks and species identification and sensitivity testing take even more valuable time. Newer radiometric culture methods can reduce the time for detection of mycobacteria to 1 to 2 weeks. DNA probe assay and high-performance liquid chromatography of mycelia acids allow identification of species within a few hours.

The next generation of rapid tests involves nucleic acid amplification techniques, such as the polymerase chain reaction (PCR), rather than growth on cultures. Although the cost is substantially higher, results are obtainable on a same-day basis and detection of drug-resistant strains at the genetic level can also be done rapidly.[9] New DNA fingerprinting methods have led to insights into the epidemiologic spread of tuberculosis and have revealed the great vulnerability of congregate living situations such as homeless shelters, prisons, and residencies for HIV-positive people. Nosocomial spread of primary tuberculosis was identified by these new techniques.

Q: When can WB leave his isolation room?

After 2 weeks of four antimycobacterial drugs, WB began to feel better. His cough had decreased, his appetite and level of energy improved, fevers and night sweats decreased, and he gained weight. AFB smears of sputum were still positive for organisms but in decreased quantities.

After effective therapy is initiated, symptoms typically improve within 4 weeks, and sputum cultures become negative within 3 months. WB's improvement in symptoms and at least a decrease in the number of organisms on acid-fast stain is reasonable evidence for lack of infectiousness. At least 2 weeks of antimycobacterial therapy is recommended prior to ending isolation precautions.[10] If the patient is infected with multi-drug-resistant (MDR) tuberculosis, the absence of organisms on AFB smear should be the indicator for ending isolation.

Accomplishing true isolation when the patient is an active substance user or has impulse control problems or poor self-discipline is often a challenge. Every effort must be made to ensure that the patient's room is hospitable. A functional radio, television, and telephone, as well as reading materials and other amenities are critical to successful isolation. When infectious patients leave their isolation room for procedures, they and the staff should be wearing particulate respirators.

WB will be discharged to a program of direct observed therapy (DOT). He will be monitored with sputum smears and cultures every 2 to 4 weeks until they are negative. Again, success in adherence to this long-term treatment plan, especially for the homeless, will require a commitment from social services and public health programs. DOT offices that are geographically and psychologically accessible to these patients, incentives (food, money, shelter), enablers, and short-course, twice-weekly therapy are prerequisites for success. Concomitant social services, attention to needs for housing and nutrition, and psychiatric and substance abuse counseling are also necessary. Education and surveillance of those exposed or at risk, and chemoprophylaxis for those infected are other ingredients of a successful program.

Case #2

JR is an intravenous drug user (IVDU) who learned that he was HIV-positive while in prison 5 years ago. At that time, his tuberculin skin test was positive, and he took a medication sporadically for 2 months. He has had no opportunistic infections and has avoided comprehensive medical care. He does know that his CD4 lymphocyte count was around 300 about 1 year ago.

At present, JR lives in a homeless shelter for men. He has been there for 3 months. Recently, he went to the Shelter Clinic complaining of a dry cough for several weeks. The physician in the Clinic started him on antibiotics and planted a tuberculin skin test. Two days later, the cough was no better, and the skin test was negative. JR was sent to the nearest emergency department.

In the ED, JR was found to be cachectic with a temperature of 102°F. He had white plaques in his oropharynx, bilateral lower lobes rales, and diffuse lymphadenopathy. The chest radiograph revealed bilateral lower and middle lobe interstitial infiltrates and significant mediastinal adenopathy.

Q: What aspects of this patient's history and presentation are clinically relevant?

JR is an immunocompromised patient with a history of presumed latent infection with M. tuberculosis that was partially treated. The profound effect of HIV immunocompromise in patients who also harbor M. tuberculosis is demonstrated by the fact that they progress to active tuberculosis at the rate of 10% per year, compared to the rate of 10% over a lifetime for HIV-negative patients.[11]

Although JR has had no opportunistic infections to date, his weight loss, oropharyngeal candidiasis, and loss of tuberculin reactivity imply a deterioration in immune status. While opportunistic respiratory infections in HIV-positive patients are uncommon with CD4 lymphocyte counts greater than 300, respiratory tuberculosis is often the first infection to appear. In a San Francisco study of patients infected with HIV, the median CD4 lymphocyte cell count at time of diagnosis of tuberculosis was 326 cells/mm^3. In comparison, pneumocystis carinii pneumonia usually does not appear until the CD4 cell count is below 200 cells/mm^3.[12]

The clinical manifestations of active tuberculosis in AIDS patients vary with the state of immunosuppression. Patients with higher CD4 counts tend to present with "typical" pulmonary tuberculosis secondary to reactivation of latent disease and chest radiographs with upper-lobe infiltrates and cavities. Patients with CD4 counts of less than 300/mm^3 are more likely to develop primary disease, have greater systemic symptoms, have an increased incidence of extrapulmonary disease, and have a tendency to have more atypical chest radiographs—for example, diffuse or miliary infiltrates as well as mediastinal and hilar adenopathy.[13]

Q: Does this patient have primary tuberculosis and of what significance is this fact?

JR was undoubtedly exposed to tuberculosis in prison, in the homeless shelters, and among his colleagues on the streets. His advanced state of immunocompromise makes him vulnerable to new infection and chances are high that this newly acquired infection is multidrug resistant.

Outbreaks of tuberculosis among HIV-positive persons have been reported from hospitals, clinics, prisons, residential facilities and homeless shelters. "DNA fingerprinting" techniques have been able to prove that these outbreaks were due to primary spread of similar or same organisms contrary to prior belief that the vast majority of new TB was due to reactivation of latent infection.[14,15] Several new studies have estimated that up to 40% of all new tuberculosis may be due to primary spread, with the predominance of these cases occurring in HIV-infected individuals.[16,17]

Q: Does homelessness increase the risk of acquiring tuberculosis?

The demographics of homelessness have shifted from a predominance of older white males with chronic alcohol abuse to younger men and women from ethnic minorities with significant rates of intravenous substance abuse, psychiatric disease, and HIV infection. Poor nutrition, crowding, and immunosuppression have led to alarming rates of tuberculosis. A survey of 244 consecutive patients with active tuberculosis admitted to a hospital in Harlem revealed that 68% were either homeless or had unstable housing, and 80% were unemployed. More than half reported significant use of alcohol, and more than 60% were intravenous drug users (IDU or IVDU's).[18] In a 1,000-bed homeless shelter on Ward's Island in New York City, 62% of the men were HIV-positive. Conversely, 90% of patients who developed active tuberculosis during their stays in the shelter tested HIV-positive.[19] In addition, tuberculosis among the homeless is resistant to medication to a far greater degree than in patients who are domiciled. Clearly, people who are homeless have a high burden of tuberculosis, have risks for HIV and other sources of immunocompromise, live in conditions that promote respiratory spread, and are often noncompliant with the long treatments required.

EPIDEMIOLOGY OF TUBERCULOSIS

Worldwide, the majority of TB cases are reported from Southeast Asia (31%), China (27%), and Africa (15%), and there are increasing trends in these areas both in absolute number and in rate per 100,000. The annual incidence is highest in Africa (220/100,000) and lowest in the industrialized nations (e.g., U.S., with 10.3/100,000) by a factor of 10 to 20. In Africa, Southeast Asia, and China, more than 50% of the adult population is infected, and the majority of the infected population is now below 50 years of age.[20] In the industrialized countries, the prevalence of infection generally is lower in young age groups but higher in older persons, reflecting the high risk of infection in the past when TB was more common in western Europe. It is fortunate that this group has a very low rate of coinfection with HIV.

In the United States, public health measures, better living conditions, enhanced natural resistance, and antibiotics contributed to declining rates of TB infection. Between 1953 and 1984, reported cases decreased 74%; the yearly incidence declined from 53 to 9.4/100,000. Since 1984, however, cases of TB have increased dramatically and in epidemic proportions.[1] From 1985 to 1991, reported cases increased 18%. At present, 10 to 15 million people in the United States are infected and over 26,000 cases of active TB were reported in 1991.

The new epidemic of TB in the U.S. is localized to pockets of poverty in our urban centers and among racial minorities. Between 1985 and 1990, rates of infection among non-Hispanic whites fell 7%, while rates among blacks and Hispanics rose 27% and 54%, respectively. Almost 70% of all TB infections in adults and 85% of infections in children occurred among racial and ethnic minorities in urban centers.[21] New York City which accounts for 15% of all cases of TB in the country, reported an increase of 38% between 1989 and 1990. Over half of the cases were in black and Latino men living in the city's poorest neighborhoods. The incidence of TB among black men in New York City between the ages of 25 and 44 is 20 times the rate in the general population and equal to the rate in sub-Saharan Africa.[22,23]

EPIDEMIOLOGY OF HOMELESSNESS

Homelessness is a product of insufficient low-cost housing and social programs and services. The increase in numbers of homeless individuals and families over the last 2 decades can be blamed on economic recession, a shift in the labor market away from unskilled jobs, an increase in pockets of poverty, a decreased commitment to public assistance and education, gentrification of our urban centers, and deinstitutionalization of the chronically mentally ill.[24] In 1991, the CDC estimated that there were 600,000 to 3 million homeless individuals and families, 80% of whom were single adult men, 20% families headed by a single adult woman, and 5 to 10% elderly.[25] While in the past single white men with a high level of chronic alcoholism predominated, the homeless population today is a heterogeneous group with heterogeneous risks. They are younger, better educated, more unemployed, and with a disproportionate number from racial and ethnic minorities. Women, families, and veterans are relatively new members of this homeless population.

The homeless are at increased risk for disease. Whether it is due to poor nutrition, substance abuse, poor hygiene, psychiatric disease, exposure to the environment, physical and sexual abuse, low immunization levels, poor access to and compliance with ongoing medical care, or their close living situations, homeless individuals have more medical problems than their domiciled counterparts. In one study, 41% identified a chronic medical problem, and one in six had a communicable disease.[26] Brickner estimates that about 30 to 40% have a major psychiatric disorder (schizophrenia or manic depressive illness); 60% are chronic alcoholics; 25% are intravenous drug users; and about 10 to 20% have dual psychiatric and substance abuse diagnoses. In one New York City homeless shelter, between 45 and 60% of inhabitants were HIV-positive; among homeless and runaway youths in San Francisco, 8% were HIV-positive. In a study of clients who attended shelter/SRO (single room occupancy hotel) clinics in New York City from 1982 to 1986, 42% had a positive tuberculin skin test and 8% had active tuberculosis.[27]

PATHOGENESIS

Koch identified the causative organism of tuberculosis in 1882.[18] Mycobacterium tuberculosis is an obligate aerobic intracellular parasite. Characteristically, it withstands decolorization with acid alcohol on routine stains—that is, it is acid-fast. It replicates slowly, about once in 18 to 24 hours (compared to an organism such as E. coli, which divides every 1 to 2 hours), making definitive diagnosis by culture a lengthy process.[28] Respiratory droplets are produced when an infected individual coughs, sneezes, or talks. The largest droplets that can be felt mostly drop to the floor and are noninfectious. Smaller droplets can be inhaled but are often trapped in the mucus of the upper respiratory tree and do not produce clinical disease. The smallest droplets, droplet nuclei that evaporate to a critical size of 1 to 3μ m, however, can circulate on room air currents, evade upper airway defenses, and reach peripheral alveoli. Tubercle bacilli within droplet nuclei can survive up to 3 hours in room air.[29,30]

Alveolar macrophages are the first cells to respond to invasion by tubercle bacilli. The ability of the alveolar macrophages to control infection is a function of the number and virulence of the organisms as well as host genetic factors. If the microbicidal activity of the alveolar macrophage is overwhelmed, replication of tubercle bacilli reaches a critical burden and organisms spread beyond alveoli to regional lymph nodes via lymphatic channels and to distant organs via the bloodstream.[30]

The regional lymph node is the site of a cell-mediated immune response, which typically develops about 4 to 8 weeks after exposure and is marked by a positive tuberculin skin test. In addition to its role as an initial responder, the alveolar macrophage processes mycobacterial antigens and presents them to T-lymphocytes within regional lymph nodes. Once exposed to this antigenic stimulation, CD4+ T-lymphocytes produce lymphokines and growth factors which promote T-lymphocyte proliferation, enhance the killing activity of tagged macrophages, and attract monocytes to sites of infection. Collections of activated T-lymphocytes, monocytes, and macrophages wall off the replicating tubercle bacilli within granulomas. A calcified granuloma within the lung and its associated draining lymph node is called a primary or Ghon's complex, which sometimes can be seen on chest radiograph. Organisms can remain viable within granulomas and become a nidus for reactivation in the future if immune function wanes. The positive tuberculin skin test is a reflection of this delayed cell-mediated immune response and a marker for recent or past infection. It is not necessarily a sign of active disease.

When host defenses are inadequate at the time of initial exposure, inflammatory infiltrates are produced usually in the middle and lower lung fields. A miliary pattern of spread occurs when large numbers of virulent organisms overwhelm the immune response and spread throughout both lung fields and the rest of the body. Activated immune cells (macrophages, monocytes, and lymphocytes) often produce frank tissue destruction via caseation necrosis at the site of infection and ultimately can lead to the formation of cavities within the lung parenchyma. Among healthy, untreated individuals who become tuberculin skin-test positive, 3.3% will develop active TB during the first year after exposure. The rest of these individuals may progress to active TB at the rate of 5% over the remainder of their lifetimes.[31] Reactivation disease usually occurs among foci of tubercle bacilli in the well-oxygenated and poorly perfused areas in the apices and posterior segments of the upper lungs, as well as at sites distant from the lungs, especially the kidneys, bones, and brain.

PPD IMMUNOLOGY

Koch discovered tuberculin in 1890 and thought it would be a cure for TB. Tuberculin PPD is a filtrate prepared from heat-sterilized broth cultures of tubercle bacilli. It contains antigenic components of the organism that can elicit a sensitivity response in an individual infected with M. tuberculosis.[32] It is the best means of detecting infection. The Mantoux intradermal skin test developed in 1910 is the preferred method for applying tuberculin PPD.

The reaction to injected tuberculin is a delayed cellular hypersensitivity reaction. The response takes greater than 24 hours to develop and is characterized by induration at the site caused by the infiltration of immune cells (CD4+ T-lymphocytes). False-positive results may indicate infection with nontuberculosis mycobacteria or prior vaccination with BCG, a live attenuated strain derived from mycobacterium bovis. In general, the larger the skin reaction, the greater the probability that the reaction represents infection with M. tuberculosis. The reaction occurs at least 4 to 6 weeks post-exposure.

A reaction greater than 5 mm is considered positive in the following groups: (1) persons at risk for or who are infected with HIV, (2) close recent contacts of infectious TB, and (3) persons with chest radiographs consistent with old healed TB.[19] For others, a reaction > 10 mm is considered positive in groups such as immigrants from high-prevalence countries, IDUs, high-risk racial and ethnic minorities, patients with diseases that suppress cell-mediated immunity, and exposed health care workers. For all others, an area of induration greater than 15 mm is considered a positive reaction.[33]

DIAGNOSIS

The initial evaluation of the patient with suspected tuberculosis should include a chest radiograph and an examination of at least three sputums for acid-fast bacilli.[34] The Ziehl-Neelsen stain is used to identify tubercle bacilli in sputum.[31] It has been estimated that a count of 10,000 organisms per milliliter of sputum is necessary for a positive smear. Fluorescent microscopy utilizes low magnification screening and is more sensitive than conventional light microscopy but it is not available in most institutions. Although the sensitivity of the test varies, positive smears are 98% specific for the diagnosis of tuberculosis. Klein compared AFB smears in tuberculosis patients with and without AIDS. He found that 45% of AIDS patients had positive AFB smears, compared to 81% of non-AIDS patients.[35] The absence of cavitary disease

among AIDS patients may account for at least part of this discrepancy.

Because of its slow growth cycle, cultures of tubercle bacilli take 6 to 8 weeks to grow on agar- or egg-based solid culture media with antibacterial additives. Newer techniques for culturing mycobacteria can confirm a diagnosis of TB in as little as 5 days. The BACTEC system utilizes a 14C-labeled substrate that is metabolized by mycobacteria to radioactive CO_2. Species-specific DNA probes directed against ribosomal RNA are used to distinguish M. tuberculosis from other Mycobacteria species.

Other modalities useful in making the expeditious diagnosis of tuberculosis include bronchoscopy with bronchial washings and transbronchial biopsy; fine needle extrathoracic lymph node aspiration; and pleural and pericardial fluid examination. The polymerase chain reaction (PCR) is a technique that utilizes DNA sequences unique to a mycobacterial species to serve as a marker for the organism in various body secretions.[23] Using PCR gene replication techniques, M. tuberculosis DNA can be rapidly and reliably detected from very small numbers of organisms (1 to 1,000) in a very short time period. Clarridge et al. reported on the utility of this technique in identifying mycobacteria from clinical specimens. They found that 94% of culture (+), smear (+) specimens were positive with their PCR.[36,37]

Other laboratory techniques for rapid diagnosis include gas chromatography mass spectrometry which tests for the presence of tuberculostearic acid (TSA), a branched-chain fatty acid present in mycobacteria. Lack of specificity, however, limits its usefulness.[38] Restriction fragment length polymorphism (RFLP) is a research tool for studying genetic mutations associated with drug resistance and for tracking various strains of M. tuberculosis in nosocomial and community outbreaks.[39] Another new technique involves inserting light-producing mycobacteriophages into cultures of tubercle bacilli for early detection and rapid determination of drug sensitivities. Testing serum antibodies against mycobacterium-specific proteins using the ELISA method may serve as a future tool for rapid diagnosis.[40]

In patients with signs of extrapulmonary tuberculosis, cultures of blood, bone marrow, liver, lymph nodes or CSF may be necessary to confirm the diagnosis. The absence of organisms on smear and the lack of granuloma on histologic exam do not exclude the diagnosis, and so cultures must be performed on all tissue specimens.

TREATMENT

Effective therapy cures tuberculosis 98% of the time. Recent guidelines published by the CDC recommend that all patients with newly diagnosed tuberculosis be started on a four-drug regimen consisting of isoniazid (INH), rifampin (RIF), pyrazinamide (PZA), and either streptomycin (SM) or ethambutol (EMB).[10] This regimen should be continued until sensitivities are known. If the organism is parisensitive, PZA and ethambutol can be discontinued after 2 months. INH and rifampin should be continued for an additional 4 months in HIV-negative patients, and for a total of 9 months in HIV-positive patients.

When organisms develop resistance to standard antibiotics, the cure rate drops to 55%. Drug resistance results from random, spontaneous genetic mutation. Failure to complete a full course of therapy encourages the growth of drug-resistant tubercle bacilli. A recent survey showed that 19% of all isolates in New York City were resistant to both isoniazed and rifampin. These individuals were predominantly less than 40 years old, male, jobless, homeless, and often had histories of drug abuse and HIV. The simultaneous use of multiple drugs over a prolonged amount of time forestalls the occurrence of a resistant population of organisms. MDR-TB has serious public health implications due to the rapid progression to life-threatening disease and the efficient transmission to others, especially among HIV positive patients, and delays to diagnosis and treatment.

THE ROLE OF HIV

In the U.S., many lines of evidence support the relationship between HIV infection and tuberculosis. First, rates of TB are highest in cities and among groups that have the highest rates of AIDS.[14,41] Second, the HIV-seroprevalence among new cases of TB is hundreds of times greater than in the general population.[42] Third, the incidence of extrapulmonary TB (found in 70% of TB/AIDS patients) has quadrupled since 1984.[43] Fourth, studies have revealed a close temporal relationship between the diagnoses of AIDS and TB in the same patient.

Cross-referencing of AIDS and TB directories revealed that 5% of AIDS cases in New York City and 10% of AIDS cases in Florida have had active TB.[44] While all HIV risk groups were represented among those dually infected, the chance of having active TB was related to the prevalence of latent infection in each group. For example, 79 to 91% of Haitians in Miami are positive tuberculin reactors, and the prevalence of TB among Haitians with AIDS ranges from 27 to 60%. The prevalence of tuberculin reactivity among injecting drug users (IDUs) in New York City is 22%, and the prevalence of TB among IDUs with AIDS is 9%.[11, 45] Conversely, in San Francisco, where homosexuals and bisexuals have a very low prevalence of tuberculin reactivity, the prevalence of dual HIV/TB is less than 2%.[46]

In a similar manner, tuberculosis is currently viewed as an early marker for HIV infection. Shafer et al. prospectively studied all patients with TB at a New York inner-city public hospital. Of those patients, 46% were HIV-positive, 30% were HIV-negative, and 24% were not assessed with respect to HIV status. Most HIV/TB cases were either IDUs or of Haitian origin.[47] Other studies revealed HIV-seropositive rates of 28% among non-Asians with TB in San Francisco, and a 31% HIV-seroprevalence among TB patients in Miami.[48,49] The median HIV-seroprevalence rate in TB clinics across the country is estimated at 11%. In most cases, tuberculosis is due to reactivation of latent foci although there are many reports of progressive primary infection, mostly after nosocomial exposure.

INFECTION CONTROL

In the beginning of the HIV epidemic, hospital infection control successfully focused on parenteral transmission of the virus to health care workers. Education of staff, new technologies, and surveillance of exposures were used to prevent transmission and safeguard workers.

Nosocomial spread of TB between patients and between patients and health care workers is today's great concern. Multiple episodes of nosocomial transmission have been documented on hospital wards,[50,51] hospital clinics,[52] prisons,[53] shelters,[54] and residential facilities.[55] Between 1990 and 1992, the CDC investigated seven outbreaks of MDR-TB across the country, which involved over 200 infections. Most cases were due to nosocomial transmission and involved HIV-seropositive patients in over 90% of cases. The time course from exposure to infection was short, and the fatality rate was over 80%. Health care workers involved in the care of these patients had high rates of tuberculin skin test conversions compared to their peers on wards where these patients did not receive care; immunocompromised health care workers were at greatest risk.[56]

In 1989, the CDC established a goal of eliminating TB by the year 2010. They recommended (1) rapid assessment, reporting and treatment of suspected cases, and screening of high-risk groups, (2) development of new technologies to expedite diagnosis and improve containment, and (3) the rapid dissemination of these technologies.[4] In 1990 and 1991, the CDC published guidelines for isolation, treatment, screening, and prevention, and, in 1993 and 1995, the CDC published recommendations to state health departments to improve compliance with treatment regimens by providing incentives, social supports, voluntary and involuntary direct observed treatment programs, and, ultimately, detention and isolation of infectious cases and noninfectious cases who refuse to adhere to treatment plans.[57]

There is a hierarchy of measures to deal with infection control of tuberculosis. Primary emphasis is on control at the source.[58] Timely identification of cases, isolation, and rapid initiation of effective therapy are the best ways to prevent the generation of infectious droplet nuclei. Delays in diagnosis were common in over half the patients with TB in two retrospective studies involving over 100 patients. Absence of symptoms, advanced age, atypical radiographs, absence of organisms on smear, and misinterpretation of skin tests were cited as reasons for poor diagnostic accuracy.[59,60]

Dual HIV/TB infection produces a wide spectrum of clinical disease. Symptoms may be confused with those of other respiratory opportunistic infections which are so common in seropositive patients. All the tools of diagnosis are less sensitive and less specific in the setting of extreme immunocompromise, and, as a consequence, time delays to diagnosis and proper treatment and isolation are common. Barnes found that 4% of his group of 105 HIV-seropositive patients with pleuropulmonary TB mimicked pneumocystis carinii infection, both clinically and radiographically. On the chest radiographs, 6/105 patients with TB were read as normal, and only 14/56 radiographs in patients who had negative smears were classic for TB (i.e., upper lobe infiltrates, cavities, or a miliary pattern). Overall, the AFB smear was positive in less than 50% of his group.[61] Another study by Klein confirmed the insensitivity of AFB smears in the setting of HIV infection. He found only a 41% positivity rate among patients with AIDS and ARC, as opposed to 81% positivity in HIV-seronegative TB patients.[35]

The tuberculin skin test also lacks sensitivity in a setting of extreme immunocompromise. Whereas 60% of patients with less than 200 CD4+ T-lymphocytes are anergic, only 16% of those with 200 to 400 CD4+ T-cells are anergic.[62] Among HIV/TB patients in Spain, 22% were PPD-positive, versus 95% of tuberculosis patients who were HIV-seronegative.[63] Delays in diagnosis lead to delays in source control. Once identified, TB patients must be properly isolated and must be started on effective therapy.

The high incidence of drug resistance among HIV/TB patients produces another delay in infectious control because effective therapy is compromised. Awareness of resistance patterns in the community is important in designing primary drug therapy. In New York City, in April 1991, one-third of all isolates were resistant to at least one antituberculous drug, and 19% were resistant to both isoniazid and rifampin. If the patients submitting isolates had been exposed to antituberculous drugs in the past, 44% were resistant to at least one, and 30% were resistant to at least two drugs.[64] This pattern of resistance is emerging as one of the most critical events in public health today.

Source control includes isolation until the patient is no longer infectious. It is generally accepted that a patient is noninfectious if he responds clinically and biologically to the treatment. An improvement in symptoms and a declining number of organisms on AFB smear is usually sufficient proof of noninfectiousness, although the absence of organisms on smear does not guarantee a noninfectious state. There are many cases of nosocomial spread of active TB by smear-negative patients, as well as documented tuberculin skin test conversions among individuals who are in contact with smear-negative patients. Generally, if a patient is on effective therapy for at least 2 weeks, he is considered noninfectious, even though it takes about 3 months of effective therapy before AFB cultures become negative.

In cases of MDR-TB however, it is wise to wait for three negative smears on consecutive days before declaring a patient noninfectious. Premature release of patients from isolation has been the source of several episodes of nosocomial spread, as has laxity in enforcing rules of isolation (e.g. allowing the patient to leave his room only for procedures and to wear at least a surgical mask at all times outside his room). EDs must develop protocols regarding the isolation of patients with known or possible TB.

ISSUES IN PUBLIC HEALTH

Homeless individuals are entitled to the same level of health care as are all others. The magnitude, geographic pervasiveness, and heterogeneous vulnerability of this population requires a response on a federal governmental level. For the safety of all, a commitment must be made to attack the root problems that force people into homelessness. Useful measures include stimulating the production of low-cost housing, providing job training and education, expanding the safety net of economic and social services for those temporarily displaced, guaranteeing universal health insurance, and investing in research to identify deficiencies and create remedies for this desperate condition.

From a medical care perspective, programs must be developed that are appropriate and accessible. The heterogeneous nature of the homeless population needs both tailored and systemic solutions. Special attention to homeless families and children because they engender advocacy groups should not preclude resources devoted to the single black intravenous drug user with HIV or tuberculosis or both diseases.

The barriers to health care experienced by homeless people must be lowered. Facilities and personnel must be available at the point of service (e.g., clinics in shelters or drop-in centers) to accommodate the migratory nature and lack of funds for transportation among homeless people. Service should be free or covered by national insurance. The health care delivery system must have suitable hours and administrative procedures that are not alienating. Comprehensive services including attention to substance abuse problems, psychiatric disease and providing a liaison to more specialized services in secondary and tertiary care centers must be made available. Finally, health care personnel must have special sensitivity to the cultures, languages, lifestyles, psychology, and financial constraints of the homeless when prescribing medications or other treatment plans.[65,66]

Clearly, the rising incidence of tuberculosis, especially drug-resistant tuberculosis, reflects a breakdown in the health care systems charged with controlling it. Its contagious nature and its emergence among a population that is notoriously noncompliant demands a renewed public health approach. In 1989, the CDC published a plan for the attack on tuberculosis. The plan called for revision of state and local laws to facilitate the treatment of persons with infectious tuberculosis, the surveillance of those at risk, and the quarantine of those who are noncompliant. The CDC adopted and funded universal directly observed therapy as its main weapon in the war against tuberculosis.[67] By recognizing the complexities of the lives of socioeconomically disadvantaged and undomiciled people, the CDC decided on a strategy of treating their patients where they live, at no cost, with incentives and other services that homeless people need. Although costly, DOT is successful.[68] The CDC reported a 5% drop in the number of new cases in 1993.

ROLE OF THE ED PRACTITIONER

In the absence of an available, accessible, easily approachable, and free community public health system, emergency physicians will continue to be the primary caregivers to the homeless. To be effective, we must recognize the heterogeneity of the group and of their medical risks. We must treat the current disease process, and then we must intervene preventively. Surveillance for tuberculosis, HIV substance abuse, sexual and physical abuse, malnutrition, low immunization levels, environmental dangers for homeless children as well as hazards to their growth and development, and chronic medical processes like hypertension or diabetes are all appropriate. The approach should be comprehensive, involving social services, governmental agencies, substance abuse counselors, psychiatric services, and so on.

Emergency physicians must be suspicious of tuberculosis in all patients, especially in the homeless. Early isolation is critical to protect staff and other patients. Anyone with a history of prior tuberculosis disease or infection should be screened for active disease. Drug-sensitive tuberculosis in an immunocompetent host is 95% curable. Drug-resistant tuberculosis is only 50% curable. Drug-resistant tuberculosis in an immunocompromised host can be fatal. Review of prior cultures for drug sensitivities and review of old charts for partial treatment is necessary. Eleven states require health care providers to report nonadherent patients. The Emergency physician must take responsibility for coordinating this comprehensive approach to the homeless. Resources will be necessary and sensitivities must be heightened, but the long-term benefits of timely intervention can be dramatic.

ENVIRONMENTAL CONTROLS

Respiratory spread of AFB is a function of the number of organisms in inspired air and the amount of time an exposed individual spends in the contaminated space. Environmental controls are designed to reduce the concentration of tubercle bacilli in the environment once they are released by the source. Standard mechanical heating, ventilating and air conditioning systems (HVAC) reduce air contaminants within a space by dilution with outside air, by mechanical filtration, and by directional air flow (i.e., negative pressure within the room compared to pressure in hallways). The concentration of tubercle bacilli in contaminated air is relatively low so large volumes of air must be pumped, heated, and filtered in order to reduce the concentration to acceptable levels. There are limits to the abilities of HVAC systems in terms of energy costs, noise and air current production, and occupant acceptance.[5] Current federal regulations recommend at least 6 air changes per hour in any area housing patients with TB. Ventilation in contaminated areas should be nonrecirculating—that is, rooms are vented to the outside and away from any inlet valves. Negative-pressure rooms are recommended to keep organisms from escaping into hallways. High-energy particle air filters (HEPA), either in the outlet duct or free standing,

is an additional method of decontaminating air without substantial engineering expense.[69]

In 1962, Riley showed that air contaminated with tubercle bacilli is infectious at a distance from the source. He vented air from a TB ward to another floor that housed guinea pigs and compared the results with guinea pigs who were not exposed to contaminated air. Over half the exposed guinea pigs developed TB over a 2-year period, while none of the nonexposed animals did. He also demonstrated that by circulating the vented air past ultraviolet (UV) lamps, acute TB could be prevented in the exposed animals.[70]

Ultraviolet germicidal lamps (UVGL) produce a narrow band (253.7-nm wavelength) of the ultraviolet portion of the electromagnetic spectrum. This wave length is lethal to microorganisms. Prolonged direct exposure can cause eye and skin irritation in humans. However, when lamps are located above people's heads in the upper part of a room, the exposure is indirect and innocuous. Normal room air currents circulate contaminated lower room air with germ-free upper room air, thus reducing the concentration of tubercle bacilli.[67] UVGL lamps are inexpensive and theoretically effective and should be used liberally in areas where patients with possible TB may congregate—for example, waiting areas, clinics, procedure suites, and isolation rooms.

CONCLUSION

M. tuberculosis is an ancient organism that has survived all efforts to arrest its spread. It accounts for more disease and death than any other single pathogen. Technologic advances and new social insights are reasons for optimism. PCR gene amplification offers the prospect of same-day diagnosis; DNA probes can identify drug sensitivities rapidly and accurately; strain identification by RFLP enables us to track nosocomial outbreaks; advances in HVAC and other engineering controls will make for a safer work environment; new vaccines promise to protect the uninfected; and wide-scale adoption of universal direct observed therapy can increase the cure rate and retard the development of resistant strains.

Continued emphasis on the following basic principles will be critical to success:

1. Tuberculosis should be suspected in any HIV infected patient who presents with fever, cough, night sweats, and weight loss, regardless of the results of the chest radiograph;
2. All patients suspected of having TB should be properly and strictly isolated at the earliest possible moment and personnel should wear respirator masks when entering isolation rooms;
3. Effective drug therapy with four antibiotics should be initiated early and resistance patterns in the community should be tracked;
4. Surveillance of health care workers and others at risk should include tuberculin skin testing on a yearly basis and more aggressive screening of health care workers who are immunocompromised or who are exposed to patients with TB who undergo invasive procedures like bronchoscopy;
5. For any particular patient, medical factors must be evaluated within the patient's socioeconomic context;
6. A medical approach must be combined with a public health approach in order to halt the spread of tuberculosis; and
7. Access to care must be improved for vulnerable populations.

NOTES

1. Centers for Disease Control. Tuberculosis morbidity in the United States: Final data, 1990. *MMWR* 1990; 40(3):23–7.
2. Barnes PF, Bloch AB, Davidson PT, Snider DE. Tuberculosis in patients with human immunodeficiency virus. *NEJM* 1991; 324:1644–50.
3. Brudneey K, Dobkin K. Resurgent tuberculosis in New York City. *Am Rev Resp Dis* 1991; 144:745–9.
4. Centers for Disease Control. A strategic plan for the elimination of TB in the United States. *MMWR* 1989; 38(3):1–9.
5. Nardell EA, Keegan J, Cheney SA, Etkind SC. Airborne infection: Theoretical limits of protection achievable by building ventilation. *Am Rev Respir Dis* 1991; 144:302–6.
6. Dunlap NE, Briles DE: Immunology of tuberculosis. *Med Clin North Am* 1993; 77:1235–51.
7. Klein NC, Duncanson FP, Lenox TH. Use of mycobacterial smears in the diagnosis of pulmonary tuberculosis in AIDS/ARC patients. *Chest* 1989; 95: 1190–1328.
8. Long R, Scalcini M, Manfreda J. The impact of HIV on the usefulness of sputum smears for the diagnosis of tuberculosis. *Am J Pub Health* 1991; 81:1326–8.
9. Crawford JT. New technologies in the diagnosis of tuberculosis. *Sem Resp Infect* 1994; 9(2):62–70.
10. Centers for Disease Control. Initial therapy for TB in the era of multidrug resistance: Recommendations of the advisory council for the elimination of TB. *MMWR* 1993; 42(7):1–80.
11. Selwyn PA, Seckell BM, Alcabes P, et al. High risk of active tuberculosis in HIV-infected drug users with cutaneous anergy. *JAMA* 1992; 268:504–9.
12. Phair J, Munoz A, Detels R. The risk of pneumocystis carinii pneumonia among men infected with HIV. *NEJM* 1990; 322:161.
13. Jones BE, Young SM, Antoniskis D. Relationship of the manifestations of tuberculosis to CD4 cell counts in patients with HIV. *Am Rev Respir Dis* 1993; 148:1292–7.
14. Edlin BR, Tokars JI, Grieco MH. An outbreak of MDR-TB among hospitalized patients with AIDS. *NEJM* 1992; 326:1514–21.
15. Daley CL, Small PM, Schechter PF. An outbreak of TB with accelerated progression among persons infected with HIV. *NEJM* 1992; 326:231–5.
16. Alland D, Kalkut GE, Moss AR. Transmission of TB in New York City. *NEJM* 1994; 330:1710–15.
17. Small PM, Hopewell PC, Singh SP. The epidemiology of TB in San Francisco. *NEJM* 1994; 330:1705–9.
18. Brudney K, Dobkin K: Resurgent tuberculosis in NYC. *Am Rev Resp Dis* 1991; 144:745–9.
19. Torres RA, Marci S, Altholy J. HIV infection among homeless men in a NYC shelter: Association with M. tuberculosis infection. *Arch Int Med* 1990; 150: 2030–6.
20. Sudre P, ten Dam G, Kochi A. Tuberculosis: a global overview of the situation today. *WHO* 1992; 70(2):149–59.
21. Centers for Disease Control. Prevention and control of tuberculosis in U.S. communities with at-risk minority populations and prevention and control of tuberculosis among homeless persons. *MMWR* 1992; 41:1–21.
22. Centers for Disease Control. Tuberculosis and AIDS—New York City. *MMWR* 1987; 36(48).
23. City Health Information, March 1991; 10(2):1–4.
24. Robertson MJ, Greenblatt M (eds). *Homelessness a National Perspective*. New York: Plenum Press, 1991.

25. Centers for Disease Control: Characteristics and risk behaviors of homeless black males. *MMWR* Aug 1991; 40:865–8.
26. Bollinger K, Goup A, Vigna G. Health Care for the Homeless: A public concern. *J of the Louisiana S Med Soc* July 1993; 145(7):321–3.
27. Brickner PW et al. *Under the safety net.* New York: W.W. Norton, 1987.
28. Weissler JC. Tuberculosis-immunopathogenesis and therapy. *Amer J Med Sci* 1993; 305(1):52–65.
29. Fauci A. Immunopathogenesis of HIV infection. *J Acquir Immunodef Syndr* 1993; 6(6):655–62.
30. Weissler JC. Tuberculosis- immunopathogenesis and therapy. *Amer J Med Sci* 1993; 305(1):52–65.
31. Des Prez RM, Heim C. Mycobacterium tuberculosis. In GL Mandell, RG Douglas, JE Bennett (eds.). *Principles and Practice of Infectious Diseases.* New York: Churchill Livingston, 1990.
32. Snider DE. The tuberculin skin test. *Am Rev Respir Dis* 1982; 125:108.
33. American Thoracic Society. Diagnostic standards and classification of tuberculosis. *Am Rev Respir Dis* 1990; 142:725–35.
34. Kramer R, Modilevsky T, Waliany A, et al. Delayed diagnosis of tuberculosis in patients with human immunodeficiency virus infection. *Am J Med* 89; 451–6.
35. Klein N, Duncanson F, Lenox T, et al. Use of mycobacterial smears in the diagnosis of pulmonary tuberculosis in AIDS/ARC patients. *Chest* 1989; 95:1190–92.
36. Clarridge JE. Large scale use of polymerase chain reaction for detection of mycobacterium tuberculosis in a routine mycobactiology laboratory. [Author's Reply]. *J Clin Microbiol* 1994; 32:274.
37. Clarridge JE, Shawar RM, Shinnick TM, Plikaytis BB. Large scale use of polymerase chain reaction for detection of mycobacterium tuberculosis in a routine mycobactiology laboratory. *J Clin Microbiol* 1993; 31:2049–56.
38. Savic B, Sjobring U, Alugupalli S, et al. Evaluation of polymerase chain reaction, tuberculstearic acid analysis and direct microscopy of the detection of mycobacterium tuberculosis in sputum. *J Infect Dis* 1992; 166:1177–80.
39. Daley CL, Small PM, Schecter GF, et al. An outbreak of tuberculosis with accelerated progression among persons infected with the human immunodeficiency virus: An analysis using restriction fragment length polymorphism. *NEJM* 1992; 326:231–5.
40. Maekura R, Nakamura Y, Nakamura Y, et al. Clinical evaluation of rapid serodiagnosis of pulmonary tuberculosis by ELISA with Cord Factor (Trehalose 6,6'dimycolate) as antigen purified from mycobacterium tuberculosis. *Am Rev Respir Dis* 1993; 148:997–1001.
41. Rieder HL, Cauthen GM, Kelly GD et al. Tuberculosis in the US. *JAMA* 1989; 262:385–9.
42. Kaminski Z, Pearce M, Lombardo J, et al. Incidence of mycobacterial infections in HIV positive intravenous drug abusers: Analysis of 246 necropsy cases. *Abstr Gen Meet Am Soc Microbiol* 1992; 170 (abstract no. U-30): 1002.
43. Onorato I, McCray E. Prevalence of human immunodeficiency: Virus infection among patients attending TB clinics in the US. *J Infect Dis* 1992; 165:87–92.
44. Rieder HL, Chaisson R, Schechter G, et al. Tuberculosis in patients with AIDS. *Am Rev Resp Dis* 1987; 136:570–4.
45. Centers for Disease Control. Tuberculosis and AIDS—New York City. *MMWR* 1987; 36(48).
46. Rieder HL. Epidemiology of tuberculosis in the United States. *Epidemiolgic Rev* 989; 11:79–98.
47. Shafer RW, Chirgwin KD, Glatt AE, et al. HIV prevalence, immunosuppression and drug resistance in patients with tuberculosis in areas endemic for AIDS. *AIDS* 1991; 5(4)399–405.
48. Theuer CP, Hopewell PC, Elias D, et al. Human immunodeficiency virus in tuberculosis patients. *J Infect Dis* 1990; 162:8–12.
49. Pitchenik AE, Burr J, Swarez M, et al. HTLV-III seropositivity and related disease among 71 consecutive patients in whom tuberculosis was diagnosed: A prospective study. *Am Rev Respir Dis* 1987; 135:875–9.
50. Beck-Saque C. Hospital outbreak of MDR-TB factors in tranmission to staff, health care worker, and patients. *JAMA* 1992; 268(10).
51. Dooley SW, Villarino, ME, et al. Nosocomial transmission of tuberculosis in a hospital unit for HIV-infected patients. *JAMA* 1992; 267(19):2632–7.
52. Kwan R, Chiliade P, Sharp V. Report of two cases of MDR-MTB pneumonia in non-immunocompromised health care workers (HCWs) at a New York City AIDS center. *Int Conf AIDS* 1993; 9(1):329 (abst no. PO-BO7-1162).
53. Braun M, Truman B, et al. Increasing incidence of tuberculosis in a prison inmate population. *JAMA* 1989; 261:393.
54. McAdam J. Letter to the editor. *Chest* 1992; 99:792.

55. Centers for Disease Control. Tuberculosis outbreak among persons in a residential facility for HIV infected persons in San Francisco. *MMWR* 1991; 40(38): 649–52.

56. Centers for Disease Control. Tuberculosis control laws—United States, 1993. *MMWR* 1993; 42(15):1-13.

57. Centers for Disease Control. Essential components of a Tuberculosis Prevention and Control Program. *MMWR* 1995; 44:1–34.

58. Mathur P, Sacks L, Auten G, et al. Delayed diagnosis of pulmonary tuberculosis in city hospitals. *Arch Intern Med* 1994; 154:306–10.

59. Scott B, Schmid M, Nettleman D. Early identification and isolation of inpatients at high risk for tuberculosis. *Arch Intern Med* 1994; 154:326–30.

60. Barnes PF, Steele MA, Young SM, Vachon LA. Tuberculosis in patients with human immunodeficiency virus infection. How often does it mimic pneumocystis carinii pneumonia. *Chest* 1992; 102(2):428-32.

61. Blatt SP et al. DTH skin testing as predictor of progression to AIDS. *Ann Intern Med* 1993; 119(3):177.

62. Martin-Casabona N, Ocana Rivera I, Vidal Pla R, et al. Diagnosis of mycobacterial infection in acquired immunodeficiency syndrome (AIDS) patients and HIV carriers. *J Hygiene, Epidemiol, Microbiol & Immunol* 1992; 36(3):293-302.

63. Frieden TR, Sterling T, Pablos-Mendez A, et al. The emergence of drug-resistant tuberculosis in New York City. *NEJM* 1993; 328:521-26.

64. Wright J, Weber E. *Homelessness and Health.* Washington DC: McGraw-Hill, 1987.

65. Goldberg L. Health and Medical Care of Homeless Persons. *West J Med* May 1993; 158(5):518.

66. Tuberculosis Control Laws—United States, 1993. *MMWR* 1993; 42 (RR-15):1-28.

67. Weis SE, Slocum PC. The effects of directly observed therapy on the rates of drug resistance and relapse in tuberculosis. *NEJM* 1994; 330(17):1179-84.

68. Centers for Disease Control. Guidelines for preventing the transmission of tuberculosis in health care settings with special focus on HIV-related issues. *MMWR* 1990; 39(17):1-23.

69. Riley RL. Infectiousness of air from a TB ward. *Am Rev of Respir Dis* 1962; 85:511.

70. Riley RL, Nardell EA. Clearing the air: The theory and application of ultraviolet air disinfection. *Am Rev Respir Dis* 1989; 139:1286-94.

3

Sexually Transmitted Diseases and Disease Surveillance

THOMAS D. KIRSCH
DONNA SUE

CONTENTS

- Differential diagnosis
- History
- Risk factors
- Treatment
- Sequelae
- Surveillance
- The broader health context
- The emergency physician's role

CHAPTER SUMMARY

Patients with STDs are commonly encountered in the Emergency Department. EDs are often the primary source of care for the urban poor who are at great risk for sexually transmitted infections.[1] As such, emergency physicians have a critical role in controlling the spread of STDs. Important measures that EPs can take include:

- Ensuring that they are up-to-date regarding the changing therapy recommendations
- Providing appropriate screening services, or presumptive treatment
- Providing patient education and discharge instructions
- Encouraging partner treatment
- Reporting cases to public health authorities.

Case #1

A 19-year-old female, G2P2, presents to the Emergency Department complaining of abdominal pain and vaginal bleeding. She states that her last menstrual period was approximately six weeks before but notes that she is often irregular. Her pain and bleeding had rapid onset approximately 2 hours prior to presentation. The pain was associated with mild nausea but no vomiting, diarrhea, or urinary symptoms. The patient denies any vaginal discharge. She reports a history of unprotected sexual intercourse during the past 6 months. She also states that she has a previous history of gonorrhea.

Physical examination: The patient is a mildly obese young female in moderate distress. She has a temperature of 99.8°F, a pulse of 100, respiratory rate of 20, and a blood pressure of 102/64. Her HEENT, chest, and cardiac exams are all normal. Her abdominal exam reveals hypoactive bowel sounds and diffuse tenderness that is markedly increased in the right lower quadrant. Voluntary guarding and local rebound are noted. No CVA tenderness was noted. Vaginal exams reveals scant blood in the vault, marked cervical motion tenderness (CMT), and marked tenderness with possible fullness in the right adnexa. Rectal exam is diffusely tender with guaiac negative stools.

Q: What is the differential diagnosis for this patient?

Rapid assessment of lower abdominal pain in women of reproductive age is needed to identify potentially life-threatening conditions. Hemorrhagic shock from a ruptured ectopic pregnancy and septic shock secondary to pelvic inflammatory disease are the two most important emergent gynecologic conditions to consider, while appendicitis is a surgical emergency. Other causes of severe lower abdominal pain included in the differential are ruptured ovarian or corpus luteum cyst, mechanical torsion of the fallopian tube or ovary around its vascular pedicle, or endometritis. A complaint of lower abdominal pain may be also be related to acute cystitis, ureteral stone, or acute gastroenteritis.

Q: What other important historical questions should be asked if pelvic inflammatory disease (PID) or an ectopic pregnancy are suspected?

There are certain behavior and health risk factors that are associated with PID that can be elicited in the history. Some of the major risk factors for acquiring a sexually transmitted disease (STD) and PID are similar. These include unmarried women from 15 to 24 years in lower socioeconomic status groups. Other shared risk factors include smoking, noncompliance with treatment, and failure to notify partner. Risk factors specific for PID include the use of an intrauterine device (IUD) for birth control; douching; and previous PID. PID that is contracted at a younger age (i.e., immediately post-menarche) is more likely to lead to complications such as tubal scarring and infertility. The risks for acquiring an STD that have not been associated with increased risk for PID include early onset of sexual intercourse, multiple (>3 per year) sexual partners, and the frequency of intercourse. Besides a history of PID, other risk factors for ectopic pregnancy include a history of infertility with the use of ovulation-inducing drugs or in-vitro fertilization, a history of previous ectopic pregnancies, tubal surgery, the use of intrauterine devices, and cigarette smoking.

Case Continuation

Initial management included starting a large-bore IV and ordering a CBC, type and screen, urinalysis, and urine pregnancy test. While waiting to pass urine, the patient developed increased abdominal pain, became light-headed, her blood pressure dropped to 70/48, and her pulse increased to 140. A repeat physical examination demonstrated a diffusely tender, rigid abdomen. A second IV line was started, and fluid resuscitation was begun with lactated ringers solution.

The patient's pregnancy test came back positive and a culdocentesis revealed frank blood. The OB/GYN physician on call was contacted. The patient was immediately brought to the operating room for an emergency laparotomy, which revealed a ruptured ectopic pregnancy in the right fallopian tube. The left tube was also noted to be scarred, which was consistent with previous PID. The patient had approximately 1,200 cc of blood in her abdomen and required transfusion of 4 units of packed red blood cells during the procedure. She had a prolonged hospital course complicated by postoperative pneumonia but was discharged on the fourteenth day after admission.

Q: What is the approach to lower abdominal pain in a sexually active female in the emergency department?

For female patients with acute abdominal pain, the emergency physician must be able to quickly recognize those who require volume resuscitation, surgery, or sepsis evaluation. The initial history should focus on current pregnancy status, vaginal bleeding, last normal menstrual period, prior pregnancies, vomiting, and the presence of postural dizziness or fever. If the patient is hemodynamically unstable, early volume resuscitation with isotonic crystalloid through two large-bore IVs is necessary. Initial laboratory tests should include a spun hematocrit, complete blood count and differential, blood type and cross-match, and a pregnancy test.

The physical exam should include vital signs, the presence of pallor, diaphoresis, and poor capillary refill to assess for signs of shock. The abdomen is examined for specific areas of tenderness or peritoneal signs, and the pelvic exam performed to look for bleeding, inflammation, or discharge. The bimanual exam localizes tenderness and identifies abnormal masses.

In a stable patient, a more detailed history is necessary to help form the differential diagnosis and should focus on the quality, onset, location, radiation, severity, duration and pattern of the pain. Associated symptoms of nausea, vomiting, diarrhea, urinary symptoms and vaginal complaints are elicited. Menstrual functioning and reproductive history should also be obtained. Risk factors for PID should be sought including history of sexually transmitted disease, multiple sex partners, use of an IUD, vaginal douching and smoking. Young age is an important risk factor for PID as sexually active teenagers are three times more likely to be diagnosed with PID than women between the age of 25 and 29.[2]

The key piece of information to obtain in the initial assessment of lower abdominal pain is whether or not the patient is pregnant. Unfortunately, the history and physical are not sensitive for the diagnosis of early pregnancy. A urine or blood pregnancy test should always be ordered in this situation. The urine hCG is detectable at 20 mIU/ml, is positive at the time of the first missed menses, and has a false-negative rate of 1%. Serum hCG is detectable at 10 mIU/ml and has a false-negative rate of 0.5%.[3] In a normal pregnancy, the quantitative B-hCG level will double every 2 days. Low values on a single assay may indicate an ectopic pregnancy that has outgrown its blood supply and is about to rupture or an early intrauterine pregnancy. If the patient is stable and the ultrasound is nondiagnostic, the hCG level should be repeated in 48 hours and the patient reevaluated. Institutions located in communities where there is a high risk for ectopic pregnancy might consider developing a joint ED-OB/GYN protocol for observation and follow-up.

Q: What is the role of pelvic inflammatory disease (PID) in the etiology of a ruptured ectopic pregnancy?

There has been a fivefold increase in the incidence of ectopic pregnancy over the past 20 years, which represents a major health risk to women of child-bearing age.[4] More than 80,000 ectopic pregnancies are reported annually in the United States.[5] Despite the decrease in the case-fatality rate due to increased physician awareness and improved diagnostic techniques, ectopic pregnancy remains the second lead-

ing cause of maternal death. African American teenagers have a mortality risk that is five times greater than the average for white women. In addition, the risk of adverse reproductive outcome following an ectopic pregnancy is high, with about 30% of women becoming infertile, and the risk of subsequent ectopic pregnancy is greatly increased.[6]

A history of sexually transmitted diseases (STD), especially gonorrhea and chlamydia, and the association with ectopic pregnancy is well documented.[7,8,9,10] A woman has a seven- to tenfold increased risk of ectopic pregnancy following one episode of pelvic inflammatory disease (PID).[11] The rise in the number of ectopic pregnancies in the past decade may be the result of the increased incidence of PID. The public health impact is reflected by the tremendous direct and indirect costs of PID and its sequelae, estimated at approximately $4.2 million in 1990.[12]

Despite the polymicrobial nature of PID, the two main causative microorganisms are Neisseria gonorrhea and Chlamydia trachomatis, contributing to up to two-thirds of all pelvic infections.[13] Chlamydia trachomatis is the most common bacterial STD in developed countries today, accounting for 3 to 4 million infections annually in the United States.[14] In women, chlamydia is an important causative agent for mucopurulent cervicitis which predisposes to acute pelvic inflammatory disease. PID from chlamydia is associated with a more indolent, less acute, less severe clinical picture than that caused by gonorrhea and has a greater potential for causing permanent tubal damage that may result in an ectopic pregnancy or infertility.[15,16] Those at highest risk for infection are unwed teenagers living in urban areas, precisely the group at highest risk for other STDs and for other adverse pregnancy outcomes.[17]

Q: What are the health consequences of STDs, specifically with regard to women and children?

Women suffer the greatest morbidity and mortality from STDs, because their primary infections are often asymptomatic and the physical findings more difficult to detect. It is estimated that more than 1 million women experience active PID each year in the United States, and 200,000 are hospitalized.[18] The complications of PID include sterility, ectopic pregnancy, tubo-ovarian abscess, pelvic adhesions, and dyspa-

Table 3-1   Estimated Incidence and Reported Cases of Selected Sexually Transmitted
Diseases in the United States, 1992

	Estimated Incidence	Reported Cases
Gonorrhea (GC)	1,100,000	501,409
Syphilis	120,000	112,581
Congenital syphilis	3,500	3,850
Chancroid	NA	1,886
Chlamydia (CT)	4,000,000	NN
Human Papillomavirus	500,000–1,000,000	NN
Genital herpes	200,000–500,000	NN
Trichomoniasis	300,000,000	NN
Urethritis (non-GC, non-CT)	1,200,000	NN
Mucopurulent cervicitis (non-GC, con-CT)	1,000,000	NN
Reported AIDS cases	45,472	45,472
HIV infection	NA	NN

Note: NA = not available.
       NN = not notifiable.

SOURCE:[37] Centers for Disease Control, Division of STD/HIV Prevention *1992 Annual Report.*
       [19] CDC. Summary of notifiable diseases, United States, 1992. *MMWR;* 41(55):3.

reunia. A single episode of PID leads to sterility in approximately 12% of women and to a sevenfold increased risk of an ectopic pregnancy.[2] Serious long-term sequelae will affect 25% of those afflicted with PID.[11] Because of this, to prevent long-term morbidity, female patients require aggressive diagnosis, treatment, and education (See Tables 3-1 through 3-3).

Children also suffer from congenital STD infections. In 1992, there were 3,850 cases of congenital syphilis reported.[19] In 40% of pregnant women with an untreated syphilis infection, the pregnancy will end in spontaneous abortion, stillbirth, or perinatal death. If the infant survives, the infection may lead to multisystemic manifestations including hepatitis, pneumonitis, osteitis, anemia, lymphadenopathy, and mucocutaneous lesions. There are also late manifestations of congenital syphilis that affect the central nervous system, skin, eyes, teeth, bone, and cartilage. Chlamydia and gonorrhea can be transmitted by direct contact to the vaginal canal during birth. These infections can

lead to neonatal conjunctivitis, which was once a leading cause of blindness in the U.S. Congenital transmission of gonorrhea can also lead to a disseminated infection with resultant bacteremia, meningitis, arthritis, and endocarditis. Chlamydia can cause pneumonia in neonates.

Intrauterine transmission of HIV disease from HIV-infected mothers is common but can be markedly reduced by AZT treatment during pregnancy. Intrauterine infection with herpes is rare, but may lead to premature delivery and to local and systemic manifestations. STDs such as gonorrhea, chlamydia, and syphilis that are contracted after the neonatal period are evidence of sexual contact and an abuse investigation should be initiated. Other infections such as vaginitis and human papilloma virus (HPV) may or may not be a result of sexual contact. It is important to accurately diagnose STDs in children and to cooperate with social workers, pediatricians, and legal authorities for long-term investigation and follow-up.

Table 3-2 The Most Common Sexually Transmitted Diseases and Their Pathogens

Pathogen	Diseases and Syndromes
BACTERIA	
Neisseria gonorrhoea	Urethritis, epididymitis, proctitis, cervicitis, endometritis, salpingitis, perihepatitis, bartholinitis, pharyngitis, conjunctivitis, disseminated gonococcal infection (DGI), premature rupture of membranes
Chlamydia trachomatis	All of above except DGI, plus pneumonia in infants, otitis media and Reiter's syndrome
Treponema pallidum	Syphilis
Ureaplasma urealyticum	Nongonococcal urethritis
Gardnerella vaginalis	Bacterial ("nonspecific") vaginosis
Haemophilus ducreyi	Chancroid
Calymmatobacterium granulomatous	Granuloma inguinale (Donovanosis)
Shigella spp	Shigellosis in homosexual men
VIRUSES	
Human immunodeficiency virus, types 1 and 2	AIDS
Herpes simplex virus	Genital herpes, aseptic meningitis, neonatal herpes
Human papilloma virus (multiple type)	Condyloma acuuminata, laryngeal papilloma, cervical neoplasms and local carcinoma
Hepatitis B virus	Acute and chronic hepatitis
Hepatitis A virus	Acute hepatitis A
Cytomegalovirus	Infectious mononucleosis; congenital CMV infection with birth defects and infant mortality
Molluscum contagiosum virus	Molluscum contagiosum
Human T-lymphotrophic retrovirus, type 1	Human T-cell leukemia or lymphoma
PROTOZOA	
Trichomonas vaginalis	Vaginitis, urethritis
FUNGI	
Candida albicans	Vulvovaginitis, balanitis
ECTOPARASITES	
Phthirus pubis	Lice infestation
Sarcoptes scabiei	Scabies

Case #2

A 19-year-old male presents to the emergency department complaining of dysuria for 3 days. He also notes that he seems to be urinating slightly more frequently than usual. His past medical history is negative. He denies fevers and chills. He denies any GI symptoms or back pain. He denies any history of urethral discharge or previous sexually transmitted disease. He has no previous history of urinary tract infection. He states that he has unprotected sexual intercourse with three different partners during the last 2 months.

Physical examination reveals a well-developed, well-nourished male with normal vital signs. His abdomen is soft, nontender, and no bowel sounds are present. He has no CVA tenderness. Genital exam reveals normally

Table 3-3 Criteria for Hospitalization for Patients with PID[30]

Uncertain diagnosis

Pelvic abscess

Pregnancy

Adolescence (because of unpredictable compliance)

HIV infection

Severe illness or nausea and vomiting precluding outpatient therapy

Inability to tolerate outpatient regimen

Follow-up within 72 hours after outpatient treatment not possible

developed circumcised male with bilaterally distended testicles with no masses. There are no lesions evident and there is scant clear discharge noted at the meatus. There are no inguinal, axillary, or cervical nodes noted.

Q: What is your differential diagnosis?

The patient clearly has symptoms of a genitourinary infection. However, simple urinary tract infections are uncommon in males in this age group. Infectious urethritis is a more likely diagnosis and is most commonly secondary to Neisseria gonorrhea or Chlamydia trachomatis. In fact, 15- to 19-year-old men have the highest incidence of gonorrhea of all age groups.

Q: What other historical points should be noted?

Because of the frequency of co-infections with other sexually transmitted diseases, it is important to question for signs or symptoms of infections. Since sexually transmitted diseases put persons at greater risk for contracting HIV, one should ask specific questions regarding signs and symptoms of AIDS as well as for previous HIV test results and any known exposures to HIV.

Further questioning of this patient revealed that he had noted a small sore on his glans approximately two weeks before. He had attributed this sore to a local injury from his zipper and it had healed without incidence. The patient denied any signs or symptoms of AIDS or any known contact with the disease, but had never been tested.

All patients with a sexually transmitted disease require additional testing because of their risk of co-infection, particularly with syphilis and HIV. However, it is difficult to conduct such testing in the emergency department because the results are not immediately available and patient follow-up is difficult. Some departments actually have policies against testing for HIV for emergency patients because of the lack of counseling and the difficulty of following these patients. Because of this, emergency physicians should establish relationships with either an inpatient department or the public health department to conduct these tests and treat positive cases. It is recommended that all departments keep a list of HIV testing clinics to offer to their patients who are diagnosed with or suspected as having a sexually transmitted disease.

Q: What type of discharge instructions and patient education should this patient receive?

Patient education is an important part of any physician-patient interaction. Discharge instructions are one valuable method of education and they are now considered a requirement in all ED charting. In 1990, the Pennsylvania Supreme Court ruled that a physician could be held liable for not instructing a patient to notify the partner about the need for treatment in a case in which the partner went on to become infected.[20]

Discharge instructions for patients with sexually transmitted diseases should focus on three areas:

1. Partner identification and treatment
2. Education about safe sexual practices
3. Proper outpatient treatment of the infection, including reasons to return.

In order to interrupt the spread of sexually transmitted diseases, it is very important to ensure that potential partners of infected patients are treated. If the partner is with the patient at the time of the ED presentation, he or she should be registered and treated immediately. If not, the patient must be instructed to have his or her partner treated. Another way to facilitate partner treatment is to ensure that the case is reported to public health authorities.

Patients also require explicit instructions regarding safe sexual practices. These practices include abstinence, monogamy, or the use of barrier contraceptives, especially condoms. Patients who remain sexually active must be warned of the dangers of contracting HIV disease through sexual contact. This is particularly true for women whose partners are IV drug abusers or bisexuals.

Because both N. gonorrhea and C. trachomatis may occur in up to 30 to 40% of patients with urethritis and PID, the CDC recommends broad-spectrum, empiric antibiotic treatment for both infections.[21] In addition, the pathogenic role of anaerobes recently elucidated in patients with tubo-ovarian abscesses, further supports the need for polymicrobial coverage. The CDC also emphasizes the need for early detection and appropriate antibiotic therapy for acute PID including admission (Table 3-3) to help prevent the potentially more damaging long-term sequelae.

Q: Should STDs be reported to public health authorities?

The identification and control of infectious diseases is an important task for all physicians and surveillance is a key component of disease control programs. The goals of surveillance are (1) early identification of epidemics; (2) to chart the disease trends for health planning; (3) to collect data for research; and (4) to demonstrate the effectiveness of health interventions.[22] Physicians contribute to surveillance programs by careful disease reporting. Reported cases allow public health authorities to contact partners, follow trends, and, if cultures are provided, to determine patterns of antibiotic susceptibility.

Emergency departments receive almost 100 million visits per year. Many of these are primary care visits by populations such as the urban poor who are most susceptible to STDs and disease outbreaks. This high volume, combined with a limited geographic care area and a high-risk population, makes the ED an ideal reporting site for infections and injuries.

All state and territorial reporting jurisdictions in the United States have legal requirements that mandate that physicians report cases of certain infectious diseases. Nationally, the Centers for Disease Control and Prevention (CDC) focuses on 49 infectious diseases, whereas 17 other diseases are reported by more than 90% of jurisdictions.[23]

Reporting completeness varies between 6% and 90%,[24] depending on the disease being reported and its severity; public awareness and concern about the dangers of the disease;[25] the availability of measures to prevent transmission;[23] the physician's knowledge of reporting methods and requirements;[26] the ease of the reporting and concerns for patient confidentiality.[27] The attending physician is ultimately responsible for assuring the completeness and accuracy of reporting. This includes emergency physicians treating outpatient cases. The penalties for failing to report a notifiable disease may include fines, the suspension of a physician's license, and even jail terms.[24] Some physicians are hesitant to report cases because they feel that it violates patient confidentiality. However, public health law not only protects physicians in these circumstances but requires case reporting.

Many physicians, especially those with hospital-based practices, rely on laboratories or hospital infectious disease staff to report the cases they treat. Unfortunately, this leads to great underreporting because only 54% of jurisdictions require laboratories to report and more than 40% will not count a laboratory-reported case without physician confirmation.[28] Relying on laboratory confirmation also misses the many STDs that are treated presumptively without testing.[29]

BROADER PUBLIC HEALTH CONTEXT

There is more to the treatment of STDs than the provision of antibiotics. The *1993 Sexually Transmitted Diseases Treatment Guidelines* by the Centers for Disease Control emphasizes measures that prevent the transmission of the diseases.[30] Prevention is even more important because a significant portion of HIV infections are sexually transmitted, and STDs, particularly syphilis, increase the risk of contracting HIV.[31,32,33] Because GC rapidly develops resistance to antibiotics, the CDC's recommendations for treatment have changed accordingly.[30,34] However, the elements of therapy that remain constant are the importance of the need for therapy for co-infections, patient education, case reporting, and the follow-up of tests and treatment outcomes. Because STDs are a common health problem encountered in the ED, emergency physicians become experts in both their treatment and prevention.

In the past, STDs were referred to by the less graphic term *venereal diseases,* a term derived from the Greek goddess of love, Venus. STDs have received much attention from the lay and medical population for centuries, particularly since the emergence of the "Great Pox" (syphilis) in Europe after the return of Columbus from the New World. Throughout history there has been a delicate balance between the perceived immorality of the nature of the disease's transmission and the need to treat and prevent infection. The intentional withholding of treatment as punishment for promiscuity has evolved to the forthright public prevention programs of today.

STD control programs in the U.S. began during World War I but were brought into national prominence with the introduction of antibiotics during World War II. Initially, control efforts were directed exclusively at GC and syphilis, and they, along with AIDS, continue to receive the greatest attention. However, there are many sexually transmitted diseases (Table 3-1) which are of significance for humans. Those with the greatest morbidity and mortality include HIV infections, hepatitis, syphilis, gonorrhea, chlamydia, and herpes.

More than 1 million Neisseria gonorrhea infections are estimated to occur each year in the United States (Table 3-2) for a rate of almost 450 cases per 100,000 population. Gonorrhea account for half of all reported cases of infectious diseases, and syphilis another 10%.[19] While incidence of gonorrhea has been decreasing overall, the rates in adolescents has been increasing.[35]

EMERGENCY PHYSICIANS' ROLE

Q: What can an emergency physician do to prevent STD infections?

The CDC has made very specific recommendations regarding the prevention of STDs and PID.[30,36] These recommendations are even more important for emer-

gency physicians who work in urban, economically depressed areas. The following are recommendations adapted for emergency physicians:

Adequate diagnosis and treatment. STDs should be diagnosed promptly. In the emergency department where it may not be possible to make a definitive diagnosis and where patient follow-up is difficult presumptive treatment is often necessary.

Treatment for co-infections. GC and chlamydia are often found together in persons diagnosed with urethritis, and the infections are impossible to distinguish clinically. Therefore suspected cases should be treated for both in all circumstances.

Seventy-two-hour follow-up examination for PID. The CDC recommends that all patients with suspected PID be reexamined at 72 hours to assess the effect of the treatment.

Testing for or referring for testing for additional infections (syphilis, HIV). Because the presence of one STD increases the risk of infection for another, it is important that patients be tested for additional, but less common co-infections. Unless the emergency department has a preestablished system to provide and follow-up on such testing, patients should be referred to a hospital or public health clinic.

Partner treatment. Generally, public health officials only trace contacts for high-yield infections, such as syphilis. Therefore, emergency physicians must emphasize to patients the importance of informing their partners of the need for treatment, or providing such treatment in the ED should the partner be present.

Patient education. Besides the importance of informing partners, patients should receive instructions on proper treatment after discharge and safe sexual practices.

Case reporting. The surveillance of diseases is an essential part of infectious disease control. Therefore, emergency physicians should report all confirmed cases of STDs. Laboratory reporting is not reliable, and each ED should develop a reporting mechanism.

CONCLUSION

Gonorrhea is the most commonly reported notifiable disease in the United States, accounting for half of all notifiable diseases. Chlamydia is estimated to have an incidence 2 to 3 times as great as gonorrhea, but is not as widely reported.

STDs are also associated with an increase risk of transmission of AIDS. Ectopic pregnancy, a life-threatening condition often associated with STDS, should be ruled out in all women of childbearing age who present to the ED with pain or bleeding.

Certain groups at high risk for infection with sexually transmitted diseases (such as the urban poor) often use the ED as their primary source of clinical care.

Emergency physicians must ensure that their patients receive proper treatment, including treatment for co-infection. They must also work with public health clinics to test for the presence of other diseases including syphilis and HIV infections, report all cases of STDs to public health authorities, and provide patient education regarding partner notification, further treatment needs, and safe sexual practices.

NOTES

1. Rice R, Roberts P, Handsfield H, Holmes K. Sociodemographic distribution of gonorrhea incidence: Implications for prevention and behavioral research. *AJPH* 1991; 81(10):1252–7.
2. Bell TA, Holmes KK. Age-specific risks of syphillis, gonorrhea, and hospitalized pelvic inflammatory disease in sexually experienced US women. *Sex Transm Dis* 1984; 11:291–5.
3. Ory SJ. New options for diagnosis and treatment of ectopic pregnancy. *JAMA* 1992; 267(4):534.
4. Centers for Disease Control. Ectopic pregnancy surveillance, United States, 1970-1987. *MMWR* 1990; 39:9.
5. Goldmer TE, Lawson HW, Xia Z, Trash HK. Surveillance for ectopic pregnancy, United States, 1970–1989. In special focus: Surveillance for reproductive health. *MMWR* 1993; 42(55-6):73–85.
6. Doyle MB, DeCherny AH, Diamond MP. Epidemiology and etiology of ectopic pregnancy. *Obstet Gynecol Clin North Am* 1991; 18(1):1.
7. Westrom L. Incidence, prevalence, and trends of acute pelvic inflammatory disease and its consequences in industrialized countries. *Am J Obstet Gynecol* 1980; 138:880–92.
8. Cates W Jr, Wasserheit JN. Genital chlamydial infections: Epidemiology and reproductive sequelae. *Am J Obstet Gynecol* 1991; 164(6 Pt.2):1771.
9. Faro S. Chlamydia trachomatis: Female pelvic infection. *Am J Obstet Gynecol* 1991; 164(6 Pt.2):1767.
10. Maccato M, Estrada R, Hammil H, et al. Prevalence of active Chlamydia trachomatis infection at time of exploratory lapartomy for ectopic pregnancy. *Obstet Gynecol* 1992; 79(2):211.
11. Westrom L. Pelvic inflammatory disease: bacteriology and sequelae. *Contraception* 1987; 36:111–28.
12. Washington AE, Katz P. Cost of and payment source for pelvic inflammatory disease. Trends and projections, 1983 through 2000. *JAMA* 1991; 266:2565–9.
13. Jossens MOR, Schachter J, Sweet RL. Risk factors associated with pelvic inflammatory diseases of differing microbial etiologies. *Obstet Gynecol* 1994; 83:989–97.
14. Toomey KE, Barnes RC. Treatment of Chlamydia trachomatis genital infection. *Rev Infect Dis* 1990; 12 (suppl 6):S645–S655.
15. Brunham RC, MacLean IW, Binns B, Peeling RW. Chlamydia trachomatis: Its role in tubal infertility. *J Infect Dis* 1985; 152:1275–82.
16. Conway D, Caul EO, Hull MGR, et al. Chlamydial serology in fertile and infertile women. *Lancet* 1984; 1:191–3.
17. Cates W Jr, Holmes KK. Sexually transmitted diseases. In Last JM, Wallace RB (ed.). *Public Health and Preventive Medicine.* Maxey-Rosenau-Last, 1992: 99–114.
18. Rolfs RT, Galaid EI, Zaidi AA. Pelvic Inflammatory disease: Trends in hospitalizations and office visits, 1979 through 1988. *Am J Obstet Gynecol* 1992; 166:983–90.
19. Centers for Disease Control. Summary of notifiable diseases, 1992. *MMWR* 1993:41(55):1–73.
20. Pennsylvania Supreme Court. *DiMarco* v. *Lynch Homes,* 1990; 583 A.2d 422.
21. Soper DE, Brockwell NJ, Dalton HP, Johnson D. Observations concerning the microbial etiology of acute salpingitis. *Am J Obstet Gynecol* 1994; 170:1008–17.
22. Thacker SB, Choi K, Brachman PS. The surveillance of infectious diseases. *JAMA* 1983; 249:1181–5.
23. Chorba TL, Berkelman RL, Safford SK, Gipps NP, Hull HF: Mandatory reporting of infectious diseases by clinicians. *JAMA* 1989; 262:3018–26.
24. Thacker SB, Berkelman RL. Public health surveillance in the United States. *Epidem Rev* 1988; 10:164–90.
25. Davis JP, Vergeront JM. The effect of publicity on the reporting of toxic-shock syndrome in Wisconsin. *J Infect Dis* 1982; 145:449–57.

26. Konowitz PM, Petrossian GA, Rose DN. The under-reporting of disease and physicians' knowledge of reporting requirements. *Pub Health Rep* 1984; 99(1): 31–5.

27. Cleere RL, Dougherty WJ, Pumara NJ, Jenice C, Lentz JW, Rose NJ: Physician's attitudes toward venereal disease reporting. *JAMA* 1967; 202:941–6.

28. Sacks JJ. Utilization of case definitions and laboratory reporting in the surveillance of notifiable communicable diseases in the United States. *AJPH* 1985; 75(12): 1420–2.

29. Kirsch TD, Shesser RS, Barron M. Factors relating to underreporting of gonorrhea from emergency departments. *AJPH*, in press.

30. Centers for Disease Control. 1993 Sexually transmitted disease treatment guidelines. *MMWR* 1993: 42 (RR-14):1–67.

31. Wasserheit JN. Epidemiological synergy, interrelationships between HIV infection and other sexually transmitted diseases. *Sex Transm Dis* 1992; 19(2): 61–77.

32. Kassler WJ, Zenilman JL. Seroconversion in patients attend in STD clinics. *AIDS* 1994; 8(3):351–5.

33. Macabe E, Jaffe LR, Diaz A. HIV seropositivity in adolescents with syphilis. *Pediatrics* 1993; 92(5):695–8.

34. Centers for Disease Control. 1989 sexually transmitted disease treatment guidelines. *MMWR* 1989:38(S-8):1–43.

35. Webster LA, Berman SM, Greenspan JR. Surveillance for gonorrhea and primary and secondary syphilis amoung adolescents, United States—1981–1991, In special focus: Surveillance for sexually transmitted diseases. *MMWR* 1993:42(SS-3):1–11.

36. Centers for Disease Control. Pelvic inflammatory disease: Guidelines to prevention and management. *MMWR* 1991:40(RR-5):1–25.

37. Centers for Disease Control, Division of STD/HIV Prevention. 1992 Annual Report.

4

Communicating an AIDS Diagnosis in an ED Setting

ERICA BERNSTEIN
JUDITH BERNSTEIN

CONTENTS

CHAPTER SUMMARY

Illnesses and deaths due to HIV are no longer rare in emergency departments, nor are they confined to big cities. Since the ED is often the only source of care for the patients at highest risk, HIV education and intervention are indicated. Risk factors are elaborated, and the ethical responsibilities associated with testing are discussed. An appropriate process for pretest counseling is suggested. A case study of an AIDS-defining illness is presented, and the difficulties of communicating this information are discussed.

INTRODUCTION

One out of every 250 persons in the U.S. is infected with HIV.[1] AIDS is the second leading cause of death among adult men aged 25 to 44, and will soon be the fifth leading cause of death for women in that age group. The number of new cases of AIDS in women is increasing by 45% each year; women are the fastest growing group.[2] At the end of 1994, the cumulative number of diagnosed AIDS cases was estimated at 535,000, and the cumulative death total at 385,000.[1]

While the majority of AIDS cases still cluster in the urban areas, the number of cases in nonmetropolitan areas is growing. Clark and others report results of a multicenter ED study conducted at a level-one trauma center in Baltimore. Among excess sera obtained randomly from 2,300 patients over an 8-month period in 1989, 186 samples (8.1%) were Western Blot positive for HIV-1 antibodies. With more than 40,000 new infections diagnosed annually in the U.S., this rate projects to around 750 persons with undiagnosed HIV infections who may seek primary health care in any given week in the United States.[3] It is no longer rare for HIV/AIDS to be diagnosed by clinical presentation in the emergency department.[4–7]

Case #1

A thin 19-year-old white woman presents to the ED in respiratory distress. She was found by hospital security lying near the entrance. The patient appears disheveled and agitated. She is tachypneic and tachycardic.

After she is stabilized, a medical student is sent in to get a history. The patient reports a persistent nonproductive cough for the past 3 weeks. The cough has been accompanied by intermittent fever. Over the past week she has become progressively more short of breath. She reports no other symptoms. She has no allergies and takes no medications.

The last thing she remembers is speed balling (intravenous injection of heroin and cocaine) with a friend earlier that day. The patient reports a past medical history (PMH) of multiple STDs for which she sought treatment at a local free clinic. Two years ago she was hospitalized for a cocaine overdose. She has smoked one and a half packs per day for the last 6 years. She has a 5-year history of polydrug use, including marijuana, cocaine (crack and injection), speed, and alcohol.

At present, she is homeless and sleeps at the women's shelter on occasion. She is still agitated, and during the interview she asks repeatedly when she can leave.

Q: Is the ED an appropriate place to begin a discussion about HIV and the patient's risk factors?

Discussion about HIV risk factors should be an automatic part of the medical interview with all adolescents and adults who are well enough to engage in discussion, regardless of the chief complaint, especially since the ED is often the sole source of medical care for patients who are at very high risk for HIV infection. These encounters may be the only opportunity for HIV education and intervention. The medical interview can be a safe context within which to discuss safe sex and addiction treatment.

Discussion about HIV should be followed with a referral to a test site and/or a drug treatment center, where pretest counseling can be offered and patients will be given all the information they need to make a good decision about whether or not to choose anonymous testing and other issues that they need to consider.

Q: What are the HIV risk factors for this young woman?

Among 58,428 AIDS cases reported in women through 1994,[1] 48% were in women who inject drugs, and 36% involved documented heterosexual transmission. This young woman's history of intravenous drug injection and documented STD exposure put her at very high risk for HIV infection.[7] In addition

to the HIV risks for this patient, the possibility of concomitant physical and/or sexual abuse should be explored. Engaging in HIV risk behaviors has been shown to be related in young adults to a history of having been beaten or raped; the young ED patient who admits to high-risk behavior should also be questioned about personal safety.[8,9]

Case Continuation

The medical student is not sure how to approach the questions of drug abuse and HIV risk and elects to present these concerns to the EM resident along with the medical history. The resident goes over the physical findings, lab results, and chest x-ray with the student and points out that the patient had no apparent abnormalities on lung auscultation in spite of tachypnea and tachycardia. Arterial blood gases demonstrate hypoxia and widened A-a gradient. The chest radiograph shows diffuse bilateral infiltrates. The resident takes some time going over the differential and discusses the treatment of suspected pneumocystis carinii pneumonia. In response to a question about how to handle the substance abuse question, the resident responds, "They'll deal with all that on the ward. Just make sure you get an HIV test. The medical student goes back into the patient's cubicle and says, "I need to draw some blood for some more tests."

Q: What are the ethical and legal obligations for HIV testing in the ED?

Urgent and emergent care settings are not exempt from the procedures prescribed by law, including pretest counseling and informed consent requirements. A noncoercive approach is necessary because of the potential for stigmatization and discrimination faced by persons who are known to be HIV-positive. If confidentiality is not adequately protected, jobs, health insurance and housing may be lost, and access to quality health care may be compromised. Persons at risk are significantly more likely to seek testing in states that have antidiscrimination laws, protection of individual rights, and anonymous voluntary testing programs.[10]

HIV testing in general carries significant advantages for the high-risk patient: (1) to assist in supporting medical diagnosis and treatment of persons who exhibit symptoms that may be AIDS-related; (2) to provide an impetus for behavior change that can improve quality of life; and, for women, (3) to give the patient the opportunity to make informed decisions about future pregnancy; and (4) during pregnancy, to have access to treatment that will decrease the chance of HIV transmission to a fetus.

Many state public health departments have established specific guidelines for HIV counseling. Physicians also need to be familiar with all applicable state laws. In general, however, the following standards apply:

1. Confidentiality of the patient should be protected. Unless documentation is necessary to confirm disability or provide eligibility for treatment, the patient's rights are probably best protected by an anonymous testing process.
2. All patients should receive pre- and post-test counseling in person, and, when possible, from the same clinician.
3. Pretest counseling should include
   - Review of reasons for testing and expectations of testing;
   - Explanation of anonymous versus confidential testing;
   - Information about risk factors and reduction measures;
   - Interpretation of results, including false positives and false negatives;
   - Assessment of support networks.
4. Post-test counseling should include
   - Test results, explanation of their meaning, and assessment of patient's understanding;
   - Provision of immediate support;
   - Assessment of reaction and ability to cope, including suicide potential;
   - Review of risk reduction;
   - Counseling about disclosure of test results to sexual partners.

The complex nature of the processes involved in pre- and post-test counseling, as demonstrated by these standards, clarifies the necessity for HIV testing to take place in a setting, unlike the ED, where there is time to explore issues and meet all requirements.

Q: Are there any circumstances in which it is appropriate for HIV testing (and pre- and post-test counseling) to take place in the ED?

When a health care worker receives a needle stick injury or any other potential exposure to HIV virus, a decision must be made as soon as possible, preferably within an hour, about AZT administration. Serostatus prior to the event must be confirmed in order to establish linkage to an occupational exposure and provide workers' compensation coverage, if the health worker later seroconverts. Under these circumstances, ED physicians routinely counsel about risks and benefits of both testing and therapy. They are still, however, held to the comprehensiveness of the standards that apply for HIV testing and counseling in all other situations[11] and must develop a plan for receiving test results and providing appropriate post-test counseling.

Q: Why is it likely that a woman will present in the ED with an AIDS-defining illness without any previous attention to risk factors or detection of HIV positivity?

Late diagnosis of HIV disease in women is the result of a combination of factors: (1) poverty and poor access to nonpregnancy related services, (2) the embarrassment and shame that are associated for many women with sexuality and sexual behavior, (3) a low index of suspicion among physicians regarding HIV disease and women, (4) the failure until recently to discern manifestations of HIV disease that are specific to women, and (5) the overwhelming predominance of men with clinically evident HIV disease in industrialized nations.[12] To date, few prospective cohort studies evaluating the course of the disease in women have published data.[13,14] Infected men tend to live longer than infected women, and the proportion of women with access to AIDS therapy is lower. Because women have until recently been excluded from most new drug trials, neither efficacy nor risk have been well established.[15,16]

Q: What are the AIDS-defining illnesses that are specific to women?

AIDS-defining illnesses that are more common in women than men include wasting syndrome, esophageal candidiasis, and herpes simplex virus. Karposi's sarcoma is rare. Gynecological conditions such as vaginal candida infections and cervical pathology are prevalent in women at all stages of HIV infection. Associations have been documented between human papilloma virus (HPV), lower genital tract neoplasia, and HIV immunosuppression. Increasing cervical pathology appears to be related to drops in CD4 counts.[17] HPV-infected women with an abnormal Pap smear appear to have the lowest CD4 counts.[18] The World Health Organization now recognizes cessation of menstrual cycling as a defining symptom of AIDS.[19]

Case Continuation

While the student is drawing blood, the resident comes into the room and tells the patient that she most likely has pneumocystis carinii pneumonia and will have to be admitted for treatment. The resident is interrupted at that minute by a nurse, who calls out that another patient has coded. The resident turns back to the patient and says, "I have to go now, but don't worry—we'll take care of you" and leaves abruptly.

The patient turns to the medical student and asks if the doctor is saying that she has AIDS. The student hesitates, and the patient begins crying and screaming. She grabs the student and screams, "I don't f— have AIDS!" The patient attempts to get up, and pulls out her IV. The student runs from the room calling for security.

Q: Should this patient be restrained?

People exposed to the intravenous drug-using culture are often very knowledgeable about signs and symptoms of AIDS and familiar with the medical terminology. In this case, the patient heard the word *pneumocystis* and understood immediately that she was being informed of an AIDS-defining illness. Such information can result in posttraumatic stress disorder-like reaction that includes severe anxiety

and intrusive ruminating thoughts about failing health, death, and dying; hypervigilance for signs of physical deterioration; and insomnia, depression, and guilt.[20] It can also result in a 17 to 35% increase in the risk of suicide.[21] Although a large number choose violent methods, many ingest toxic substances, especially antidepressants. The typical profile for a suicidal attempt is the younger person who is recently diagnosed.

Because of the high risk of suicide, this patient should be prevented from leaving the hospital, including temporary restraint if necessary. A psychiatric consult should be called to explore with her how the diagnosis will affect her life, who she might rely on for support, and how she might cope with immediate and long term sequelae. Dilley and Forstein[22] have formulated the following diagnostic and treatment issues: exploring how the patient previously coped with trauma, stigma, and loss; the meaning of the HIV disease in the patient's culture and community; the patient's understanding of the disease process; evaluation of suicide potential, and the meaning of suicidal ideation as a coping mechanism for loss, grief, and control issues; and assessment of cognitive impairment. Suicidal ideation should also be evaluated as a neuropsychiatric marker for the direct effect of HIV on the nervous system.[21]

Q: If we could change the way this patient was told, and model the right way to give bad news, what are some of the principles we might adapt?

It is not unusual for the first AIDS diagnosis to occur in the ED. The most important tool for a good outcome is patient support. Patients need to be told clearly the implications for mortality of an AIDS-defining illness but also offered hope of the life-prolonging effects of certain treatments. Examples might be shared of ways in which people in similar circumstances have been able to turn their lives around and achieve quality of relationships and meaning that they had previously thought beyond their reach. Interactions begun in the ED must be continued during the hospital admission and followed by referrals to a support program on discharge.

The principles involved in breaking bad news effectively need to become a standard part of emergency medicine residency training. When news is broken badly, the consequences for the patient can include misunderstandings, compromised decision making, emotional pain, acting out behavior, wrecking of relationships within a social network, and suicide. For the practitioner, too, the experience can be traumatic, leading to decreased professional satisfaction and an aversiveness to emotional interactions with patients in the future.[23] Some of the reasons for doctors' difficulty in breaking bad news include lack of training, poor awareness of patient's feelings, fear of being blamed, fear of unleashing an emotional outburst and not knowing how to deal effectively with emotion, fear of displaying emotion oneself and being labeled inappropriate, and personal fears of illness and death. There is a consensus that the process of telling can be improved by

- Careful preparation, including planning among care givers about who will say what;
- Attention to privacy;
- Tailoring the method of presentation, whenever possible, to the patient's cultural milieu;
- Making sure the patient knows who you are, and who is in charge;
- Bringing in family and/or friends to be present during the discussion to provide support where appropriate;
- Allowing time for the news to sink in, and the patient to react;
- Dividing the process into two phases, so the news can sink in before decisions must be made;
- Avoiding false reassurance;
- Providing practical support and information and describing options and offering choices;
- Explaining that someone else will be by later to provide referrals and make plans for future care.

There are no easy answers or cookbook formulas, and there will always be some patients who will react violently to being told they have a fatal disease no matter how well the information is communicated. This case study, however, could have ended quite differently:

Alternative Case Continuation

The resident listened quite carefully to the medical student and realized that the medical student could grasp the pathophysiology of the problem quite easily, but was daunted by the human suffering aspects of the physician-patient encounter. Together they planned how to tell the patient what they suspected; any further testing issues would be dealt with once the patient was transferred upstairs to the floor. They asked a nurse to talk with the patient and find out if there were any relatives or friends who might be called. The patient said "my mother, if she will come." The mother was called and came to the ED to be with her daughter.

The resident and medical student went in to talk to the patient together. The resident sat on the bed and began by saying, "It looks like there's good and bad news today. The good news is that you're having trouble breathing because you have an infection in your lungs, and we can probably get that cleared up fairly easily with antibiotics. The bad news is that this infection looks like it might be pneumocystis carinii. Have you heard of that?" The patient broke out in a sweat. Shaking and sobbing, she asked, "Are you talking about AIDS? Are you telling me I'm going to die?" The resident and medical student explained together that the diagnosis was possible but not certain, and reassured the patient that a whole team of people would be working together to get to the bottom of the problem and start the right treatment. The patient was told that if she did have AIDS, there was a good chance she might die of it in time; she was also told that there were drugs that might prolong life, and new discoveries might happen at any time. The medical student explained that it would be necessary for the patient to stay in the hospital overnight for a complete evaluation and for treatment of her lung condition. The student also informed the patient that a psychiatrist would be in shortly to talk with her and help her sort out what she was feeling. The medical student promised to come by later to answer any questions, and they left the patient alone for a while, as she requested, with her mother.

CONCLUSION

Under the pressures of practice in a busy ED, the physician-patient relationship is often reduced to its medical bare bones: to elicit and organize biological data, generate hypotheses, and develop a plan for testing them. But there is another critical component of the medical interview that cannot be sacrificed without compromising quality of care—the interest, respect, support, and empathy that are as necessary as professional expertise for achieving desired outcomes.

The AMA Council of Ethical and Judicial Affairs sums up clearly what is required:

> AIDS patients are entitled to competent medical service with compassion and respect for human dignity and to the safeguard of their confidences within the constraints of the law. Those persons who are afflicted with the disease or who are seropositive have the right to be free from discrimination. . . . Physicians should respond to the best of their abilities in cases of emergency . . . and physicians should not abandon patients whose care they have undertaken.[24]

NOTES

1. CDC. *AIDS information: Cummulative cases.* Atlanta: Centers for Disease Control Document No. 320200, 1995.

2. CDC. The second 100,000 cases of acquired immunodeficiency syndrome—United States. *MMWR* 1992; 41:28–29.

3. Clarke SJ, Kelen GD, Henrard DR, Daar, ES, Craig S, Shaw GM, Quinn TC. Unsuspected primary human immunodeficiency virus type I infection in seronegative emergency department patients. *J Infect Dis* 1994; 170:194–97.

4. Baker JL, Kelen GD, Sivertson KT, Quinn TC. Unsuspected human immunodeficiency virus in critically ill emergency patients. *JAMA* 1987; 257:2609.

5. Kelen GD, Fritz S, Quqish B, et al. Unrecognized human immunodeficiency virus in emergency department patients, *NEJM* 1988; 318:1645.

6. Kelen GD, DiGiovanna T, Bisson L, Kalainov D, Sivertson KT, Quinn TC. Human immunodeficiency virus infection in emergency patients: Epidemiology, clinical presentations, and the risk to health care workers—the Johns Hopkins experience. *JAMA* 1989; 262:516.

7. Strumm JT. HIV prevalence in a midwestern emergency department. *Ann Emerg Med* 1991; 20:272.

8. Wasserheit JN. Epidemiological synergy: Interrelationship between HIV infection and other sexually transmitted diseases. *Sex Trans Dis* 1992; 19:61–77.

9. Cunningham RM, Stiffman AR, Dore P, Earls F. The association of physical and sexual abuse with HIV risk behaviors in adolescence and young adulthood: Implications for public health. *Child Abuse and Neglect* 1994; 18:233–45.

10. Angell M. A dual approach to the AIDS epidemic. *NEJM* 1992; 324: 1498–1500.

11. Oddi LF. Disclosure of human immunodeficiency virus status in health care settings: Ethical concerns. *J Intraven Nurs* 1994; 17: 93–102.

12. Hankins CA, Handley MA. HIV disease and AIDS in women: Current knowledge and a research agenda. *J Acq Imm Def Synd* 1992; 5:957–71.

13. Anzala DA, Nagelkerke NJ, Bwayo JJ, Holton D, et al. Rapid progression to disease in African sex workers with HIV virus type I infection. *J Infect Dis* 1995; 171:686–9.

14. Cozzi LA, Pezzotti P, Dorrucci M, Phillips AN, Rezza G. HIV disease progression in 854 women and men infected through injecting drug use and heterosexual sex and followed for up to nine years from seroconversion. *BMJ* 1994; 309:1537–1542.

15. Bernstein E, Goldfrank LR, Kellerman AL, et al. A public health approach to emergency medicine: Preparing for the twenty-first century. *Acad Emerg Med* 1994; 1:277–87.

16. Corea G. *The invisible epidemic: The story of women and AIDS.* New York: HarperCollins, 1992.

17. Anastos K, Marte C. Women: The missing persons in the AIDS epidemic. *Healthpac Bulletin* 1989; 19:6–13.

18. Vernund SH, Kelley KF, Keihe RS, et al. High risk HPV infection and cervical squamous intraepithelial lesions among women with symptomatic human immunodeficiency virus infection. *Am J Obstet Gynecol* 1991; 165:392–4.

19. Lombardo J, Kloser P, Chung R, Jenson A, Rska K. Cervical human papilloma virus (HPV) infection in HIV positive females. VII International Conference on AIDS, Florence 1991: Abstract TU.C.97: 47.

20. Daniolos PT, Holmes VF. HIV public policy and psychiatry. *Psychosomatics* 1995; 36:12–21.

21. Goldfrank LR, Flommenbaum NE, Levin NA, Weisman RS, Howland MA, eds. *Goldfranks's Toxicology Emergencies.* Englewood Cliffs, NJ: Appleton & Lange, 1990.

22. Dilley JW, Forstein M. Psychosocial aspects of the HIV epidemic. In E Tasman, SM Goldfinger, CA Kaufman (eds). *American Psychiatric Press Review,* vol 9. Washington DC: American Psychiatric Press, 1990.

23. Fallowfield LJ, Lipkin ML, Jr. Delivering sad or bad news. In M. Lipkin Jr., S. Putman, A. Lazare (eds.). *The medical interview: Clinical care, education and research.* New York: Springer Verlag, 1995.

24. Council on Ethical and Judicial Affairs. Ethical issues involved in the growing AIDS crisis. *JAMA* 1988; 259:1360–1.

5

Alcohol-Related Health Problems

GAIL D'ONOFRIO
ERIC S. FREEDLAND
NIELS K. RATHLEV

CONTENTS

- Magnitude of the problem
- Identification of the alcoholic or problem drinker with high risk behavior
- Indications for Blood Alcohol Concentrations (BAC)
- Use of physical and chemical restraints
- Medicolegal implications
- Safety plans for evaluation, discharge, and referral
- The emergency physician's role in future legislation and public health initiatives

CHAPTER SUMMARY

Alcohol use and abuse is a major health threat to society that costs billions of dollars every year in lost productivity and employment. This chapter describes markers for alcoholism and the process of identification of the problem drinker with high-risk behavior. Management of the intoxicated patient is outlined with emphasis on the use of blood alcohol levels, repeated examinations, and use of chemical and physical restraints. The medicolegal implications for screening and reporting the problem drinker and/or impaired driver as well as appropriate treatment and referral are discussed. Finally, the

role of the emergency physician is explored in lobbying for future legislative changes and assisting in community activism to prevent further alcohol-related illnesses, injuries, and deaths.

Case #1

Mr. S, a 37-year-old male, presents to an urban ED at 10:00 p.m. with a chief complaint of fatigue. He is a truck driver and just completed a trip from Atlanta to Boston. He parked his 18-wheeler full of frozen chickens approximately one-half mile away and walked to the ED. He denies pain, shortness of breath, fever, weight loss or history of similar feelings of fatigue. He has no significant PMH. He admits to several drinks prior to presenting to the ED. He denies other drug use. On PE he is alert and oriented. VS are slightly abnormal; pulse 110, BP 150/94, T 99TM, RR 12. There is a question of an odor of alcohol on his breath. His chest, heart, abdominal and brief neurological exam are within normal limits.

Q: What should be included in the initial work-up of this patient?

The above case illustrates many potential problems and raises serious medical and legal implications. The Emergency Physician is faced with an interstate truck driver who by his own admission has been drinking alcohol and is fatigued. A thorough history, physical examination and laboratory tests are warranted.

Case Continuation

The history is a crucial part of this patient's evaluation. Further questioning reveals that he has three to four drinks on most weekend days. Within the last hour, he has had "several" drinks that he will not quantify, but he adds that he is drinking less than usual. He vehemently denies other drugs. He also denies abdominal pain, vomiting, diarrhea, BRBPR, or melena. However, he has had episodes of epigastric pain and nausea during the past few weeks, which have caused him to decrease his alcohol intake. He does have a history of blackouts, described as periods when he is unable to account for his whereabouts or actions when he has had "a bit too much to drink." He denies seizures or major withdrawal symptoms. Finally, he admits to sleep deprivation, having been driving most of the last 2 days.

A more detailed physical exam reveals a very slight unsteadiness in his gait, a mild tremor, and brown stool that is guaiac positive for occult blood.

Blood samples are drawn for a complete blood count, electrolytes, blood sugar, creatinine, blood urea nitrogen, liver functions tests, clotting studies, and a blood alcohol concentration. An ECG reveals normal sinus rhythm with normal axis and intervals and no signs of ischemia.

Q: What is the magnitude of the problem of alcohol use and abuse?

Alcohol is the single most common recreational drug used by Americans. Approximately one-half the population over 12 years of age drink alcohol regularly.[1] There are an estimated 22 million alcoholics in the U.S. and more than 107,000 alcohol-related deaths each year.[1,2] Up to one-third of adult inpatients have problems related to alcohol, and 20% of the total national expenditure for hospital care is related to alcohol abuse.[3,4] Alcoholism is the leading cause of morbidity and mortality in the U.S. Chronic liver disease, about half of which is caused by alcohol abuse, is now the eleventh leading cause of death in the U.S.[5,6] It permeates all levels of society and is one of its most devastating problems.[7] The tragic results of alcohol abuse not only affect the individual drinker but have far-reaching implications for the family, community, and workplace. These effects and the widespread incidence of alcoholism are well

known to the emergency physician. One study determined that 40% of all patients presenting to the ED in the evening had been drinking and had blood alcohol concentrations (BAC) greater than 80mg/dl.[8] The economic impact of alcohol abuse and alcoholism is monumental. It is estimated that the cost to the nation is anywhere from $130 to $200 billion dollars a year, mostly in lost productivity and employment.[4,9]

Q: What is the relationship between alcohol and injury?

The above case immediately brings to every EP's mind the relationship between alcohol and injury. The prevention of injury is fast becoming an important public health initiative in EM. Effective screening and intervention for high-risk drinking behavior have the potential to benefit the patient as well as the community at large, preventing future injury, illness, and death.

Alcohol and trauma are inextricably linked. Independently, the tragic effects of both are numerous; in combination, they are staggering. Injury is the leading cause of death between the ages of 1 and 44.[10] It accounts for more than 140,000 deaths per year, and, for each death, two patients suffer permanently disabling injuries.[11] The resultant medical costs and loss of productive years are astronomical. In the U.S., alcohol is a major risk factor for both intentional and unintentional injury. Alcohol increases the frequency and severity of injury, and significantly complicates the management of the trauma victim. It is the major risk factor for virtually all categories of injury, including motor vehicle crashes (MVC), pedestrians, cyclists, burns, drownings, suicides, crimes including assault, rape, and murder, and all forms of domestic violence including spousal battering and sexual assault.[2,12–24] Traumatic injuries are responsible for 41% of all years of potential life lost (measured as patient's actual age subtracted from 65).[25] In the U.S., motor vehicle crashes (MVCs) are the single greatest cause of death between the ages of 5 and 34. Nearly one-half of the approximately 35,000 fatal MVCs are alcohol-related, according to the National Highway Traffic Safety Administration definition that includes any participant (driver, pedestrian, bicyclist, etc.) who is intoxicated.[26] Traffic accidents account for approximately 40% of all teenage deaths.[26] In a single MVC between midnight and 6 a.m., the chance of a driver being under the influence of alcohol is 94%.[27] In one U.S. national survey, 6.1% of adults responded positively when asked if they had driven "when you've had perhaps too much to drink" during the previous month.[28] It has been shown that victims of MVCs with higher BACs have poorer survival rates, even accounting for the speed of the vehicle, type of crash, and use of restraints.[29]

Q: How can the emergency physician identify the patient with alcohol problems?

The ED is often the point of entry for patients with acute intoxication or alcohol-related illnesses. Studies have shown that 10 to 38% of ED patients are legally intoxicated at the time of the visit.[13,15] The emergency physician is in a unique position to recognize, diagnose, intervene, and refer patients with alcohol-related injuries or illnesses and has a responsibility to do so both for the management of the individual patient and to society at large. While the physician may often be alerted to alcohol abuse by a clinical assessment, equally often the chronic alcoholic may have developed tolerance to alcohol levels, and it may not be so readily apparent on physical exam that alcohol is a factor.[30] Certain presentations, such as trauma/injury mentioned above, or blackouts, seizures, psychiatric symptoms, or change in mental status should always prompt further questioning regarding alcohol use and or a BAC. Alcohol intoxication associated with injury may be a marker of alcoholism. The American Psychiatric Association, in its *Diagnostic and Statistical Manual of Mental Disorders* (DSM III-R) and the World Health Organization Expert Committee on Drug Dependence both define alcoholism as "consumption of alcohol in quantities sufficient to damage or impair physical health."[31,32]

Other medical diagnoses or past medical history of diseases such as cirrhosis, hepatitis, esophageal varices, gastritis, gastrointestinal bleeds, macrocytic anemia, pancreatitis, peripheral neuropathy, holiday heart, dilated cardiomyopathy, or dementia should alert the physician of the possibility of alcohol use and abuse.

A genetic predisposition to alcoholism has been clearly demonstrated, especially in the sons of men with early-onset alcoholism,[2,33,34] and a family history of alcoholism should always raise a red flag. It is estimated that one-third of any sample of alcoholics will have at least one parent who is also an alcoholic.[35]

Although the specific gene has yet to be identified, research has produced evidence that both genetic and environmental factors contribute to alcoholism.[2] Possible biological markers of susceptibility have been identified. These include electrophysiological markers such as alterations in event-related electroencephalographic potentials on EEG,[36] endocrinological markers such as decreased ethanol-induced stimulation of cortisol and prolactin,[37] and biochemical markers such as increased inhibition by ethanol of monoamine oxidase(MAO) in platelets,[38] and an increased frequency of an antigen, CW3, part of a group of human leukocyte antigens (HLA).[39] Genetic variance of enzymes of alcohol metabolism such as alcohol dehydrogenase (ADH) and aldehyde dehydrogenase (ALDH), common in Asian populations, cause such an unpleasant reaction or the so-called alcohol flush reaction, that their presence may actually be a protective factor against heavy drinking and the development of alcohol dependence.[40] Subjective responses to alcohol may also be a potential marker of susceptibility, as sons of alcoholic fathers have been shown to exhibit mood patterns such as higher measures of tension, depression, and fatigue, independent of the amount of alcohol consumed, and they reported less perceived intoxication at all levels.[41]

Eliciting a social history regarding alcohol use is an imperative screening tool for patients presenting with any injury, family violence, suicide ideation, or multiple medical problems potentially related to alcohol. Having had a drink within the last 24 hours and answering positively to the question "Have you ever had a drinking problem?" provides a greater than 90% sensitivity and 85% specificity as a screening tool for identifying the alcoholic when combined with ≥ 2 positive answers on the CAGE.[42] All emergency physicians should know the CAGE questions as a simple, rapid, and respectful screening test for alcoholism.[43,44]

Have you ever felt you should **C**ut down
on your drinking?   **C**

Have people **A**nnoyed you by criticizing
your drinking?   **A**

Have you ever felt **G**uilty about your
drinking?   **G**

Have you ever had a drink first thing in
the morning to steady your nerves or
get rid of a hangover: **E**ye opener?   **E**

Positive answers to two or more of these questions are sufficient to identify individuals who require more intensive evaluation.

CASE DISCUSSION

There are several reasons for the physician to be concerned that Mr S may chronically abuse alcohol. He has recently ingested alcohol, and he has had four or more drinks on more than one occasion during the past month. A history of epigastric pain with a guaiac positive stool on physical exam is also suggestive of alcohol-induced gastritis. His slightly elevated pulse and blood pressure along with his mild tremor should raise the question of early mild withdrawal symptoms. At this point, the EP is obligated to collect more information and pursue this diagnosis.

Case Continuation

Laboratory results are available. The patient has a macrocytic anemia with a HCT of 34, Hgb of 11, and MCV of 100. His SGOT (AST) is 65, SGPT (ALT) is 40. The blood alcohol concentration is 250mg/dl. The remainder of his labs are within normal limits.

Mr S is asked the CAGE questions and responds positively to questions one (C) and four (E), but he adamantly denies that he has a problem. In fact, he becomes annoyed with the trend of questions related to his drinking instead of what he perceives as his medical problem of fatigue, a positive response to question (A). At this point, the nurse notifies the physician that Mr. S is becoming more uncooperative and belligerent. He has pulled out his intravenous line. After some discussion with the nurse, he agrees to return to his stretcher and have another IV inserted. However, she is worried that he will attempt to leave the department shortly if not restrained.

Q: What is the value of the blood alcohol concentration (BAC) in patient management?

While the diagnosis of acute ethanol intoxication can sometimes be made clinically by observing the combination of impaired judgement, unsteady gait, slurred speech, and an unmistakable odor of alcohol on the patient's breath, the physician may often be misled by more subtle presentations. The chronic alcoholic may be very tolerant to high levels of alcohol and often appears alert and oriented without neurologic deficits on a brief exam. However, the patient's response times and coordination may be severely affected, making him an impaired driver.

Determining the BAC in many situations is critical for management and discharge plans, and it is a useful screening tool for alcoholism. It should be considered for all presentations of trauma/injury, domestic violence, suicide, homicide, altered mental states, and multiple related illnesses. It has been suggested that a BAC above 150mg/dl in a patient without evidence of intoxication is pathognomonic of alcoholism.[45]

While emergency physicians are aware of the relationship between alcohol and trauma, and the body's altered response to alcohol, they often fail to obtain a BAC and thus miss an opportunity for referral. Although two-thirds of trauma centers in a national survey estimated that the majority of their patients had consumed alcohol, only 55% routinely conducted BAC tests upon admission.[46] Even with a concerted effort, up to one-third of trauma patients admitted to EDs are not tested.[47,48] One recent study by Becker and colleagues revealed that 20% of patients who presented to the ED with subacute injuries were noted to have been intoxicated in triage by the use of a Saliva Alcohol Test (SAT). Only 52% of these patients had subsequent documentation of clinical intoxication by either the nurse or physician.[49]

In addition to obtaining the BAC, the physician should be knowledgeable concerning the pharmacokinetics of ethanol and utilize the results in patient management. Ethanol is absorbed within 30 to 60 minutes on an empty stomach and is, therefore, usually at or beyond peak at the time of evaluation.[50] In most clinically relevant scenarios, the elimination of ethanol follows zero order kinetics; in other words, the BAC declines in a linear fashion, independent of concentration. In nontolerant patients, ethanol is eliminated at a rate of approximately 13 to 25 mg/dl per hour. However, in the chronic, tolerant alcoholic, this rate is increased to up to 37mg/dl per hour.[51]

The BAC should be measured when the cause of a patient's neurological impairment is unclear. It is important to determine whether alcohol intoxication is the sole explanatory factor for the patient's mental status, or whether other etiologies such as CNS injury or coingestion should be considered. For example, an additional etiology should be considered in patients who are deeply somnolent or comatose with a BAC less than 100mg/dl. On the other hand, a BAC of 200mg/dl may result in no obvious impairment in the chronic, tolerant drinker. Several factors can modify the relation between the blood ethanol concentration and the neurologic impairment.[52] The severity of intoxication at a given ethanol concentration is greater when the concentration is rising than when it is falling, known as the Mellanby effect.[53] Even among highly intoxicated patients, a search for other causes such as subdural or epidural hematoma, diffuse brain injury, or ingestion of other CNS suppressant drugs such as benzodiazepines and barbiturates should be considered, when a discrepancy exists between the BAC and the patient's clinical status.

Q: Are there alternative tests to the BAC that measure alcohol levels and how accurate are they?

In addition to the BAC, there are two alternative methods of measuring alcohol content: the breath analyzer and saliva content. Both methods have limitations. Use of a breath analyzer for ethanol has been demonstrated to correlate highly with blood level (R = .963, p = .001) in cooperative patients.[54] The correlation, however, is clearly decreased in patients who are unable or unwilling to cooperate (although it remains significant). It has been demonstrated that exhaled air is a reliable means of measurement due to an equilibrium of approximately 2,100 to 1 between ethanol in the blood and in alveolar air. It is estimated that the result obtained with the breath analyzer is approximately within 10% of the BAC. Falsely elevated results occur if blood or emesis is

present in the oral cavity.[55] This method of estimating the BAC is particularly useful when rapid determination is necessary. Patients in whom acute brain injury or coingestion of CNS depressants are suspected are prime candidates. Its use is limited either by the patient's ability to cooperate or by technical problems such as the recalibration required prior to each use.

A newer method involves the measurement of ethanol content in the saliva—the SAT (saliva alcohol test). An excellent correlation between saliva and BAC was found in volunteers in the range of 0 to 150mg/dl (R = .98).[56] Sample collection is easy on a cooperative patient, and the test result is available in minutes. However, vomitus in the mouth can falsely elevate the results. Its use is limited by the fact that patients may not have sufficient saliva available for sampling, and it has a relatively low upper limit for estimating blood alcohol content.

A recent study by Keim compared blood ethanol estimation by BAC with breath and saliva analysis. Many patients were excluded because of inability to cooperate or because of their lack of sufficient saliva. Forty-four (56%) of the 78 patients enrolled completed the study. K values for the breath test and saliva test as compared to BAC were .69 and .84 respectively, with Pearson coefficients of .77 and .90.[57] While SAT is a more reliable estimation of BAC, its use is limited.

Case Continuation

The nurse informs the physician that Mr S insists on leaving and that he had actually tried to take a swing at her when she attempted to obtain an additional set of vital signs. She insists that he be restrained for his protection as well as hers. The physician attempts to speak with Mr. S, who becomes extremely agitated and will not allow the physician to continue. Security is called to restrain the patient.

Q: When should the emergency physician institute physical/chemical restraints?

Reasonable restraint should be instituted when it is necessary to prevent the patient from potentially harming himself or others. This includes unruly behavior that prevents an adequate physical evaluation. If an intoxicated, impaired patient is released and subsequently injures himself or others, the physician who released the patient may be liable to third parties as well as the patient. Although the restrained patient may later assert a claim for "false imprisonment," the theoretical liability for detention by reasonable restraint is far less than the potential liability for injury sustained by the alcohol-dependent patient or an innocent bystander after inappropriate discharge. The restrained and sedated patient must have continuous pulse oximetry and cardiac monitoring with frequent vital signs recorded. Ideally, a medical aid should provide one-to-one observation. Physicians' orders and documentation should reflect that a less restrictive means had been tried (see Chapter 13, "Cycle of Violence: Emergency Department Staff As Victims").

The key to avoiding medical malpractice claims is to establish that the actions taken are indeed *reasonable* for the protection of the patient and provider. Meticulous documentation is the best defense.

Case Continuation

Mr. S received 2mg of IV Lorazepam, as the physician felt that part of his behavior could be related to alcohol withdrawal, since he has been in the ED for several hours without a drink. A careful further exam revealed no other immediate concerns. Mr S slept for the next 4 hours, during which time his heart rate, blood pressure, and oxygen saturation were continuously monitored. The physician did a brief neurological exam every hour. He is now awake, cooperative, oriented × 3 with normal speech. The restraints are removed and his gait is normal.

Q: When is it time for discharge? Is a repeat BAC necessary?

The intoxicated patient may be discharged when he or she is sober. Direct patient observation, however, is an unreliable means of determining sobriety for clinical or medicolegal purposes. The appearance of sobriety does not correlate well with safe motor vehicle operation, which has been shown to be impaired at BACs below 100 mg/dL.[58] In the case of drivers, therefore, waiting for a specific repeat BAC may be necessary. The safest course is to evaluate the patient for trauma and, if suspected, a metabolic disorder. The patient diagnosed with acute alcohol intoxication and without significant cardiorespira-

tory or neurologic impairment may be discharged with a responsible, sober adult who will stay with the patient for the next 24 hours, or the patient can be transferred to a detoxification facility. In addition, documented instructions must state specifically how long to wait before attempting to drive or engage in other activities again. If the emergency physician is concerned, he or she should observe the patient, involve social service, and if necessary, restrain the patient physically and chemically, as noted previously, to protect the patient and society.[12]

Case Continuation

The EP conducts a Brief Negotiation Interview with Mr S (see chapter 31). Further discussion reveals that he is depressed, but not suicidal. He feels that he is ready to change his behavior and agrees to remain in the ED until the morning to speak with psychiatry and a counselor.

Q: What are the medicolegal implications for treatment, discharge, and referral of the alcohol impaired patient?

Physicians should familiarize themselves with the particulars of laws in the states in which they practice regarding the following: an intoxicated patient's right to make decisions for himself; patient dumping; antidiscrimination and physician comments; obtaining blood alcohol levels; confidentiality and informing third parties (e.g., parents, spouse, police, etc.) regarding a patient's intoxicated state; and liability for premature release or false imprisonment versus forced confinement of intoxicated patients.[59] The best defense against a malpractice claim is to take precautions in order to avoid one altogether. Alcohol intoxication can mask serious underlying disease, and it behooves the physician to avoid the cynical "frequent flier" mentality and search diligently to rule out dangerous entities every time in every intoxicated patient, no matter how familiar he or she may be. A meticulously documented history, physical, treatment, hospital course, and disposition is your best defense.

Physicians should advocate for patients to the best of their ability, while respecting their individual rights. An intoxicated patient with multiple stab wounds sued a physician and a New York hospital for having had to undergo a negative exploratory laparotomy even though he had refused to consent. The patient was determined to be incompetent under life-threatening circumstances, and consent from the administrator was obtained. The decision for the plaintiff was overturned on appeal, but the assault claim was determined to be a viable theory of recovery for a jury to consider, especially if it could be proven that no emergency situation existed. Patients have the right to make treatment decisions for themselves and to be allowed "sobering up" time to regain competency in order to make their own health care decisions—assuming that no actual life- or limb-threatening condition exists in the interim. Similarly, take caution when family members or friends urge treatment of the intoxicated patient (e.g., surgery, invasive diagnostics, or medications to be administered) before he or she is sober enough to be competent.[59]

Providers should avoid expressing discriminatory attitudes and derogatory expressions toward the alcoholic patient, especially within earshot of accompanying family and friends. State and federal laws prohibiting discrimination against the handicapped have been broadened to preclude discrimination against alcoholics.[60,61]

The emergency physician may be liable for negligent care if the alcohol-impaired patient is discharged and injures himself or others. Attorneys were surveyed regarding a case of a patient who was treated in the ED for a wrist sprain following a fall.[62] He was noted to have alcohol on his breath and admitted to alcohol ingestion, but he was cooperative and was released without obtaining a BAC. He subsequently was involved in a serious automobile crash and was found to have a BAC beyond the legal limit for driving. Overall, 64% of the lawyers advised suing. Another study[63] indicated that 88% of physicians surveyed would not obtain BACs in patients who had alcohol on their breath but were coherent and cooperative, with most physicians citing legal considerations as the basis for their decisions. The impaired, intoxicated patient must not be allowed to leave by himself or herself and must be restrained if necessary (see above). In 1982, the U.S. Supreme Court, after ruling *Youngberg* v. *Romeo*, deferred to professional judgment the management of incompetent patients, which includes restraining them in order to assure their safety.[64] Most states have enacted statutes regulating restraints. However, in *Youngberg*, the Court recognized that professionals, rather than courts, are best able to determine the needs of patients, including the use of restraints.[65]

While there is federal legislation that mandates employers to screen and report employees who serve in safety sensitive functions, such as pilots, train engineers, and interstate truck drivers as in our present case, there is currently no mandate for physicians to report such incidences.[66] In fact, as alluded to above, the physician who reports may be violating the patient's right to privacy. Only a few states, such as Maine, have legislated immunity laws for physicians who report drinking and driving behavior. Yet the physician can certainly be liable for allowing an impaired driver to leave, if he is later involved in some form of injury either to himself or others.

If in the above case Mr. S appeared sober and refused to stay for counseling, the EP would be faced with a major dilemma. Although the BAC may be low enough for Mr S to be sober, we know that the short term physiologic effects of alcohol may decrease coordination and balance, increase reaction time, impair attention, perception, and judgment, all of which may increase the risk of accidental injury. Alternatives may include threatening to call police if he leaves and attempts to drive; asking the patient for keys to the vehicle until sobriety is assured; calling a friend or family member; or allowing Mr. S to leave the ED and then notifying the police, who may place him under arrest for attempting to drive under the influence and require that he submit to a BAC. Negotiating with the patient and giving strict options may yield results for both parties. The physician may decide to notify the employer, and/or the state department of driver registration. Ideally, each institution should discuss these issues and have a hospital or departmental policy that establishes appropriate procedures for documenting discharge instructions and reporting to authorities.

Q: What is the emergency physician's role in screening, intervening, and promoting legislative change for the patient presenting with high-risk drinking behavior?

Alcoholism must be identified as a disease and treated accordingly. One would never discharge a patient with chest pain, hypertension, or diabetes without appropriate referral and follow-up instructions. However, individuals with alcohol problems are less likely to receive help. In one study, 45% of patients under a physician's care at the time of a documented drinking problem were discharged without having their problem addressed. Only one-fourth of those were encouraged to reduce intake or warned about health hazards; only 3% of these heavy drinkers were referred for treatment.[67]

Unfortunately, in spite of the fact that EPs know the relationship of alcohol and injury and the high incidence of alcohol-related diseases in the hospitalized patient, numerous studies document the failure of the emergency department staff to recognize and refer patients for counseling and rehabilitation.[14,46,47,49,68–70] Lowenstein et al.[14] reported that out of 153 intoxicated patients only 13% received referral for counseling and/or rehabilitation, and only 15% were instructed to stop drinking. Reasons cited for lack of recognition and referral include inadequate time, education, and resources as well as disinterest, avoidance, disdain, or pessimism when confronted with a hostile, manipulative, or combative patient.[71–76] This is particularly unfortunate, as programs instituted for persons apprehended for driving under the influence of alcohol have had success in changing the behavior of some intoxicated drivers.[49,77–81]

The ED offers an ideal opportunity for screening and initiating treatment and referral of patients with alcohol problems. The goal of identification and early intervention can be accomplished by the use of easily administered and inexpensive screening procedures to identify people at risk for alcoholism and those who may develop alcohol problems.[2] Remembering to routinely screen the patient with acute trauma, change in mental status, or obvious psychiatric diagnosis may not be a problem, since the BAC is important patient management. However, screening the asymptomatic or subacutely injured patient poses more difficulties. Ethical concerns suggest that these patients would most likely need to consent to such testing and documentation. And, of course, patient confidentiality and reporting of results are issues in either case. Should—and can—the physician report the results to employers or other third parties? Could this practice of routine screening, if known by the public, potentially prevent individuals from seeking care in a timely fashion, or at all?

The ED visit is often a crisis encounter, where patients are most receptive to education.[82] Gentilello reported that 17 of 19 hospitalized trauma patients agreed to immediate counseling and accepted referral to a treatment facility after discharge.[68] Another study initiated intervention with patients who were injured and found a 50% decrease in alcohol consumption.[20] Data suggest, however, that police and courts do not usually intervene when patients are injured, and if the EP does not initiate the process of detection, referral, and treatment, possibly no one else will.[83]

Many physicians may be unaware that even simple advice-giving to the patient to decrease or stop drinking may have a somewhat beneficial effect,[84] or a brief intervention may trigger a change in behavior or encourage patients to seek further treatment.[85,86] Treatment of alcohol dependency also significantly reduces health care costs. Individuals involved in some form of alcohol treatment had decreased ED visits, hospitalizations, work-related problems, criminal arrests, and a lowered risk of injury and motor vehicle crashes.[87] One should remember that success may be measured in even a few days or weeks of abstinence that may result in fewer ED visits and fewer potential injuries, although not necessarily in total rehabilitation.

The typically hectic ED may present many real barriers to identification and referral of the problem drinker. The EP has a responsibility, however, to identify potential markers for alcoholism and high-risk drinking behavior and offer brief intervention and referral. Appropriate personnel should be available for a lengthier, more inclusive assessment 24 hours a day, and policies must be in place to deal with situations when referral for assessment is not available. The EP also has the opportunity to educate other professionals regarding the identification and referral of high-risk patients. The EP can offer educational programs in combination with other team members from areas such as nursing, social work, and psychiatry. These programs should extend into the community and involve schools, other health care programs such as HMOs and clinics, and community centers.

As a specialty, EM is in a powerful position to mandate change. Knowledge of the magnitude of the problem to society, current research, and firsthand experience enables EPs to be leaders in lobbying for change and new legislation. The impaired driver must be taken off the road. In addition to mandatory counseling and education sessions, the intoxicated driver must have strict penalties such as license suspension, fines, possible imprisonment, and revocation of license on second offense. Some have suggested revoking car registrations or impounding the cars of repeat offenders.[88] States such as New Jersey have reported a decrease in alcohol-related motor vehicle crashes because of the use of widespread roadblocks for stopping and testing drivers for intoxication.[89] Legislation at both the local and federal levels can restrict liquor licensing in depressed areas, reduce the availability of cheap beverages with high alcohol content, and prohibit the concurrent sale of alcohol and gasoline. Increasing taxes on alcohol potentially will limit access to teenagers, particularly when a six-pack of beer may cost less than a six-pack of cola.

Legislation is also necessary to mandate inpatient treatment for chronic alcoholic patients, particularly those with underlying psychiatric illnesses. Placement in an institutionalized setting may be necessary, instead of permitting homelessness in our major cities. Recourse to the courts may be required in situations in which a legal guardian must be appointed.

CONCLUSION

Alcoholism is pervasive in our society and a major risk factor for injury, medical illness, and family violence. The acutely intoxicated patient presenting to the ED provides an opportunity for therapeutic intervention and referral that should not be missed. The emergency physician has a responsibility to the individual patient and the community at large to identify patients with high-risk drinking behavior and prevent subsequent injury, illness, or death. Emergency physicians are in a unique position to educate other professionals and the public, as well as to lobby for future legislative changes for screening, reporting, referring, and treating patients with alcohol problems. In addition, EPs can impact public health legislation by assisting the community to insist on stricter laws for the impaired driver and limiting access to alcohol.

NOTES

1. Substance Abuse and Mental Health Services Administration, Office of Applied Studies. *1993 National Household Survey on Drug Abuse. Advance Report no. 7.* Rockville, MD: Department of Health and Human Services, 1994.
2. Department of Health and Human Services. *Eighth Special Report to Congress on Alcohol and Health: National Institute on Alcohol Abuse and Alcoholism.* Rockville, MD: Department of Health and Human Services, 1993.
3. Rice DP, Kellman S, Miller LS, Dunmeyer S. Estimates of economic costs of alcohol and drug abuse and mental illness, 1985 and 1988. *Pub Health Rep* 1991; 106(3):280–92.
4. Burke TR. The economic impact of alcohol abuse and alcoholism. *Pub Health Rep* (1988); 103 (6):564–8.
5. Centers for Disease Control and Prevention, National Center for Health Statistics. Advance report of final mortality statistics, 1991. *Mon Vital Stat Rep* 1993; 42:1–64.
6. McGinnis JM, Foege WH. Actual causes of death in the United States. *JAMA* (1993); 270:2207–12.
7. Martinez, R. Alcoholism and society. *Emerg Med Clin North Am* 1990; 8(4):903–12.
8. Holt S, Stewart I, Dixon J, et al. Alcohol and the emergency service patient. *Br Med J* 1980; 281:638.
9. Duke SB, Gross AC. *America's Longest War; Rethinking Our Tragic Crusade against Drugs.* New York: Putnam, 1993.
10. Baker S, O'Neil B, Karpf R. *The Injury Fact Book.* Lexington, MA: Lexington Books, 1984.
11. Committee on Trauma Research. *Injury in America: A Continuing Public Health Problem.* Washington, DC: National Academy Press, 1985.
12. Freedland ES, McMicken DB, D'Onofrio G. Alcohol and trauma. *Emerg Med Clin of North Am* 1993; 3(1): 225–339.
13. Peppiatt R, Evans R, Jordan P. Blood alcohol concentration of patients attending an accident and Emergency Department. *Resuscitation* 1978; 6(1):37–43.
14. Lowenstein SR, Weissberg MP, Terry, D. Alcohol intoxication injuries, and dangerous behaviors and the revolving Emergency Department door. *J Trauma* 1990; 30(10):1252–7.

15. Teplin LA, Abram KM, Michaels SK. Blood alcohol levels among emergency room patients: A multivariate analysis. *J Studies Alcohol* 1989; 50:441–7.

16. Wechsler H, Kasey E, Thumb D, Demone H. Alcohol level and home accidents: A study of emergency service patients. *Pub Health Rep* 1969; 84:1043–50.

17. Shepherd J, Leslie I. Alcohol intoxication and severity of injury in victims of assault. *Brit Med J* 1969; 296:1299.

18. Cherpitel CJ. Alcohol and violence-related injuries: an emergency room study. *Addiction* 1993; 88:79–88.

19. Cherpitel CJ. Alcohol and injuries: A review of international emergency room studies. *Addiction* 1993; 88:651–65.

20. Antti-Poika I, Karaharju E. Heavy drinking and accidents—A prospective study among men of working age. *Injury* 1988; 198–200.

21. Howland J, Hingson R. Alcohol as a risk factor for injuries or death due to fires and burns: Review of the literature. *Pub Health Rep* 1987; 102(5):475–83.

22. Hingson R, Howland J. Alcohol as a risk factor for injury or death resulting from accidental falls: A review of the literature. *J Studies Alcohol* 1987; 48(3):212–19.

23. Hingson R, Lederman R, Walsh DC. Employee drinking patterns and accidental injury: A study of four New England States. *J Studies Alcohol* 1985; 46(4):298–303.

24. Brewer RD, Morris PD, Cole TB, et al. The risk of dying in alcohol related automobile crashes among habitual drunk drivers. *N Eng J Med* 1994; 331(8):513–17.

25. United States Department of Health and Human Services PHS Center for Disease Control. Premature mortality due to alcohol-related motor vehicle traffic fatalities—United States. *MMWR* 1985; 37: 753.

26. Department of Transportation, National Highway Traffic Safety Administration. *Alcohol involvement in fatal traffic crashes—1991.* Springfield, VA: National Technical Information Service, 1993.

27. Terhune D, Fell J. The role of alcohol, marijuana, and other drugs in the accidents of injured drivers. In *Proceedings of the 25th Annual Meeting of the American Association for Automotive Medicine.* San Francisco, October 1–3, 1981.

28. Bradstock M, Marks J, Forman M. Drinking-driving and health lifestyle in the United States: Behavioral risk factors surveys. *J Stud Alcohol* 1987; 48:147.

29. Waller P, Stewart J, Hansen A, et al. The potentiating effects of alcohol on driver injury. *JAMA* 1986; 256:1461.

30. Urso T, Gavaler JS, Van Thiel DH. Blood ethanol levels in sober alcohol users seen in an emergency room. *Life Sci* 1981; 28:1053–6.

31. American Psychiatric Association. *Diagnostic and Statistical Manual of Mental Disorders,* 3rd ed.(DSM-III-R). Washington, DC: American Psychiatric Press, 1987.

32. Kramer JF, Camera DC (eds.). *A Manual on Drug Dependence.* Geneva: World Health Organization, 1975.

33. Cloninger, CR, Bohman M, Sigvardsson S. Inheritance of alcohol abuse. *Arch Gen Psychiatr* 1981; 38:861–8.

34. Cloninger, CR. Neurogenetic adaptive mechanisms in alcoholism. *Science* 1987; 236:410–16.

35. Cotton, NS. The familial incidence of alcoholism: A review. *J Study Alcohol* 1979; 40:89–116.

36. Begleiter H, Porjesz B, Bihare B, Dissin B. Event-related brain potentials in boys at risk for alcoholism. *Science* 1984; 225:1493–6.

37. Schuckit, MA. Differences in plasma cortisol after ethanol in relatives of alcoholics and controls. *J Clin Psychiatr* 1984; 45:374–8.

38. Tabakoff B, Hoffman PL, Lee JM, Saito T, Willard B, DeLeion-Jones F. Differences in platelet enzyme activity between alcoholics and nonalcoholics. *N Engl J Med* 1988; 318:134–9.

39. Shigeta Y, Ishii H, Takagei S, Yoshitake Y, Hirano T, Takata H, Kohno H, Tsuchiya M. HLA antigens as immunogenetic markers of alcoholism and alcoholic liver disease. *Pharmacol Biochem Behav* 1980; 13 (Suppl 1):89–94.

40. Agarwal EP, Harada S, Goedde HW. Racial differences in biological sensitivity to ethanol: The role of alcohol dehydrogenase and aldehyde dehydrogenase isozymes. *Alcoholism* 1981; 5:12–16.

41. Moss HB, Yao JK, Maddock JM. Responses by sons of alcoholic fathers to alcoholic and placebo drinks: Perceived mood, intoxication, and plasma prolactin. *Alcoholism* 1989; 13:252–7.

42. Cyr MG, Wartman SA. The effectiveness of routine screening questions in the detection of alcoholism. *JAMA* 1988; 259:51.

43. Ewing J. Detecting alcoholism: The CAGE questionnaire. *JAMA* 1984; 252:1905.

44. Mayfield D, McLeod G, Hall P. The CAGE questionnaire: Validation of a new alcoholism screening instrument. *Am J Psychiatr* 1974; 31:1121.

45. Waller, JA. Management issues for trauma patients with alcohol. *J Trauma* 1990; 30(12):1548–53.

46. Soderstrom C, Cowley R. A national alcohol and trauma center survey: Missed opportunities, failures of responsibilities. *Arch Surg* 1987; 122:1067.

47. Chang G, Astrachan B. The emergency department surveillance of alcohol intoxication after motor vehicle accidents. *JAMA* 1988; 260:2533.

48. Roizen J. Alcohol and trauma. In Giesbricht N, Gonzales R, Brant M, et al. (eds.). *Drinking and casualties:*

Accidents, poisonings, and violence in an international perspective. London: Routledge, 1988.

49. Becker BM, Woolard RH, Longabaugh R, Minugh PA, Nirenberg TD, Clifford PR. Alcohol use among subcritically injured emergency department patients and injury as a motivator to reduce drinking. *Acad Emerg Med* 1995; 2:784–90.

50. Winek DL, Murphy KL. The rate and kinetic order of ethanol elimination. *Forensic Sci Int* 1984; 25: 159–166.

51. Gershman H, Steeper J. Rate of clearance of ethanol from the blood of intoxicated patients in the emergency department. *J Emerg Med* 1991; 9:307.

52. Charness M, Roger S, Greenberg D. Ethanol and the nervous system. *N Eng J Med* 1989; 321:442–54.

53. Goldstein DB. *Pharmacology of alcohol.* New York: Oxford University Press, 1983.

54. Gibb KA, Yee AS, Johnston CC, et al. Accuracy and usefulness of a blood alcohol analyzer. *Ann Emerg Med* 1984; 15,3:349–53.

55. Gibb KA. Serum alcohol levels, toxicology screens, and use of the breath alcohol analyzer. *Ann Emerg Med* 1986; 15,3:349–53.

56. Christopher TA, Zeccardi JA. Evaluation of Q.E.D. saliva alcohol test: A new rapid, accurate device for measuring ethanol and saliva. *Ann Emerg Med* 1992; 21(9):1335–7.

57. Keim ME, Bartfield J. Blood ethanol estimation: A comparison of three methods. (Abstract). *Ann Emerg Med* 1995; 25,1:140.

58. Sullivan JJ, Hauptman M, Bronstein A. Lack of observable intoxication in humans with high plasma alcohol concentrations. *J For Sci* 1987; 2:1660–5.

59. Lydon D, Miller C. Legal considerations for attending alcoholic or intoxicated patients. *Emerg Med Reports Legal Briefings* 1990; 1(1):1–8.

60. Ohio Rev. Code Chapter 4112; Fla. Stat. Ann. #396.022(1).

61. Federal Rehabilitation Act of 1973, 29 U.S.C. 794 (prohibiting discrimination in programs or activities governed by federal laws); comprehensive Alcohol Abuse and Alcoholism Prevention and Rehabilitation Act, 42 U.S.C. 290dd-2.

62. Simel D, Feussner J. Does determining serum alcohol concentration in emergency department patients influence physicians' civil suit liability? *Arch Intern Med* 1989; 149:1016–18.

63. Simel D, Feussner J. Blood alcohol measurements in the emergency department: Who needs them? *AJPH* 1988; 78:1478–9.

64. 457 U.S. 307 (1982) on remand, *Romeo v. Youngberg,* 687 F2d33 (3rd Cir 1982).

65. Simon R. *Psychiatry and law for clinicians.* Washington, DC: American Psychiatric Press, 1992.

66. U.S. Department of Transportation. *Alcohol & drug rules: An overview.* Washington, DC: Federal Highway Administration, Publication No. FHWA-MC-94-013, 1994.

67. Bowen OR, Sammons JH. The alcohol abusing patient: A challenge to the profession. *JAMA* 1988; 260: 2267–70.

68. Gentilello LM, Duggan P, et al. Major injury as a unique opportunity to initiate treatment in the alcoholic. *Am J Surg* 1988; 156:558–61.

69. Moore RD, Bone LR, Geller G, et al. Prevalence, detection, and treatment of alcoholism in hospitalized patients. *JAMA* 1989; 261:403–7.

70. Reyna TM, Hollis HW, Hulsebus RC. Alcohol-related trauma; The surgeon's responsibility. *Ann Surg* 1985; 201:194–7.

71. Kamerow EB, Pincus HA, MacDonald DI. Alcohol abuse, other drug abuse, and mental disorders in medical practice: Prevalence, costs, recognition and treatment. *JAMA* 1986; 255:2054–7.

72. Lewis DC, Niven RG, Czechowicz E, et al. A review of medical education in alcohol and other drug abuse. *JAMA* 1987; 257:2945–8.

73. Niven RG. Alcoholism: a problem in perspective. *JAMA* 1984; 252:1912–14.

74. Chappel JN, Schnoll SH. Physician attitudes: Effect on the treatment of chemically dependent patients. *JAMA* 1977; 237:2318–19.

75. Clark WD. Alcoholism: Blocks to diagnosis and treatment. *Am J Med* 1981; 71:275–88.

76. Yates, EW, Hadfield JM, Peters K. The detection of problem drinkers in the accident and emergency department. *Br J Addiction* 1987; 82:163–7.

77. Foon AE. The effectiveness of drinking-driving treatment programs: A critical review. *Int J Addiction* 1988; 23(2):151–74.

78. Hoffman NG, Ninonuevo F, et al. Comparison of court-referred DWI arrestees with other outpatients in substance abuse treatment. *J Stud Alcohol* 1987; 48(6):591–4.

79. Wells-Parker E, Anderson BJ, et al. Interactions among DUI offender characteristics and traditional intervention modalities; a long-term recidivism follow-up. *Brit J Addiction* 1989; 84(4):381–90.

80. Eutzelman HG. The irrefutable benefits of courses for alcohol intoxicated drivers. *Blutalkohol* 1990; 27(2): 106–9.

81. Jensch M. Remedial courses for alcohol apprehended drivers are effective, *Blutalkohol* 1990; 27(4):285–8.

82. Booth RE, Grosswiler RA. Correlates and predictors of recidivism among drinking drivers. *Inter J Addiction* 1978; 13:79–88.

83. Soderstrom CA, Birschback JM, Dischinger PC. Injured drivers and alcohol use: culpability, convic-

tions, and pre- and post-crash driving history. *J Trauma* 1990; 30(10):1208–12.

84. Walsh D, Hingson RW, Merrigan DM, et al. (1992). The impact of a physician's warning on recovery after alcoholism treatment. *JAMA* 1989; 267:663–7.

85. Skinner HA. Spectrum of drinkers and intervention opportunities. *Can Med Assoc J* 1990; 143(10):1054–9.

86. Bien T, Miller WR. Brief interventions for alcohol problems: A review. *Addiction* 1993; 88:315–36.

87. Hoffman NG, Miller NS. Perspectives of effective treatment for alcohol and drug disorders. *Psychiatr Clin N Am* 1993; 16(1):127–40.

88. Angell M, Kassirer J. Alcohol and other drugs—toward a more rational and consistent policy. *N Engl J Med* 1994; 331(8):537–9.

89. Levy D, Shea D, Asch P. Traffic safety effects of sobriety checkpoints and other local DWI programs in New Jersey. *Am J Pub Health* 1989; 79(30):291–3.

6

Dual Diagnosis: Substance Abuse and Psychiatric Illness

EDWARD BERNSTEIN

CONTENTS

CHAPTER SUMMARY

Patients with dual diagnosis of psychiatric illness and substance abuse are especially difficult management problems for the ED practitioner. Detection and treatment are complicated by behavioral challenges, and placement in an appropriate facility for inpatient care is difficult to achieve. Prognosis depends on a comprehensive approach; substance abuse issues must be directly addressed at the same time that psychotherapy and pharmacologic control of psychiatric symptoms are instituted. Research is just beginning to elucidate the complicated causal interrelationship between the two diagnoses.

INTRODUCTION

The 1988 National Household Survey on Drug Abuse estimated that 28 million people over the age of 12 in this country have used illicit drugs one or more times in the past year and reported that 21 million have used marijuana, 1 million had used crack in the last year, and 600,000 had used heroin. Two million people are hospitalized yearly, and over 6,100 deaths attributed to drug abuse were reported in 1985. The economic costs to society for all drug abuse were estimated at 58.3 billion for 1988, including the cost of crime, which amounts to 75% of the total amount.[1]

According to 1991 data, cocaine has become the most commonly used illicit drug, with 24 million people using cocaine at least once in their lives and 5 million persons using it regularly. Visits to EDs for cocaine related complications have increased rapidly. In the past decade, Emergency departments experienced a 20-fold increase in the number of cocaine related complaints. Chest pain was the most frequent complaint, and myocardial infarction occurred in about 6% of these patients.[2]

In 1994, it was estimated that $37.6 billion was spent by consumers of cocaine. Although the number of light users declined over a 20-year period, the number of heavy users increased. Heavy users consume eight times that of light users, canceling out any downward trend in consumption. The four main interventions during the "war on drugs" included source-country control, interdiction, domestic enforcement, and treatment of heavy users. Of the $13 billion spent on these programs, treatment received only 7%. The war on drugs has been lost, and in retrospect the money would have been more effectively spent on treatment of heavy users than on supply-control programs.[3] The money saved could also have been invested in economic development for high-risk communities. The merits of a rational policy of decriminalization are being seriously debated among professionals, and the governments of the cocaine-producing countries are looking toward the U.S. population to reduce both demand and consumption. Supporting preventive programs and facilitating access to treatment are important community roles for the country's 5,000 emergency departments and their staff. The crisis and consequences related to cocaine use affords emergency physicians an opportunity to intervene.

The drug-using population has a vast array of unmet needs that may include lack of primary care access, STD and HIV testing and treatment, victimization, and social and mental health services. Among the polydrug heavy users, there is a large subset of patients who are self-medicating serious undiagnosed and untreated mental illness. These patients with dual diagnosis of polysubstance abuse and psychiatric illness are often poorly understood and inadequately treated.

Management of these patients in the ED, if and when the complexity of the problem is indeed recognized, poses an enormous challenge for detection, treatment, and referral. Because dual diagnosis patients are frequently noncompliant with treatment, disruptive, and a drain on resources and time, they are often rejected by both the traditional substance abuse treatment system and by psychiatric facilities. It is difficult to arrange an appropriate disposition.

The patient with dual diagnosis is not new to us. These are the repeat visitors who have frustrated ED providers for years, because of the challenge they present and the lack of resources and solutions. The difference today is that there is a clearer explanation for their behavior and a definite movement to provide this population with more effective and appropriate services.

Case #1

Steve, a 30-year-old young male, walked into the ED triage at 5:17 a.m. The patient was scared and thought he was going to die. He had severe diffuse chest tightness, numbness in his arms and around his lips, and shortness of breath. He felt his heart pounding so hard he thought it would burst out of his chest. After repeated questioning, he admitted to smoking crack cocaine over the last few days. After developing the pain, he walked from his friend's house to the ED. He denied nausea, vomiting, loss of consciousness, muscle weakness. He had no history of diabetes, hypertension, peptic ulcer disease or kidney or heart disease. He had a history of asthma, migraine headaches, and seizures. His father and mother were divorced but both alive.

His vital signs were pulse 130, BP 140/90, respirations 18, temperature 98.6°F, and O₂ saturation 99% on room air. On the physical examination no trauma was noted about face or head. His pupils were 5mm bilaterally; the remainder of the neurological examination was within normal limits. He had no jugular venous distention. There were no rales or wheezes on auscultation of the lungs. No friction rub was heard, and there were no murmurs, rubs, or gallops on cardiac examination. The chest wall was diffusely tender, but no point tenderness was noted, nor was his pain reproducible. There were no signs of trauma. His abdomen was nontender and bowel sounds were hyperactive. He had no pedal edema or calf tenderness. Skin showed no lesions, track marks, or bruises.

Q: What is the initial approach to this patient?

Everything begins with the ABC's (Airway, Breathing and Circulation).

Case Continuation

An IV was started with D5W TKO, and 2 liters/min of oxygen were administered. Continuous monitoring was instituted of O₂ saturation, cardiac rate and rhythm, and blood pressure. An ECG and chest x-ray were ordered. A urinalysis and serum toxicology screen were ordered; a bedside blood glucose was 105. The ECG showed a sinus tachycardia rate of 130 with no ST or T wave abnormalities. The chest x-ray revealed no cardiomegaly, infiltrates, effusions, pneumothorax or pneumomediastinum, or rib fractures. Ativan 1mg IV was given. Ten minutes following treatment, the patient's heart rate was noted to be 96 on the monitor, and he no longer complained of chest pain. His urinalysis *was negative for blood and myoglobin, and electrolytes including the BUN and creatinine were within normal limits. The toxicologic screens were positive only for cocaine.*

Q: What are the cardiac complications of cocaine use?

Cocaine has multisystem pathologic effects; among the most life-threatening are toxic psychosis, ventricular arrhythmias, myocardial infarction, cardiomyopathy, aortic dissection, tonic clonic seizures, subarachnoid hemorrhage, intracerebral hemorrhage, cerebritis, renal failure associated with rhabdomyalysis, and, for the pregnant patient, spontaneous abortion and placental abruption.

A review of 91 cases of cocaine-related myocardial infarction found that the event was independent of the route of administration. Previous chest pain was reported in 44%; 87% smoked cigarettes regularly; myocardial infarction occurred within 3 hours of using the drug; and, of those undergoing cardiac catheterization, 30/54 were abnormal.[4]

Sudden death in cocaine users has been postulated to be related to cocaine's proarrhythmic properties as a potent sodium channel-blocking drug.[5] Cocaine's cardiotoxic effects include arrhythmias, suppression of contractility, coronary artery constriction and reduction of flow, and increased blood pressure. Myocardial ischemia results from the oxygen demand outstripping the supply. Also noted is platelet aggregation contributing to thrombus formation.

Chronic use has been associated with microscopic changes of myocyte necrosis and fibrosis, resulting in the generalized damage of cocaine related myocardiopathy. In addition to blocking sodium channel uptake, cocaine may have a direct effect on calcium channels leading to contraction of vessels and heart muscle. Cocaine's ability to block the reuptake of catechoamines results in increased levels of circulating catecholamines like norepinephrine, which are responsible for spasm of coronary arteries. Therapeutic intervention includes calcium blockers, alpha-adrenergic blockers, nitrates, and thrombolytic therapy.[6] Although patients with risk factors and abnormal coronary arteries represent the majority of patients with cocaine-related myocardial in-

farction, the otherwise healthy cocaine user is also at risk for a myocardial infarction.

Q: Does our patient have cardiac chest pain?

A decision has to be made about whether the reported pain is cardiac in origin. Once cardiac etiology is ruled out, ED staff can begin to plan for referral for substance abuse treatment and safe discharge. New recommendations that take the prevalence of dual diagnosis into account suggest that ED staff consider the appropriateness of a psychiatric referral for patients with substance abuse problems as part of the discharge process. Detection of dual diagnosis is critical, because these patients will not be "safe" if they are returned to their own communities without a plan for psychiatric evaluation and follow-up.

Case Continuation

The patient was recognized by the ED physician who had admitted him to the CCU a month before for similar complaints. At that time, myocardial infarction was ruled out. With this history of prior CCU admission and today's presentation of palpitation, diffuse chest tightness, increased respiratory rate, and numbness in hands (similar to several episodes associated with smoking crack and a normal ECG), it was elected to treat him with a benzodiazepam rather than nitroglycerine because of the noncardiac origin of pain. After a 4-hour pain-free period of observation, the patient wanted to go home to sleep. He was concerned about losing a janitorial job he just started.

After gaining the patient's permission to discuss the relationship between the chest pain and crack use, the attending physician asked him how ready he was to stop his use of crack. When he hesitated, the physician explored with the patient the pros and cons of his drug use. The patient admitted that he used cocaine to handle his feeling of sadness. He was angry and sad about a relationship with his girlfriend. When asked what he needed in order to stay safe and healthy, he said he had no interest in an inpatient program because of his job. He also had recently been in such a program following a psychiatric hospitalization for suicidal ideation and homicidal feelings toward his girlfriend. Just 2 days before the current visit, he had been discharged and referred for outpa-

*tient drug and mental health counseling. He reported
that he had gone to his girlfriend's house yesterday and
gotten in a fight with her. He was angry with her for
leaving him for another man and not allowing him to see
his 2-year-old daughter. At this point, tears came to his
eyes. He denied any current thoughts of harming himself. After further discussion of his options, he agreed to
an outpatient referral. He was given a taxi cab voucher
to an alcohol and drug evaluation unit for appropriate referral.*

*After the patient was discharged, the old medical re-
cord was finally retrieved. The documentation dated
back to his birth in 1964. In March 1974, he visited pediatrics for school problems. At age 10, a penile discharge
was treated. At one point, he and his parents were referred for psychiatric evaluation. During his teen years,
he was seen for loss of consciousness, a chipped tooth
and knee injury from a trail bike crash, a left eye injury
in a fight, and a right middle finger contusion after getting kicked. In his early twenties, over a 4-year period,
he had eight ED visits for grand mal seizures attributed
to using cocaine by multiple routes, including injection.
In his late twenties, he continued using cocaine in combination with alcohol and had more than a dozen ED visits for on the job injuries, cocaine-related seizures, and
for polydrug overdoses, because, as he told the emergency physician, "I was tired of living." The drugs he ingested on various ED visits during this period were
dilantin, tegretol, motrin, imipramine, corgard, theo-
phyline, xanax, and lithium. On one occasion, he required hemodialysis. This was a period of great turmoil
with his girlfriend, the mother of his child. His record reports a number of psychiatric admissions. The information in his record was communicated to the referral
agency so that they might appreciate his long history of
psychiatric problems. The patient was subsequently referred for a short inpatient stay followed by outpatient
services at a unit that specializes in both substance
abuse and mental illness.*

Q: How common is the combination of alcohol and other drug abuse with depression or other mental illness? What challenge does dual diagnosis represent to the clinician?

Weiss et al. in 1990 studied 149 cocaine abusers to
determine the prevalence of psychiatric illness and
found that 21% had a lifetime diagnosis of depres-

sion. In another study, two-thirds of 501 patients
seeking alcohol and drug treatment had evidence of
a current psychiatric diagnosis. In the Epidemiologic
Catchment Area survey, 9% of 19,571 people surveyed reported drug abuse with a concomitant lifetime psychiatric diagnosis by DSM-III criteria, and
6% had a current diagnosis. Galanter and colleagues
pointed out that one-third of general psychiatry admissions have illnesses influenced or precipitated by
drug abuse. It is often difficult to differentiate primary depression from mood disorders secondary to
long-term use of drugs.[7] Bipolar affective disorder is
most likely to be associated with substance abuse or
dependence, and cocaine abuse or dependence and
alcoholism are more common in this Axis I category
than in the general population.[8]

Both deinstitutionalization and changing patterns of drug use in our culture have contributed to
an increased prevalence of the comorbid condition
now called *dual diagnosis*. A recent review on the
subject points out that an entire generation of young
adults who have major mental illness and easy access
to alcohol and other drugs have grown up with few
skills, many deficits, diverse symptoms, and extensive needs for psychiatric and support services. Unlike the previous generation, whose long-term
treatment needs were met in psychiatric hospitals,
this generation's needs must be met by the community, but today's community mental health services
are limited and seriously underfunded. Homelessness compounds the problem.

Persons with major mental illness use alcohol
and drugs for the same reasons as other users: mood
alteration, socializing, and availability. The high rate
of substance abuse among mental health patients
also represents factors such as homelessness, and
poverty—life in poor, urban, marginalized neighborhoods in which frequent use is common and the drug
trade is a cottage industry.

Yet these reasons do not explain sufficiently the
association of heavy use with psychiatric symptoms.
Chronic heavy drugs may cause psychiatric disorders. Alternatively, undiagnosed internal mental
states may provide specific vulnerability and risk.[9]
McClellan found that among substance abusers who
had been in treatment, their continued use was associated with personality change on a 6-year follow-up.
He followed up stimulant, depressant, and opiate
users who, on entering drug treatment, had exhibited
few psychological symptoms. Six years later, the

chronic use of stimulants was associated in the same patients with paranoid schizophrenia and mania requiring long-term treatment on locked wards. The chronic use of depressants was associated with suicidal ideation, suicide attempts and cognitive impairment, while the opiate users had no personality changes on testing.[7] The changes in symptomatology that he noted may represent a progression of a major psychiatric illness, the long-term effects of substance abuse, or some combination of both entities.

In truth, we lack extensive and solid research with which to elucidate the relationship between substance abuse and mental illness. Are they independent and autonomous from one another, causally related, or interdependent? Improvement in one disorder may mean no improvement in the other, or a worsening of symptoms. McClellan, using the (ASI) Addiction Severity Index, observed that in patients with substance abuse problems, the severity of psychiatric status is a predictor of treatment response. Patients in substance abuse treatment with fewer psychiatric symptoms showed greater improvement.

Patients with "dual diagnosis" are more likely to demonstrate disruptive, hostile, criminal and suicidal behavior. They are not very compliant as psychiatric patients, and, because of unstable living situations, they are hard to follow up, if they engage at all with services. They have very high rates of recidivism for their substance abuse, which is very frustrating for service providers. They require more intensive and numerous services. They do not fit into the traditional mental health or substance abuse treatment system and often fall through the cracks because neither system wants to take care of them. They are thus more likely to be found in jails and hospitals than on the inpatient psychiatric units, and they often present to the ED with injuries and serious illnesses.

These are the most time and resource consuming, and disruptive of our patients. They are often chemically and physically restrained because of their disruptive and threatening behavior. It is almost impossible to arrange for adequate follow-up or admission for this special population, because neither psychiatric facilities nor substance abuse treatment programs will accept them. Coordinated and integrated systems with a case management model that addresses housing and multiple service needs are needed urgently for the care of patients with dual diagnosis. Over the course of the last 5 years, the

substance abuse treatment community has developed some specialty clinics and programs for this population, but the number of available slots is clearly inadequate. And, there has been increased research interest in the subject, and a doubling of articles on the subject from 1980.[7]

Case Conclusion

The patient called on several occasions over the next 2 weeks to report to the referring emergency physician that he had returned to the program that he had been involved in previously. He returned to seeing his same counselor, and reported that he had not been using crack or other drugs. He was staying away from his girlfriend, living with his mother, and had returned to work. This information was corroborated by his mother, who confided to the physician that she was less anxious about her son now that he was actively in treatment.

Q: What is the prognosis for our patient?

The prognosis for all three presenting problems—chest pain, substance abuse and mental illness—is interconnected. A recent study by Hollander suggests that once a first episode of chest pain is ruled out for M.I. (myocardial infarction), subsequent risk for M.I. and death from cardiac causes appears to be low. "Although continued cocaine use may induce subsequent episodes of chest pain, necessitating further evaluation, greater emphasis should be placed on halting continued cocaine use." Among those in the study who continued to use, there were two nonfatal M.I.s and four cardiac-related deaths.[3]

McClellan writes that substance abuse patients with severe psychiatric problems show greater improvement when their psychiatric problems are addressed in therapy rather than in counseling. Furthermore, psychiatric therapy of any type will be inadequate unless substance abuse issues are also directly confronted.

As part of the original assessment, the Addiction Severity Instrument (ASI) was administered to Steve, and many psychiatric symptoms were detected, as supported by his extensive medical history and psychiatric hospitalizations. The ASI assesses problem severity in seven areas that are often affected by drug and alcohol dependency: medicine, law, family, employment, psychiatric function, and drug and alcohol abuse. The instrument can also be administered at 6 months follow-up to assess improvement.

This patient was referred to a program for patients with dual diagnosis and appears to be making progress. Although long-term follow-up will be required to evaluate the efficacy of the intervention, in the short term, he has not recorded an ED visit in several months, and, if reports from the family are correct, he has become less of a burden by working, staying off drugs, continuing to see his counselor, and getting legal assistance to see his daughter. These are realistic expectations for short-term goals. In order to prevent relapse, Steve most likely will require psychotherapy and medication to complement his substance abuse recovery program.

CONCLUSION

The phenomenon of co-occurring mental illness and substance abuse has been widely recognized since 1984.[10] Recent data confirm the extent of the problem; as many as 47% of individuals with a diagnosis of schizophrenia have been shown to meet criteria for substance abuse. And, similarly, two-thirds of those seeking alcohol or drug abuse treatment may demonstrate a current psychiatric disorder on standardized testing.[11] Outcomes are worse for patients with dual diagnosis, yet there are administrative barriers, resistances, and gaps within both the mental health and substance abuse service systems,[12] and caretakers are typically trained in either one discipline or the other, but not both.[9]

These are the patients for whom the ED is a continuously revolving door. Each of these ED visits represents an opportunity to identify the complex polydiagnostic nature of the presenting problem and provide referral for treatment that addresses *both* illness categories. Successful treatment of the patient with dual diagnosis provides a dual benefit—improved quality of life for these individuals and reduction in the drain on ED resources. In order to achieve these positive outcomes, a team approach must be developed among ED physicians, substance abuse counselors, and mental health service providers.

NOTES

1. Rice DP, Kelman S, Miller LS. Economic costs of drug abuse. In WS Cartwright, JM Kaple, (eds.). *Economic Costs, Cost Effectiveness, Financing, and Community-Based Drug Treatment.* Rockville, MD: U.S. DHHS PHS NIDA (ADM) 91-1823, 1991.

2. Hollander JE, Hoffman RS, Gennis P, Fairweather P, Feldman JA, Fish SS, et al. Cocaine-associated chest pain: One year follow-up. *Acad Emerg Med* 1995; 2:179–84.

3. Rydell PC, Everingham SS. *Controlling Cocaine: Supply versus Demand Programs.* Santa Monica, CA: Rand Drug Policy Research Center, ISBN:0-8330-1552-4, 1994.

4. Hollander JE, Hoffman RS. Cocaine-induced myocardial infarction: An analysis and review of the literature. *J Emerg Med* 1992; 10 (2):169–77.

5. Bauman JL, Grawe JJ, Winecoff AP, Harriman RJ. Cocaine-related sudden cardiac death: A hypothesis correlating basic science and clinical observations. *J Clin Pharmacol* 1994; 34(9):902–11.

6. Kloner RA, Hale S, Alker K, Rezkalla S. The effects of acute and chronic cocaine use on the heart. *Circulation* 1992; 85(2):407–19.

7. McClellan T. Dual Diagnosis: Drug abuse and psychiatric illness. In *Drug abuse and drug abuse research: The third triennial report to Congress from the Secretary DHHS.* U.S. DHHS PHS ADAMHA (DHHS Publ No. (ADM) 91-1704): Maryland, 1991.

8. Brady KT, Lydiard RB. Bipolar affective disorder and substance abuse. *J Clin Psychopharmacol* 1992; 12(1 suppl):17S–22S.

9. Drake RE, McLaughlin P, Pepper B, Minkoff K. Dual diagnosis of major mental illness and substance disorder: An overview. In K Minkler and RE Drake (eds.). *New Dir Ment Health Serv* 1991; 50:3–11.

10. Regier DA, Meyers JK, Kramer M, et al. The NIMH Epidemiological Cachement Area Program: Historical context, major objectives, and study population characteristics. *Arch Gen Psychiatr* 1984; 41:934–41.

11. Regier DA, Farmer ME, Rae DS, et al. Comorbidity of mental disorders with alcohol and other drug abuse. *JAMA* 1990; 246:2511–18.

12. Ridgely MS, Goldman HH, Talbot JA. *Chronic mentally ill young adults with substance abuse problems: Treatment and training issues.* Baltimore: Mental Health Policy Studies, University of Maryland School of Medicine, 1987.

7

Tobacco Use in the U.S.: The Role of the Emergency Physician

RICHARD GOLDBERG

CONTENTS

- Epidemiology of tobacco use
- Adverse health consequences
- Effects of passive and in utero exposure
- Use of smokeless tobacco
- Relevance to emergency medicine
- Counseling and treatment options
- Advocacy issues

CHAPTER SUMMARY

With emergency departments (EDs) currently receiving close to 100 million patient visits annually, emergency physicians (EPs) have an opportunity to play a pivotal role in the promotion of a number of public health initiatives. Prominent among them is the effort to reduce and ultimately eliminate the use of tobacco products in this country. Current national objectives call for a reduction in the prevalence of cigarette smoking among people aged 20 or more from a baseline of 29% in 1987 to 15% by the year 2000. These objectives are seen by public health authorities as a prelude to the creation of a smokeless society.[1]

Case #1

A 64-year-old Caucasian man presented to the ED complaining of difficulty breathing. Despite appearing to be in some respiratory distress, he greeted the examining physician with a grin, saying "Hey, Doc, I'm your classic blue bloater!" Smoking history revealed a one-to-two-pack-per-day habit since age 16. The patient was treated in the ED over the next 2 hours with oxygen by Venturi mask, nebulized bronchodilators, intravenous steroids, and antibiotics. He was subsequently admitted to the intensive care unit with a diagnosis of chronic bronchitis and respiratory failure. He was discharged from the hospital 9 days later, and arrangements were made for continuous low-flow oxygen, home nebulizer treatments, and daily visits by a home health nurse.

Q: What is chronic obstructive pulmonary disease (COPD), and what relation does it have to cigarette smoking?

The term *COPD* refers to lung conditions characterized by permanent airflow obstruction. Among the disorders resulting in COPD are chronic bronchitis, asthma, and emphysema. Cigarette smoking accounts for 82% of deaths from COPD, which is the fifth leading cause of death overall in the United States.[2] COPD is also a major cause of chronic disability, as illustrated by the case presentation. Between 1979 and 1981, chronic bronchitis and emphysema caused 169 million days of restricted activity per year, or nearly 2 months of restricted activity per year, for each affected person.[3]

This patient had chronic bronchitis and was indeed a classic "blue bloater," as opposed to patients with chronic emphysema, the so-called "pink puffers." While patients with pure bronchitis or emphysema are relatively rare, many patients have clinical and laboratory features that are clearly referable to one or the other syndrome.

Q: Given this patient's self-diagnosis as a "blue bloater," can you predict generally the features of his history, physical, and laboratory examination? What do you predict for the frequency of bronchial infections, sputum production, general appearance, findings on chest auscultation, extremity examination, chest x-ray findings, and arterial blood gases? Contrast these findings to the typical patient with chronic emphysema.

As is often the case in patients with chronic bronchitis, this patient gave a history of chronic cough with frequent bouts of bronchial infection and recent copious purulent sputum production. Examination revealed a corpulent, plethoric individual who was somewhat lethargic but appropriately responsive to questions and commands. While obviously tachypneic, he appeared to be resting comfortably in bed. Blood pressure was 180/110 mmHg., pulse 116/minute, respirations 26/minute, and temperature 99.4 orally. Other pertinent physical findings included moderately tight expiratory wheezes bilaterally and 2+ pretibial edema.

Chest x-ray showed cardiomegaly and increased bronchovascular markings. Arterial blood gases on room air revealed a pH of 7.23, pO_2 of 48 mmHg., PCO_2 of 68 mmHg., and an electrocardiogram showed findings consistent with cor pulmonale, including right axis deviation with right atrial and ventricular hypertrophy.[4]

In contrast to patients with chronic bronchitis, patients with chronic emphysema typically are cachectic individuals who present with severe air hunger. They give a history of relatively infrequent bouts of infection with scanty sputum production. Examination of the chest reveals diminished breath sounds and a notably increased AP diameter. Chest x-ray examination shows evidence of hyperinflation and a small heart. The arterial blood gases reveal a low pO_2 as well as a chronically high pCO_2. EKG may show

evidence of right atrial enlargement. Cor pulmonale is usually noted only as a terminal finding.[4]

Q: Other than COPD, what other health risks does he face?

The patient has a 48 pack/year history of heavy tobacco use. Tobacco use is a major risk factor for coronary artery and peripheral vascular diseases, cancer of the lung, larynx, pharynx, oral cavity, esophagus, pancreas, and bladder. The incidences of both acute upper and lower respiratory tract infection and ulcer disease are also increased.[2]

Case #2

A 32-year-old Caucasian female presented to the ED with a 4-week history of cough that was productive of green sputum that had become streaked with blood earlier in the day. She had also noted intermittent episodes of wheezing and dyspnea on effort. There was no history of chest pain, chills, or fever. Her husband and 14-year-old son were asymptomatic. She had no prior history of similar symptoms, though she stated that she got one cold a year "and it always goes to my lungs." She apparently had been reluctant to seek medical attention because she was 3 months pregnant and did not want to be taking medications. She gave a history of smoking one pack of cigarettes per day since age 18.

Physical examination revealed a well-developed woman in no distress. Blood pressure was 110/70, pulse 84, respirations 18, temperature 99° orally. Pertinent physical findings included a moderately inflamed oropharynx and a brassy cough with scattered rhonchi and rare wheezes bilaterally. Examination of the extremities revealed no pretibial edema and Homan's sign was negative bilaterally. Laboratory evaluation consisted of oximetry (O_2 saturation) on room air and a PA view of the chest, obtained with the abdomen shielded. These studies were normal. After consultation with her obstetrician, the patient was begun on a course of antibiotics and a beta agonist inhaler was also prescribed for prn use. At the time of discharge, the patient was able to relate her symptoms to her smoking habit and expressed a determination to quit. She declined a referral to a smoking-cessation clinic. Her obstetrician also advised against a prescription for nicotine gum. A number of issues relating to smoking were discussed with her.

Q: What health risks are associated with maternal smoking?

The patient was 3 months pregnant. Smoking during pregnancy has been shown to retard fetal growth and is associated with an increased incidence of miscarriage, stillbirth, sudden infant death syndrome, and infant mortality. In the United States, 20 to 30% of low-birth-weight infants and up to 14% of premature deliveries are attributable to maternal cigarette smoking.[5]

Q: What are the health risks associated with passive exposure to smoke? Regarding her son, what warnings might she give him as to the problems of smoking in adolescence?

Neither the patient's husband nor her 14-year-old son smoke. Exposure to smoke in infancy and childhood appears to pose risks for the development of chronic airflow obstruction later in life.[6] Middle ear infection is also considerably more common among children whose parents smoke.[2] Passive or involuntary smoking also appears to be associated with higher incidences of lung cancer and airway obstructive disease in nonsmoking adults.[6–8]

The patient's son is at an age when experimentation with cigarette smoking is common. A recent adolescent health survey found that 51% of eighth-graders (ages 13 to 14) and 63% of tenth-graders (ages 15 to 16) reported having tried cigarettes. Adolescent boys comprised the single highest category of new users of tobacco. It is estimated that 80% of smokers and 66% of users of smokeless tobacco develop their habit before the age of 21.[2]

Q: What is smokeless tobacco and what are the health consequences of its use?

Smokeless tobacco includes primarily wet or dry snuff and chewing tobacco. Oral cancers have been shown to occur several times more frequently among smokeless tobacco users and may be 50 times as frequent among long-term snuff users.[7–9]

DISCUSSION

Epidemiology

Tobacco use is responsible for more than one of every six deaths in the United States and is the most important single cause of preventable death and disease in our society; 30% of all cancer deaths, 87% of lung cancer deaths, and 21% of all coronary deaths are attributable to smoking.[2] Additionally, smoking costs this country $52 billion annually in health care and other costs.[10] Despite such statistics, there are significant obstacles to efforts by public health agencies to reduce the use of tobacco products. These include the addictive nature of tobacco, the high rate of relapse, the fact that tobacco products are so heavily advertised, and the prominent role of tobacco in the agricultural economy of several states.

Nevertheless, there has been a significant decline in the prevalence of smoking over the past 25 years, with the number of smoking adults going from 40% in 1965 to 29% in 1987. It is notable that the decline has been substantially lower in women than in men, and the prevalence of smoking remains disproportionately high among blacks, blue-collar workers, and people with fewer years of education.[2] However, public health planners are optimistic that progress in the reduction of tobacco use can continue to be made, ultimately resulting in a smokeless society for future generations. There are two major challenges to further progress at this time: (1) young people must be discouraged from starting to smoke, and (2) there must be an increase in the number of people who break the smoking habit.[1]

Relevance to the Emergency Physician

Smokers may be particularly susceptible to receiving advice to quit when they visit a physician. In fact, brief smoking-cessation counseling by primary care physicians has been shown to be effective in several clinical trials.[11–15] Unfortunately, there is a tremendous disparity between the magnitude of the health problems caused by smoking and the efforts of physicians to identify and treat this addiction. Fewer than half of all smokers report that they have ever

---

Figure 7-1   The Four *As* of Smoking Intervention

- *Ask* all patients about smoking
- *Advise* all patients to stop
  - State health risks to patient
  - State health risks to others
- *Assist* patients who want to stop now
  - Help patients select a quit date
  - Provide self-help materials
  - Consider prescribing nicotine gum or transdermal patches
- *Arrange* follow-up with local smoking cessation agencies

SOURCE: Glynn T, Manley M. *How to help your patient stop smoking: A National Cancer Institute manual for physicians.* Bethesda, MD: U.S. Department of Health and Human Services National Institutes of Health Pub. 89-8064, 1989.

---

been advised by their physicians to quit or cut down.[16] Young smokers, in particular, fail to receive cessation advice, despite evidence that initiates are more sensitive to intervention efforts than are long-time smokers.[1]

Emergency physicians, by virtue of the large number of patients they encounter, are in a unique position to participate in efforts to reduce use of tobacco products. It should be noted that smoking cessation is not a single event. Smokers often move through stages, from being uninterested in stopping, to thinking about change, to making a concerted effort to stop, to finally maintaining abstinence.[17,18] Thus, smoking cessation is a process that takes place over time. As detailed below, emergency physicians and ED staff have a role to play in this process.

- Based on the results of several clinical trials,[11–15] the National Cancer Institute (NCI) has produced a manual of practical smoking cessation counseling techniques for use by clinicians.[19] Supplementing the manual is an optional 3-hour course for physicians and nurses. The NCI-recommended approach is outlined in Figure 7–1. Often referred to as "the four As," the recommendations comprise an intervention plan easily adapatable to the ED, particularly when nursing and ancillary staff are also enlisted in delivering the antismoking message.

- *Ask* all patients about smoking. Seventy percent of smokers visit a physician each year.[20] It has been recommended that the smoking status of patients be identified and documented routinely as vital signs are being taken.[21]

- *Advise* all smokers to stop. The advice should be stated clearly and should include information on the effects of passive smoking on family members and friends.

- *Assist* patients who want to stop. Help patients select a quit date, provide educational materials[22] and consider prescribing nicotine gum or transdermal patches. Guidelines for use of nicotine products include: (1) Smokers should stop smoking completely before they start using the product. (2) Nicotine is more likely to be an effective adjunct if combined with counseling. (3) If using gum, patients should be instructed to chew it slowly and intermittently, allowing for better nicotine absorption. (4) Because smokers have a substantial risk of relapse, the nicotine product should be used for at least three months.[23]

- *Arrange* follow-up. Follow-up is an essential element in the smoking cessation process. Most communities have follow-up resources available; these may include local hospitals, public health clinics, and local cancer societies.

Advocacy Issues

Emergency physicians can add a fifth "A" to the four already recommended by the NCI: *Advocacy*. Through involvement at community, state and federal levels of government, EPs have an important role to play as public health advocates in promoting the adoption of a number of antismoking initiatives currently promulgated by the Public Health Service:[1]

- Establish tobacco-free environments and include tobacco use prevention in the curricula of all elementary, middle, and secondary schools.

- Increase to at least 75% the proportion of worksites with a formal smoking policy that prohibits or severely restricts smoking at the workplace.

- Enact in 50 states comprehensive laws on clean air indoors that prohibit or strictly limit smoking in the workplace and enclosed public places.

- Enact and enforce in 50 states laws prohibiting the sale and distribution of tobacco products to youths younger than age 19.
- Increase to 50 the number of states with comprehensive plans to reduce tobacco use, especially among youth.
- Eliminate or severely restrict all forms of tobacco product advertising and promotion to which youth younger than age 18 are likely to be exposed.
- Increase to at least 75% the proportion of primary care and oral health care providers who routinely advise cessation and provide assistance and follow-up for all their tobacco-using patients.

CONCLUSION

In summary, emergency physicians and ED staff have an important role to play in the ongoing effort to reduce and ultimately eliminate the use of tobacco products. By identifying tobacco users, delivering brief anti-tobacco messages, providing educational materials and medication supplements, and by providing appropriate follow-up, emergency personnel are in a position to greatly increase the number of people receiving professional cessation counseling and, in the process, perform a critical public health service.

NOTES

1. Public Health Service. *Healthy people 2000: National health promotion and disease prevention objectives.* Washington, DC: U.S. Department of Health and Human Services, Public Health Service; DHHS Pub. No. (PHS) 91-50212, 1991.
2. Office on Smoking and Health. *Reducing the health consequences of smoking: 25 years of progress. The report of the Surgeon General.* Washington, DC: U.S. Department of Health and Human Services; DHHS Pub. No. (CDC) 89-8411, 1989.
3. National Center for Health Statistics. Prevalence of selected chronic conditions: United States, 1979–81. In *Vital and health statistics Series 10, No. 155.* Hyattsville, MD: U.S. Department of Health and Human Services DHHS Pub. (PHS) 861583-10155, 1986.
4. Ingram RH Jr. Chronic bronchitis, emphysema, and airways obstruction. In Wilson JD, Braunwald E, Isselbacher KJ, et al. (eds.). *Harrison's principles of internal medicine,* 12th ed. New York: McGraw-Hill, 1991.
5. Kleinman JC, Madans JH. The effects of maternal smoking, physical stature and educational attainment on the incidence of low birthweight. *Am J Epidem* 1985; 121:843–55.
6. National Research Council, Committee on Passive Smoking. *Environmental tobacco smoke: Measuring exposure and assessing health effects.* Washington, DC: National Academy Press, 1986.
7. Office on Smoking and Health. *The health consequences of involuntary smoking. A report of the Surgeon General.* Washington DC: U.S. Department of Health and Human Services DHHS Pub. No. (CDC) 87-8398, 1986.
8. White JR, Froeb HF. Small air-ways dysfunction in nonsmokers chronically exposed to tobacco smoke. *NEJM* 1980; 302:720–3.
9. National Institute on Drug Abuse. *National household survey on drug abuse, 1988. Population estimates.* Hyattsville, MD: U.S. Department of Health and Human Services DHHS Pub. No. (PHS) 89-1501, 1989.
10. National Institute on Drug Abuse. *National household survey on drug abuse, 1988. Population estimates.* Rockville, MD: U.S. Department of Health and Human Services DHHS Pub. No. (ADH) 89-1636, 1989.
11. Ockene JK, Kristellar J, Goldberg R, et al. Increasing the efficacy of physician-delivered smoking interventions: A randomized clinical trial. *J Gen Intern Med* 1991; 6:1–3.
12. Cohen SJ, Stookey GK, Katz BP, Droop CA, Smith DM. Encouraging primary care physicians to help smokers quit: A randomized, controlled trial. *Ann Intern Med* 1989; 110:648–52.
13. Cummings SR, Coatee TJ, Richard RJ, et al. Training physicians in counseling about smoking cessation: A randomized trial of the "quit for life" program. *Ann Intern Med* 1989; 110:640–7.
14. Wilson DMC, Taylor DW, Gilbert JR, et al. A randomized trial of a family physician intervention for smoking cessation. *JAMA* 1988; 260:1570–4.
15. Kottke TE, Brekkle ML, Solberg LI, Hughes JR. A randomized trial to increase smoking intervention by physicians: Doctors helping smokers, round one. *JAMA* 1989; 261:2101–6.
16. Frank E, Winkelby MA, Altman DG, Rockhill B, Fortmann SP. Predictors of physician's smoking cessation advice. *JAMA* 1991; 266:3139–44.
17. Prochaska J, DiClimente C. Stages and processes of self-change in smoking: Toward an integrative model of change. *J Consult Clin Psychol* 1983; 51:390–5.
18. Rollnick S, Kinnersley P, Stott N. Methods of helping patients with behaviour change. *BMJ* 1993; 307: 188–90.
19. Glynn T, Manley M. *How to help your patient stop smoking: A National Cancer Institute manual for physicians.* Bethesda, MD: U.S. Department of Health and

Human Services National Institutes of Health Pub. 89-8064, 1989.

20. Ockene JK. Smoking intervention: The expanding role of the physician. *Am J Public Health* 1987; 77:782–8.

21. Fiore MC. The new vital sign: Assessing and documenting smoking status. Editorial. *JAMA* 1991; 266:3183–4.

22. Available through the American Cancer Society. 1-800-ACS-2345.

23. Cummings SR, Hansen B, Richard RJ, Stein MJ, Coates TJ. Internists and nicotine gum. *JAMA* 1988; 260:1565–9.

8

Childhood Injury and Abuse

JOHN F. MARCINAK
ANITA L. HURTIG
KYRAN P. QUINLAN

CONTENTS

CHAPTER SUMMARY

Child maltreatment, which includes abuse and neglect, is a significant public health problem. Injuries that occur in children can be unintentional or caused by physical abuse. Two cases of intentional injuries are presented in children at risk for child abuse. The diagnosis of intentional injury is based on discrepancies in the history regarding how the injury occurred and the presence of physical findings inconsistent with the explanation of the injury. The combination of physical abuse and neglect can occur in the same child. The child's social, emotional, and educational history are important features in the evaluation of injuries because risk factors for abuse are related to these areas. Prevention of physical abuse in the emergency department (ED) setting has focused on tertiary prevention or interventions after the condition of

physical abuse has been identified. The ED physician's advocacy role in cases of intentional injuries includes assessment and evaluation of the injury followed by identifying the possibility of abuse, reporting the injury, and validating maltreatment. The advocacy role of the ED physician for children also includes assuring the immediate safety of the child and identifying children at risk. The ED physician can also be a valuable member of child death review panels that investigate suspicious deaths of children.

Case #1

A 9-year-old African American male was brought to the ED with a fracture of the clavicle. His mother reported that he had fallen down the stairway as he was rushing off to school. An interview with the mother and child failed to elicit evidence of intentional abuse. The mother reported that this was not the first injury the child sustained—indeed, this was the third or fourth ED visit for fracture, sprain, or laceration. She attributed this pattern to the child's behavioral problems, specifically hyperactivity.

The interview in the ED focused on the etiology of the injury because of the history of repeated injuries. The incident was described as one of many where the child's clumsiness, specifically running too fast and tripping, caused a major fall. X-rays revealed lesions suggestive of previous upper and lower extremity fractures. However, because the child was noted to be "hyperactive" by the examining doctor, it was assumed that this condition was the cause of this and previous injuries.

Given this pattern of behavior, the parent was referred to the pediatric psychosocial clinic for an assess-

ment of the child's behavioral status and recommendations for treatment. The parent and child did not show for the scheduled appointment. The family was called to indicate the need to comply with the follow-up recommendation and told of the possibility of having to report the case for neglect. The parent rescheduled and did appear. A subsequent interview and testing revealed a history of physical abuse of the child by the father. The Department of Children and Family Services (DCFS) was notified.

Case #2

A 5-month-old white female infant was admitted to the hospital from the ED because of an enlarged head. There was a history of sudden enlargement of the head over the 3 days prior to admission. Additionally, the infant's 15-year-old mother reported a fall, about 1 week before the visit, from a couch that was 18 inches above the ground to a concrete floor. A swelling of the right lower thigh was present and first noted about 3 to 4 weeks prior. The swelling was attributed to a local reaction to a DTP vaccination.

Past medical history was pertinent for the infant being born prematurely at 25 weeks gestation with a birth weight of 900 grams. There was no history of intraventricular hemorrhage.

Physical exam was remarkable for an alert infant with an enlarged head with the head circumference greater than 95th percentile. The height was at the 25th percentile and weight less than the 5th percentile when corrected for gestational age. A 2 cm bluish discoloration over the left temporal scalp was noted, and a hard swelling of the right distal thigh was present without erythema or tenderness. There were no retinal hemorrhages present.

A skeletal survey revealed a fracture of the distal right femur and a left parietal skull fracture. A CT scan of the brain showed bilateral subdural collections of fluid. A neurosurgical procedure was performed to drain the subdural collection of fluid, which proved to be hemorrhagic. The infant showed good weight gain in the hospital after the operation. Social Service was consulted, and DCFS was informed. In the hospital, DCFS took temporary custody of the child. The investigation of the home revealed a history from a maternal cousin that the mother beat the infant. The infant was discharged under DCFS supervision after a 2-week hospitalization. The child continues to be a ward of the state. The case

against the mother is still pending in court after 4 months.

Q: Are there any inconsistencies about the history of the child's injuries in either of the two cases?

The history of how an injury has occurred is the first step in trying to distinguish an unintentional from an intentional injury. An important feature of intentional injuries is a discrepant history.[1] Five examples include (1) no history given for an injury, (2) partial history given, (3) history changes, (4) history of injury not developmentally appropriate, and (5) lack of history of behavioral response to injury. The ED physician must consider whether the history given of how an injury occurred is consistent with the injury sustained. In case 1, the occurrence of multiple injuries over time was incorrectly attributed to the child's hyperactivity. In case 2, there was no history of fussiness or crying in the infant, who had both a severe head injury and femur fracture. In addition, the explanation of the occurrence of the injuries was not consistent with the physical findings. Specifically, the explanation for the head injury was a fall of 18 inches. Falls from the height of 3 feet do not result in serious injury to children.[2,3] Falls of less than 10 feet in young children less than 3 years old witnessed by a second person other than the caretaker are also unlikely to produce serious or life threatening injury.[4] In addition, when deaths occur in children who have a history of a fall from 4 feet or less, the best explanation is that the history is incorrect.[5] These studies suggest that physical abuse should be considered with serious head injuries in children who fall from low heights.

The child in case #1 suffered a clavicular fracture, and the infant in case #2 was found to have a linear skull fracture and femur fracture. Radiologic imaging for intentional injuries must be combined with documentation that the observed injury is the result of abuse, because alone these types of fractures have a low specificity for physical abuse.[6] However, the specificity increases when a history of trauma is absent or the history is inconsistent with the injuries.[7] Femur fractures can be secondary to unintentional trauma but are more likely to be caused by intentional trauma in children less than 1 year of age.[8] A subdural hematoma, as was found in case #2, has been found to be common in inflicted injury in young children and uncommon in unintentional injuries, except for children as passengers in collisions.[9]

Q: What further information about the medical condition of the children would be helpful in clarification of the two cases?

The child's past medical history is important in making an assessment of whether the injury sustained is intentional. When the ED physician sees a child with an injury, a history suggesting a pattern of increased severity of injuries over time raises the suspicion of intentional trauma.[1,10] Does the child have an underlying medical or surgical problem that is not being taken care of? Has the child received appropriate immunizations? Answers to these questions may indicate that the child was neglected. This is important because the same child may experience a combination of physical abuse and neglect.[11]

A complete physical examination is essential in all cases of suspected physical abuse. In addition to the fractures and head injuries resulting from child abuse that are illustrated in the two cases, many other organ systems can be involved with resulting injury. These conditions include injuries to the head and neck region;[12] injuries to the skin because of burns, bruises, and bite marks; and hair loss;[13,14] and injuries to the genitalia[15] and abdomen.[16,17] Assessment of general appearance and growth parameters is essential, because failure to thrive and physical abuse can exist in the same child.[1] This point is illustrated by case #2 in which the infant demonstrated poor weight gain.

Q: What further information about the psychosocial history of the children would be helpful in clarification of the two cases?

The relevant data that influence management decisions in the ED must include not only a thorough review of the history of the specific event and the more global medical history of the child but also the equally important factor of the child's psychosocial history. This would include relationships with caretakers and current and past emotional status. With sensitive probing, the ED physician can often ascertain the nature and quality of the family situation. Some of the questions to be considered are (1) Who brought the child in? Is this the primary caretaker or a substitute, possibly indicating unavailability or avoidance? (2) Who lives with the child? Is there an appropriate responsible adult caretaker? (3) Is this a foster placement? If so, of what duration? Foster parent status may indicate reduced investment in the care of the child or inconsistent caretaking and the need for follow-up contact with a legal or, at least, official supervisor.

The physician must always be alert to the sociocultural bias he or she may bring to this line of inquiry. Do chaotic or nontraditional families evoke a negative bias which may lead to less careful treatment and follow-up or to a hostile and therefore less effective interaction with parent or caretaker? Because the ED physician may be the only professional to maintain contact with the family, it is as important to maintain a positive therapeutic alliance as it is to detect child abuse, and these competing needs should be consciously balanced.

Q: What might be an association among hyperactivity, physical injury, and physical abuse?

The child's social, emotional, and educational history is crucial information to be considered in management decisions. Children who are in special programs, such as classes for the behaviorally or emotionally disturbed, may have particular problems coping with the ED, both in terms of long waits and painful procedures. This is particularly true of children with Attention Deficit Hyperactivity Disorder (ADHD), whose special handling may require behavioral management techniques such as rewards for compliance and more specific, clear-cut, and immediate guidelines for control. The presence of impulsive or hyperactive behavior in the ED may clue the physician in to chronic behavioral problems and the possibility that the family has reacted in punitive and aggressive ways.

The ED physician must be alert to these social, emotional, and educational factors. Children whose impulsivity, overactivity, or low frustration tolerance place high demands on the skills and patience of their adult caretakers are particularly vulnerable to physical abuse. The additional complications of chaotic family situations or cross-generational care-taking place these children at even higher risk for abuse. At the other end of the spectrum, the family may claim hyperactivity when it does not exist. Parents who abuse children often externalize responsibility and blame them for the events leading up to the incident; infants "cry too much" and older children "misbehave." Allegations of hyperactivity in a child who does not exhibit this behavior should trigger further investigation.

BROADER PUBLIC HEALTH CONTEXT

Child maltreatment is a significant public health problem for which recognition and scientific study have increased in the past half-century. Inquiry into abuse was first spurred by radiologist John Caffey's report of intentional trauma to six infants in 1946.[18] "The battered child syndrome" was applied to this condition in 1962 by Henry Kempe and his coworkers.[19]

The true incidence of child abuse is not known. An estimate of between 949 and 2,002 deaths from abuse and neglect each year in children less than 18 years old for the period 1979 through 1988 has been reported.[20] More than 90% of these deaths were in children less than 5 years of age, and more than 40% were in infants less than 1 year of age.[20] Fatal child abuse and neglect appear to have a geographic variation, with highest death rates seen in the southern and western United States and the lowest rates in the northeast.[21] Homicide is the leading cause of injury death for infants in this country.[22] Hands and fists are the weapons used in 50% of homicides of 0 to 4 year olds.[23]

Fatal cases of abuse, like fatal injuries in general, represent the tip of the iceberg. Rates of nonfatal abuse and neglect increase with age.[24] A 1988 U.S. Department of Health and Human Services study reported that a total of more than 1.4 million children nationwide experienced abuse or neglect and over 1 million children experienced serious or moderate nonfatal injuries due to abuse and neglect in 1986.[24] As a result, 140,000 children suffered life-threatening conditions or potential long-term impairments in that year. According to the most recent annual 50-state survey of the National Committee to Prevent Child Abuse, 2,989,000 reports of child abuse and neglect were made in 1993.[25] Of these, an estimated 1,016,000 children were confirmed as victims of maltreatment. The rate of reports (number of reports/1,000 children) has increased 50% since 1988. These changes must be interpreted with caution, because increases in reporting may represent increases in rates of incidence, rates of recognition, or rates of reporting.

As previously noted, the work of Caffey and Kempe forced mental health workers and physicians to confront the reality of the severity of the child abuse problem in our society. Physical and emotional abuse of children is well documented in the literature of the nineteenth century, exemplified in Dickens' stories of hungry, neglected, and violated children. Recent epidemiological and case studies have moved the abused child out of the group home and into the family setting.

The horror of child abuse lies not only in the pain and danger involved but also in the emotional and cognitive sequelae.[26] There is substantial evidence that child abuse, most often in the form of severe parental punishment, leads to later aggressivity and delinquency in the older child, adolescent, and adult.[27] Research on those variables which may contribute to abuse of children has focused on adult/parent characteristics, child characteristics, and the interplay between the two. Among the parent characteristics noted are depression and emotional distress in mothers,[28] young maternal age and unwanted pregnancy,[29] and impulsivity in fathers.[30] Most recently, the role of substance abuse in maltreatment cases has been substantiated, with data indicating that 26% of such cases involve substance abuse.[25] Within the family, foster care and poverty,[29] isolation from family and community resources,[31] as well as marital discord[32] have also been noted.

A review of research on the coexistence of spouse abuse and child abuse points to the importance of recognizing this association. A dramatic overlap between the victimization of mothers and abuse of their children has been reported,[32–35] providing further evidence that information about the domestic status of the mother may offer clues to the presence of violence against children. To this end, it is important for emergency department staff to have basic knowledge of the legal rights of domestic violence victims.[34]

While some studies have found an association between abuse in childhood with abusive parenting,[36] these findings have not been consistently supported.[32] A study of multigenerational patterns of abuse has suggested that severely punitive acts experienced in childhood increased the risk of violence in parenting and that being reared in a family characterized by marital violence and conflict increased the risk of violent parenting more than having had the personal experience of violent discipline.[37]

The role of the child in the experience of physical abuse has also been studied with evidence that certain childhood characteristics place children at increased risk for experiencing abuse. These include hyperactivity,[38] as illustrated by case #1. Prematurity and low birth weight, as seen in case #2, are other child characteristics associated with physical abuse; these factors may be reflective of the socioeconomic status, the possibility of maternal substance abuse, and the age of the mother, rather than causative in themselves.

From the perspective of the cases noted above, there is general consensus that there is a relationship between children who are difficult to control and discipline[39] and children who are aggressive[40] and are at risk for injury. Parental abuse may be the force behind the injury, a relationship not always recognized in the ED setting. The ED physician must be sensitive to the potential for caretaker abuse of children with a wide range of behavioral problems such as ADHD, oppositional defiant disorder and conduct disorder. These are children who are noted or reported to be aggressive to the point of causing physical harm to others, destructive of property (their own or others), violators of home and school rules, consistently negativistic and defiant, angry, resentful, and vindictive.[41] This awareness should lead to appropriate follow up with the state child protection agency or hospital interdisciplinary team, which evaluates these children and provides services to them and their families. Most important from the perspective of the ED physician is the willingness to recognize the presence of the abusive relationship while still maintaining an empathetic but objective role with the parent or caretaker.

While recognition of abuse in the ED is crucial, the public health challenge is prevention. Prevention of physical abuse is possible in many cases. The use of public health nurses in a home visitation program for poor, single, teenage mothers, for example, resulted in a reduction of physical abuse and neglect as well as fewer ED visits of children in the first 2 years of life.[42]

The prevention of child abuse can occur at three levels.[43] These are primary, which is directed to the population in general; secondary, which is directed to groups at high risk for abuse; and tertiary, which are interventions after the condition is identified.

Child maltreatment warrants a public health response appropriate to the impact of this problem. Carefully collected national epidemiologic data from both fatal and nonfatal cases of maltreatment of children is needed to guide allocation of limited resources. Future efforts would likely be boosted by the wide acceptance of operational case definitions for each form of child maltreatment. Both passive and active surveillance systems could then be put in place to monitor this public health problem and help assess the impact of intervention efforts.

Much work remains to be done to understand and reduce the impact of child abuse and neglect. Emergency department physicians are in a unique position to participate in this work in the coming years. The Division of Violence at the recently established National Center for Injury Prevention and Control at the Centers for Disease Control and Prevention will likely play a major role in coordinating efforts in reducing child maltreatment. A worthwhile aid to clinicians is a recent summary by the American Academy of Pediatrics of national and regional resources for providers caring for children with suspected or potential child abuse and neglect.[44]

EMERGENCY DEPARTMENT/ PROVIDER'S ROLE

As well as delivering medical care for the physical injuries, the role of the ED provider in cases of maltreatment includes identifying and reporting suspected abuse to child protection services. Identification and reporting of abuse in the injured child is a four-step process:[45] (1) *assessing and evaluating* the injury and explanation for it; (2) *identifying* the *possibility* of abuse based on the physician's judgement; (3) *reporting*, which involves contacting the appropriate agency and providing necessary information; and (4) *validating* maltreatment, which involves definitive diagnosis following a report of suspected abuse. The ED physician may be required to testify in either civil court, where most child abuse cases are heard, or in criminal court. Guidelines to assist physicians preparing to testify in child abuse cases in order to improve the accuracy and credibility of expert testimony have recently been published.[46]

Since injured children who have been abused are likely to be seen in an emergency department, the ED physician has the opportunity to be the child's advocate. It is important in this regard to work in collaboration with professionals in mental health, social work, and law enforcement.[43]

Based on a careful and sensitive evaluation, the ED physician who suspects the presence of abuse must deal with both follow-up for the physical injury and referral for the psychological and social sequelae of abuse. The physician must consider how best to treat the child in the moment, as well as how to protect the child and the family from further occurrences. In the case of suspected abuse, the physician is not only responsible for hot-line contact but also for guidance to the family. This might be in the form of referral to the ED social worker, the hospital's Child Protection Team, or a specific Adolescent or Child Guidance Center. The ED physician should be familiar with human care services available within the hospital setting and the community.

The role of whistle-blower is often a difficult one for the ED physician. There may be concerns about lost time, uncertainty about sufficient expertise in making the assessment, and underlying fear of angering an already anxious or potentially explosive parent. The ED physician who recognizes the potential for danger to the child and who recognizes that the ED physician may possibly be the only advocate for the child at that moment may more easily make the decision to report or to hospitalize, pending further evaluation.[1]

The ED physician is in an excellent position to identify children at risk and make an appropriate referral, with a goal of tertiary prevention (preventing recurrence of abuse or negative outcomes associated with abuse). The ED physician can also become involved with child death review panels in the community to investigate suspicious deaths of children. A model created in Missouri in 1991 has provided for multidisciplinary child death review panels in every county of the state as well as urban models for major urban areas.[47] The findings of the panels provide important information to determine trends, target prevention strategies, identify family and community needs, and support criminal prosecution, if indicated.

Because children injured as a result of maltreatment are likely to present to the ED, physicians in this setting are confronted with and must learn to recognize and evaluate these young victims. The ED physician has the role of the child's advocate and coordinates a multidisciplinary team of professionals in the case of abused children. While important insights in this area have been gained in the last few decades, much remains to be learned regarding the epidemiology of child maltreatment and the development of effective intervention strategies to reduce this public health problem.

CONCLUSION

A discrepant history is an important feature of physical abuse in childhood injuries. The psychosocial history of family and child gives direction to management decisions with the injured child. Physical abuse has emotional, cognitive, and behavioral sequelae. Homicide is the leading cause of injury death among infants in the United States, and rates of nonfatal injuries from child maltreatment increase with age. Advocacy for the child with intentional injuries in the ED includes identifying and reporting to protect the child and prevent further maltreatment.

NOTES

1. Sirontak AP, Krugman RD. Physical abuse of children: An update. *Pediatr Rev* 1994; 15:394–9.
2. Helfer RE, Slovis TL, Black M. Injuries resulting when small children fall out of bed. *Pediatr* 1977; 60:533–5.
3. Nimityongskul P, Anderson LD. The likelihood of injuries when children fall out of bed. *J Pediatr Orthoped* 1987; 7:184–6.
4. Williams RA. Injuries in infants and small children resulting from witnessed and corroborated free falls. *J Trauma* 1991; 31:1350–2.
5. Chadwick DL, Chin S, Salerno C, Landsverk J, Kitchen L. Deaths from falls in children: How far is fatal? *J Trauma* 1991; 31:1353–5.
6. Merten DF, Carpenter BLM. Radiologic imaging of inflicted injury in the child abuse syndrome. *Pediatr Clin North Am* 1990; 37:815–37.
7. Kleinman PK. Diagnostic imaging in infant abuse. *Am J Radiol* 1990; 155:703–12.
8. Thomas SA, Rosenfield NS, Leventhal JM, Markowitz RI. Long-bone fractures in young children: Distinguishing accidental injuries from child abuse. *Pediatr* 1991; 88:471–6.

9. Duhaime AC, Alario AJ, Lewander WJ, et al. Head injury in very young children: Mechanisms, injury types and ophthalmologic findings in 100 hospitalized patients younger than 2 years of age. *Pediatr* 1992; 90:179–85.

10. Krugman RD. Child abuse and neglect: The role of the primary care physician in recognition, treatment, and prevention. *Prim Care* 1984; 11:527–34.

11. Ney PG, Fung T, Wickett AR. The worst combinations of child abuse and neglect. *Child Abuse Neglect* 1994; 18:705–14.

12. Willging JP, Bower CM, Cotton RT. Physical abuse of children: A retrospective review and an otolaryngology perspective. *Arch Otolaryngol Head Neck Surg* 1992; 118:584–90.

13. Feldman KW, Schaller RT, Feldman JA, McMillon M. Tap water scald burns in children. *Pediatr* 1978; 62:1–7.

14. Ellerstein NS. The cutaneous manifestations of child abuse and neglect. *Am J Dis Child* 1979; 133:906–09.

15. Slosberg EJ, Ludwig S, Duckett J, Mauro AE. Penile trauma as a sign of child abuse. *Am J Dis Child* 1978; 132:719–20.

16. Cooper A, Floyd T, Barlow B, et al. Major blunt abdominal trauma due to child abuse. *J Trauma* 1988; 28:1483–7.

17. Coant PN, Kornberg AE, Brody AS, Edwards-Holmes K. Markers for occult liver injury in cases of physical abuse in children. *Pediatr* 1992; 89:274–78.

18. Caffey J. Multiple fractures in long bones of children suffering from chronic subdural hematoma. *AJR* 1946; 56:163–73.

19. Kempe CH, Silverman FN, Steele BF, et al. The battered child syndrome. *JAMA* 1962; 181:17–24.

20. McClain PW, Sacks JJ, Froehlke RG, Ewigman BG. Estimates of fatal child abuse and neglect, United States, 1979 through 1988. *Pediatr* 1993; 91:338–43.

21. McClain PW, Sacks JJ, Ewigman BG, Smith SM, Mercy JA, Sniezek JE. Geographic patterns of fatal abuse or neglect in children younger than 5 years old, United States, 1979–1988. *Arch Pediatr Adolesc Med* 1994; 148:82–86.

22. Waller AE, Baker SP, Szocka A. Childhood injury deaths: National analysis and geographic variations. *Am J Publ Health* 1989; 79:310–15.

23. Division of Injury Control, Center for Environmental Health and Injury Control, CDC. Childhood injuries in the United States. *Am J Dis Child* 1990; 144:627–46.

24. National Center on Child Abuse and Neglect. *Study Findings: Study of National Incidence and Prevalence of Child Abuse and Neglect.* Washington, DC: U.S. Department of Health and Human Services, 1988.

25. McCurdy K, Daro D. *Current Trends in Child Abuse Reporting and Fatalities: The Results of the 1993 Annual Fifty-State Survey.* Chicago: National Center on Child Abuse Prevention Research, National Committee to Prevent Child Abuse, 1994.

26. Goldson E. The affective and cognitive sequelae of child maltreatment. *Pediatr Clin North Am* 1991; 38:1481–96.

27. McCord J. A 40-year perspective on effects of child abuse and neglect. *Child Abuse Neglect* 1983; 7:265–70.

28. Lahey BB, Conger RD, Atkeson BM, Treiber FA. Parenting behavior and emotional status of physically abusive mothers. *J Consult Clin Psychol* 1984; 52:1062–71.

29. Christoffel KK. Intentional injuries: homicide and violence. In Pless IB (ed.). *The Epidemiology of Childhood Disorders.* New York: Oxford University Press, 1994:392–411.

30. Green A. Child abusing fathers. *J Amer Acad Child Psych* 1978; 18:270–82.

31. Elmer E. A follow-up study of traumatized children. *Pediatr* 1977; 59:273–9.

32. Berger AM. Characteristics of child abusing families. In L'Abate L (ed.). *Handbook of Family Psychology and Therapy,* vol 2. Homewood, IL: Dorsey Press, 1985, pp. 900–36.

33. McKay MM. The link between domestic violence and child abuse: Assessment and treatment considerations. *Child Welfare* 1994; 73:29–39.

34. McKibben L, DeVoe E, Newberger EH. Victimization of mothers of abused children. *Pediatr* 1989; 84:531–5.

35. Stark E, Flitcraft A. Women and children at risk: A feminist perspective on child abuse. *Int J of Health Serv* 1988; 18:97–118.

36. Kempe CH, Helfer RE. *Helping the Battered Child and His Family.* Philadelphia: Lippincott, 1972.

37. Strauss MA. Stress and physical child abuse. *Child Abuse Neglect* 1980; 4:75–88.

38. Freidrich WN, Boriskin JA. The role of the child in abuse: A review of the literature. *Am J OrthoPsychiatry* 1976; 46:580–90.

39. Bijur P, Golding J, Haslum M, Kurzon M. Behavioral predictors of injury in school-age children. *Am J Dis Child* 1988; 142:1307–12.

40. Langley J, McGee R, Silva P, Williams S. Child behavior and accidents. *J Pediatr Psychol* 1983; 8:181–9.

41. American Psychiatric Association. *Diagnostic and Statistical Manual of Mental Disorders,* 4th ed. Washington, DC: American Psychiatric Association, 1994.

42. Olds DL, Henderson CR, Chamberlin R, Tatelbaum R. Preventing child abuse and neglect: A randomized trial of nurse home visitation. *Pediatr* 1986; 78:65–78.

43. Dubowitz N. Pediatrician's role in preventing child maltreatment. *Pediatr Clin North Am* 1990; 37: 989–1002.

44. Section on Child Abuse and Neglect. *A guide to references and resources in child abuse and neglect.* Elk Grove Village, IL: American Academy of Pediatrics, 1994.

45. Warner JE, Hansen DJ. The identification and reporting of physical abuse by physicians: A review and implications for research. *Child Abuse Neglect* 1994; 18:11–25.

46. Chadwick DL. Preparation for court testimony in child abuse cases. *Pediatr Clin North Am* 1990; 37:955–70.

47. Schulze C. *Missouri Child Fatality Review Program Annual Report 1993,* July 1994.

9

African American Youth and Violence

DON WESLEY MOUNDS
PETER H. MOYER

CONTENTS

- Scope of the problem
- Causes
- Strategies
- The role of emergency practitioners

CHAPTER SUMMARY

We are a violent society. Our homicide rate is the highest by far of any industrialized nation. Particularly hard-hit are young African American males. While most interpersonal violence is still between friends and acquaintances, growing numbers of injuries and deaths are gang-related.

This chapter highlights the gunshot death of a 9-year-old boy, the innocent victim of what was probably a gang-related, drive-by shooting. The boy was African American. His family was poor, headed by a single mother, had lost other relatives and friends to violent death, and lived in a housing project known for its gang activity. These circumstances are all too familiar to ED practitioners.

The survivors are struggling. Community programs are trying to help them with their grief and their efforts to make sense out of a loss of this magnitude and, at the same time, prevent other members of this family from experiencing similar disasters.

The causes of violence in our society are discussed. TV violence, the market for illegal drugs, and the ready availability and increasing lethality of guns in our society are obvious culprits and are taking a front-and-center position in political debates. The American public does not yet grasp the linkage between inner-city violence and its root causes, poverty and racism. There is much work to be done to promote this understanding and develop a public will to redress the fundamental social inequalities that give rise to misdirected rage and aggression.

Finally, a response is proposed. Community violence prevention programs are presented, and a role for ED practitioners is described. Suggestions are made for advocacy activities to curtail TV violence and control the sale of handguns. Most important, and most difficult, is a call to improve inner-city economies and combat racial inequities.

INTRODUCTION

According to the World Health Organization, the U.S. ranks third among nations in its rate of intentional homicide (12.7/100,000 men and 3.9/100,000 women in 1985). Among men aged 15 to 24, the rate is even higher (18.5), and, in absolute numbers, the U.S. has the distinction of being at the top of the list.[1] As former Surgeon-General Everett Koop described, this is *the* public health challenge for our century, as smallpox, tuberculosis, and syphilis were for our predecessors. Sims et al., reporting a patient series from Detroit in the *Journal of Trauma*, call urban trauma a chronic disease with a recurrence rate of 44% and a 5-year mortality rate of 20%.[2]

We are a violent society, far more violent than any other industrialized nation. In 1991, 26,513 people died from homicide in the U.S.[3] And, we are becoming *more* violent. The number of incidents of violence in our society jumped from 161/100,000 people in 1960 to 758/100,000 people in 1992, an increase of 371%.[4] During this period, our homicide rate also doubled.

Homicide is the leading cause of death among young black men (85.6/100,000). Half of all victims of homicide are African Americans (who make up 12% of the population). Young black men die of homicide seven times more frequently than do whites. According to the Centers for Disease Control, a black male born in 1989 has a 1 in 27 chance of dying of homicide.[5] Most homicides occur among the poor, half of whom are black. The following case illustrates some of the harsh realities that families face and the consequences that arrive all too regularly at the emergency department door.

Case #1

MG, a 9-year-old, fun-loving, high-spirited young black child, was out trick-or-treating with his brothers (Christopher, age 13, and Jerome, age 11) on Halloween, 1994. They were two doors away from his grandmother's home in Boston's Academy Homes Housing Development when an automobile turned into Weaver Terrace, a short, dead-end street, and made a U-turn. On the car's way out, someone from within fired a hand gun several times into a group of trick-or-treaters. As the shots rang out, everyone ran and ducked, for the children were all too familiar with the sound of gunfire.

When it was over, when everyone came out of hiding, there lay MG, shot and dying. The children ran screaming, "He's been shot, get his mom." The mother, Ms. H., couldn't go to her son, couldn't bear to see him lying there helpless and dying. Within minutes, Boston EMS arrived. The patient was transported to Boston City Hospital, where he died of a gunshot wound to the left chest. Autopsy revealed a fractured spleen, holes in the stomach and diaphragm, pulmonary contusions, and a left hemothorax.

This is not the first tragedy that this very strong black family has suffered. In 1980, Ms. Haskins lost a 2-month-old son. In 1993, in Atlanta, her 14-year-old nephew was accidentally shot dead by his best friend. In April and July 1994, her oldest son, Christopher, was treated at Boston City Hospital for stab wounds in the leg and back. In July 1994, her children's father had died accidentally, falling four floors from a porch while walking in his sleep.

Q: How representative is MG's death?

A 9-year-old African American boy living in a housing project known for its heavy gang activity is at risk. The average age of homicide victims is dropping. In Massachusetts, for example, the percent of homicide victims who were teenagers or younger averaged 15% from 1977 through 1982; from 1991 through 1993, it averaged 23%.[6]

Mercifully, the murder of a 9-year-old (MG's age) is still uncommon. The June 1993 weapons injury report of the Massachusetts Department of Public Health reported that only 2% of Boston's 1992 gunshot and stab wound victims were less than 14 years old. The largest group (20%) was between 15 and 19 years old.

The report also notes, however, that younger individuals tend to use handguns instead of knives, resulting in a higher level of fatality. For black youth, 54% of injuries were by guns. For Hispanic youth, 27% of penetrating injuries were caused by guns.[6] These trends hold for both small and large cities throughout the U.S.

The Academy Homes Housing Development is known for its heavy gang activity. There are African American, Puerto Rican, and Dominican gangs (Heath Street, Academy 1&2, Goya Boys, Latin Kings, and Humbolt). There is an ongoing feud between the Heath Street and Academy gangs. Whether MG's homicide was gang-related is unknown, although the drive-by nature of the incident is suggestive. Forty to fifty percent of all homicides are still between individuals who know each other (family, friends, and acquaintances), but gang-related homicides make up a growing percentage of homicides, particularly among youth.[7]

Case Continuation

That tragic evening was not the end of the involvement of the medical staff in this case. The Violence Prevention Counselor was contacted when Mrs. H. brought MG's brother, CG to Boston City Hospital for a rash and asked for assistance. This was the same counselor who had been consulted when CG was stabbed in April 1994.

The two became reacquainted, and the counselor was able to offer friendship and support to Ms. H., who he saw as a brave and strong mother. He reported back to the ED staff to tell them how she was doing and described some of the problems she faced.

MG's mother and grandmother are both single parents. Female-headed households are now the rule for the majority of inner-city children. Many single-parent households are actually subunits of strongly bonded extended families that include connections with both blood relations and involved nonrelatives, and children in those families receive love, nurturing, and a protective environment.

But the difficulty of the struggle to do so cannot be denied. In the inner city, many children are deprived of a positive male role model. Even more importantly, the biggest consequence of growing up in a single-parent family is the likelihood of growing up in poverty, without economic resources, adequate housing and health care, and a chance for a good education or access to opportunity. Female-headed households, in 1991, earned less than half the average for all families ($16,692 compared to $35,939) and less than one-third of the earnings of families with two wage earners.[8]

Case Continuation

On December 1, the Violence Prevention Counselor at Boston City Hospital called Ms. H. to confirm the next counseling session. She wasn't home, so he spoke with the grandmother. She seemed upset and said that she had just found out that her two remaining grandsons, CG and JG, had been suspended from visiting her. She had been visited by police, who informed her that these grandsons, (MG's two older brothers), had been involved in several fights with a neighbor's children. She said that the police, trying to avoid the suspension because they were aware that the younger brother had been murdered, had warned them several times. The grandmother really felt terrible because she knew that this was an important time for her to be with her grandsons. When the boys have to appear in court, the counselor plans to act as advocate to help the boys gain the right to visit their grandmother on weekends.

As part of his role, the counselor also met with the mother, Ms. H., at the LAMP (Life After Murder Program), at Roxbury Community Health Center and ob-served while Ms. H. explained to the LAMP director how she and her family were doing. The mother said that her two sons were enrolled in counseling, both privately and through school. Counseling was individual, because the mother didn't feel the oldest son, CG, would show any emotions around the younger brother. She realized the importance of counseling for the whole family, and hopes to enroll herself with LAMP as well.

On December 4, 1994, the family dedicated a Christmas tree lighting ceremony to the memory of MG. It was held at his grandmother's home near the site where he was murdered. The ceremony, which was televised by several local channels, ended with prayers by a neighborhood minister from People of Color Against Homicide. The ED counselor stays in touch with this family and hopes to connect them with mentors for the remaining boys.

Q: What potential effects might MG's death have on his mother and brothers?

Rosenberg and Mercy write that "Homicide can have a crippling effect on surviving family members that affects several generations . . . (and) have a devastating impact . . . in terms of fear, anxiety and subsequent restrictions in activities and movements."[7] They also report that children who are victims of violence have delayed emotional, physical, and social development, and many experience posttraumatic stress syndrome, especially if they have to testify in court.

Q: What are the causes of interpersonal violence among youth?

Kellermann and Holliger, in Chapter 25, characterize gunshot injuries as complex interactions between victim, assailant, weapon, and the immediate environment, not just the result of being in the wrong place at the wrong time, and not an accident at all. We live, after all, in a culture of violence, where violence is entertainment, and guns are readily available. By the age of 18, the average U.S. child has seen 200,000 acts of violence on TV, including 40,000 murders.[9] Numerous studies have shown a statistically significant correlation between viewing TV violence and the viewers' aggressiveness and tendency to murder. Viewers of TV violence become desensitized to violence, especially since the pain and aftermath for the individual, family, and society are rarely depicted on TV. The effects are particularly strong on preschool children, for whom fact and fantasy are blurred. An acceptance of violence and its ubiquitous presence in both the background and foreground of our lives certainly contributes to the grim statistic that today more teenagers die from gunshot wounds than from all natural diseases combined.[10]

The 187% increase in homicide by firearms among 15-to-19 year-old men from 1985 to 1991 (source: National Center for Health Statistics) is paralleled by an increasing availability of guns. Firearms are common in the U.S., and half of our households have them. In 1990, 4,371,000 guns were produced for the U.S. market.[11] Minimal federal restrictions on firearm sales have facilitated the proliferation of guns, gun owners, and gun dealers. In one U.S. city, 1 out of every 15 eleventh-grade boys has carried a handgun to school at some point. Over one-half of these eleventh-graders said they could obtain handguns easily.[12] Guns—80% of the time, handguns—are responsible for 80% of all teenager homicides and 68% of homicides for all ages in the U.S.[13] The firearm homicide rate for 15-to-19-year-olds increased 61% from 1979 to 1989.[14] Nationally, handgun homicide has been the leading cause of death for young black men since 1969.[15] If current trends continue, the number of firearm-related deaths will surpass that of motor-vehicle-related deaths by 2003.[3]

But guns alone do not kill. In her book *Deadly Consequences*, Deborah Prosthrow-Stith points out that all men in Switzerland are, for reasons of military preparedness, required to bear arms. Yet few Swiss use their guns to kill one another. Guns need to be controlled; they do increase the lethality of an argument many-fold. But gun control alone is no magic solution to the problem of teen violence. The fundamental social problems which lead to interpersonal violence must be recognized and addressed by whatever means necessary. "Such an approach," says the sociologist David Gil, "is consistent with the public health concept of *primary* prevention of diseases and destructive conditions, which involves identification and eradication of sources rather than mere neutralization of symptoms." Gil proposes a useful typology of violence, in which he distinguishes between what he calls *initiating structural violence* and *reactive counterviolence.*[16]

We live in a structurally violent society, one in which there is domination of some individuals and social groups by others that results in social and economic exploitation and an inability for large numbers of people to meet their needs for material sustenance, creativity, security, self-actualization and meaning in life—the basic drives described by Maslow and Fromm, among others, as motivators for human behavior. Blockage of these needs, according to Gil, is the initiating structural violence. Reactive counter violence, often enacted by oppressed peoples against each other, is an outbreak of violent feelings, attitudes, and actions of rage against these barriers. It is the expression of blocked developmental energy, transformed destructively and aimed at substitute targets. This typology helps explain why the sector of society that suffers the most interpersonal violence—black youth—is that which suffers the most from the two fundamental problems of poverty and racism.

Federal guidelines classify a family of three with an income of less than $745 per month ($9,000 per year) as poor. Using this measure, the Children's Defense Fund estimated that in 1989, one-half of African American children were poor. Black families typically earn just more than one-half that of their white counterparts. Black individuals suffer twice the unemployment as whites; black youth have an unemployment rate twice that of the rest of the black population. Black poverty has become more concentrated in inner cities. Between 1970 and 1980, the combined populations of New York, Chicago, Los Angeles, Philadelphia, and Detroit declined by 9%. Over the same period, the number of poor people living in these cities—disproportionately black—increased by 22%.[5]

Racism has been experienced by people of color in the U.S. since the early 1600s, when slaves were first brought to the colonies and the first Native American territories were seized. The genocide of the slave trade was one of the most violent acts in our history. Violence continued in the form of the omnipresent whip and sundering of families during plantation slavery. Post–Civil War lynchings were a mass celebration of violence; up to 15,000 white people would travel miles to see a lynching. Brown estimates that 3,437 lynchings of black people occurred between 1882 and 1951.[17]

In *Frantz Fanon and the Psychology of Oppression,* Bulham describes Manichean psychology, the ideological underpinnings used to justify racism. "A Manichean view is one that divides the world into components, and people into different species. This division is based not on reciprocal affirmation, but rather on irreconcilable opposites cast into good vs. evil, beautiful vs. ugly, intelligent vs. stupid, white vs. black, human vs. subhuman modes. . . . The oppressed is full of self-doubt; he is made to feel inferior; his self-worth is undermined; his confidence and bond with others are weakened. His history is obliterated; he cannot control what happens to him."[18] The black person is called stupid, ignorant, weak, crazy, lazy and good for nothing. *He often believes it.* Lack of ownership of housing and community enterprises and lack of educational opportunities lead to despair. Generations of hard work produce only a subsistence existence. Black youth respond with hopelessness, depression, loss of pride, loss of dignity, and anger. They believe society has nothing to offer them and they have nothing to offer it. They are angry at adults—all adults, including their parents. Parents working at low-paying jobs are seen as sell outs with no sense of self-respect. Youth vow not to follow their footsteps. "Why should I work hard? It won't get me anywhere." They ask how can adults demand respect when it's mainly adults who buy drugs from them.

The victim of oppression, Bulham says, has no other escape, and so he internalizes his oppression and turns on his own people. DuRant et al., writing in the *American Journal of Public Health,* surveyed inner-city youth and found a statistically significant correlation between violent behavior, lack of purpose, and expectation not to be alive at 25.[19] While blacks are 12% of the population, they comprise half of those arrested for murder and half the homicide victims.

Closely linked to poverty and racism are the changes in structure of the inner-city family. In 1965, 25% of black children grew up in female-headed households. By 1990, the figure had approached 60 to 75% for many inner-city black children.[20] How did this happen?

During the 1970s and 1980s, many inner-city middle-class blacks left their neighborhoods, and many more of the remaining working-class black men lost their jobs when high-wage manufacturing industries moved abroad, and government, a major source of jobs for the black community, downsized. "Entire neighborhoods were depopulated of laboring men—blue collar and white collar—who earned enough to support their families. Black men, demeaned by the economic conditions that made them economically superfluous, withdrew from the family scene."[20] The result was more and more inner-city families headed by a remaining mother and men left standing on the street corner with "nothing to do and nowhere to go."

As manufacturing jobs have left the cities a new industry has moved in to take their place—drug trafficking. The illegal drug trade is now the number-one industry in our inner cities. In this climate of female-headed, poor inner-city families, gangs are making a comeback. More and more youth—black, Hispanic, white, and Asian—are caught up in well-organized gangs; organized, at times across multiple states, around turf protection and drug sales.

In the last decade, we have seen health professionals broaden their definitions of illness and begin to pay attention to violence and other public health issues. This has represented a major advance. But the medical model with which the consequences of violence have been evaluated has shone only a narrow light on the results and not paid enough attention to the causes. It is people, not guns, that kill people, and the death of so many young black men is a social phenomenon, related to the structure of our institutions, not a problem of individuals or family values.

Q: What strategies might be utilized to reduce the rate of firearm homicides among youth?

Our response must be multifaceted. Rosenberg and Mercy suggest that we develop policies and programs to (1) decrease cultural acceptance of violence; (2) reduce racial discrimination and its effects; (3) teach conflict resolution; (4) support families with services; (5) increase recognition in the medical setting of risk for violence; (6) educate professionals to understand that consequences extend beyond the purely medical; (7) create links between medical settings and community violence prevention programs; (8) improve management and treatment for victims of violence and their families; (9) identify and train high-risk adolescents and make jobs available to them; (10) focus on prevention.[7] In the broadest of senses we must build the inner-city economy, and oppose racism.

Many believe in the need to develop an Afrocentric approach to understanding and combating violence in African American communities, and "emphasize the need for enhancement of Afrocentric values and culture, in order to combat the American system that leads to powerlessness, self-hatred and lowered self-esteem for so many African American youngsters, especially males."[21] William Oliver, a professor of Criminal Justice at the University of Delaware, suggests that "institutional racism—that is, the systematic deprivation of equal access to opportunity—has prevented a substantial number of African American males from achieving manhood through legitimate means. African American males who adhere to the compulsive masculinity alternative define manhood in terms of overt toughness, sexual conquest, manipulation and thrill seeking."[22]

Oliver believes institutionalized racism is responsible for the high rate of African American interpersonal violence. To counter, he suggests that black people redefine themselves as African American with Afrocentric (not Eurocentric) worldview. This worldview emphasizes love of self, respect of the African heritage, and commitment to African American unity and progress, in place of the self-perpetuating pathology of academic failure, adolescent pregnancy, substance abuse and black-on-black crime. African American churches, organizations, and professionals must recommit themselves to the survival and progress of African Americans. African Americans must develop their own business and access to the media[22] and promote black education—especially as we move into a global economy where only the educated will qualify for the better paying U.S. jobs. We must defend affirmative action in school and at work. We must fight to maintain and improve day care and proven programs such as Head Start. We must have drug detoxification on demand and a willingness to look at new solutions such as drug legalization.

What about incarceration—prisons, boot camps, and mandatory sentencings (three strikes and you're out)? It does keep criminals off the street (at least for a while); it doesn't prevent crime. Over the last decade, the number of federal and state inmates has doubled; local jail populations have tripled. During the same 10 years violent crimes have doubled.[20]

The U.S. has the dubious distinction of being the world's number-one jailer. There are more African American men in jail than in college. The average annual cost of incarceration is $23,500. California now spends more on prisons than it does on schools. Recidivism is high—averaging 35% nationally per year. Clearly, we cannot look to jails as the only or main solution to adolescent homicide in particular, or crime in general.

All parents are encouraged to limit their children's total TV hours (school-age children now average 4 hours a day), know what their children are watching (watch TV with their children), lobby the TV industry to reduce violence and push for new TVs to have the technical capacity to "lock out" channels that parents do not want their children to see.

Throughout the United States, community organizations are developing violence-prevention programs. Schools are developing ways to reduce the number of weapons brought onto campus. Changes in the environment such as better lighting of playgrounds, speed bumps, ID badges, and dress codes are being implemented. Youth can be taught about situations "that are likely to result in violence . . . such as associating with violent peers, using alcohol or drugs, and possessing a firearm or other weapons."[23] They can be helped to develop the self-esteem needed to solve differences without violence. They can be taught conflict resolution using nonviolent techniques. Such teaching began in the Boston Violence Prevention Project and has spread to 45 states. Teachers and students are taught that conflicts often arise from prejudices, competition, miscommunications, inability to constructively express feelings, and a lack of respect for oneself and others. Youth can be provided with mentors who can serve as role models. Young parents can be provided with training and support. One example of a parenting program is Project STEEP (Steps Toward Effective Enjoyable Parenting) in Minneapolis, Minnesota.[24] The program serves low-income, first-time, mostly single parents. It begins in the first trimester of pregnancy and continues until the baby is at least 1 year old. The program focuses on child care skills, infant development, and infant—mother communication. Support and recreation are provided in many communities by the church, Boys and Girls Clubs, and the YMCA and YWCA.

Q: What role can emergency department practitioners play?

At the emergency department level, the Massachusetts Department of Health runs a weapon-related Injury Surveillance System. All 90 of Massachusetts' emergency departments participate. For every gunshot and stab wound, the emergency physician or surgeon completes a form detailing the circumstances of the incident. Data is fed back to the Department of Health, which periodically issues a newsletter summarizing statewide trends.

Physicians can learn brief intervention techniques that facilitate productive discussion with youth at risk (see Figure 9-1). They can also help to set up programs to deal directly with interpersonal violence. Project Direction is a violence-prevention program for youth ages 14 to 21 seen in the Boston City Hospital Emergency Department for gunshot wounds, stab wounds, and other assaults. The project's counselor is an African American man who lives in BCH's catchment area and is familiar with violence not only through his community, but also from his youth in Hartford, his experience in the Vietnam War, and his work as a BCH security officer. His counseling involves an emergency department talk with the victim (unless the patient is too sick to talk), follow-up counseling with the victim, family, and friends, and referral to community agencies (following the African proverb, "it takes a village to raise a child"). Some of the guidelines used in approaching adolescent victims of interpersonal violence are outlined in Table 9-1.

Agencies that may cooperate or provide services to clients of a violence prevention project include hospitals and medical schools, community youth outreach projects, community health centers, public health department programs, school-based programs, and private organizations such as church groups and Vietnam Veterans Against Violence. The take away message is that resources *can* be mobilized, and young people's lives *can* be turned around.

Table 9-1 Project Direction Youth Violence Prevention Program: Guidelines

1. Be patient. The first meeting should be seen as a start, and accomplishments may be minimal. The young person may be afraid to talk (may think you're a policeman), and may be angry or in pain, or may not trust adults and may give bogus telephone numbers and addresses.
2. Give the victim a sense of control of the initial and future meetings.
3. Be nonjudgmental, open-minded, and a good listener; don't preach or parent; explain to the patient what you understand about the situation and how this violent act may have happened.
4. Show the patients that you care, during the time in the emergency department, and afterwards, when they leave the hospital and are back in their "hood running with the boys." One way to demonstrate that you care is to relate something that you have in common with them, a parallel between your life and theirs.
5. Realize that advising nonviolence may seem unreal when the only model the patient knows for protection and conflict resolution may be violence.
6. Involve siblings, parents, and friends. People live in social networks and make judgments and decisions within that context.
7. Explain that you think you can help, then introduce strategies for safety and prevention from further violence.
8. Develop relationships with community agencies and refer patients to them.

YOUTH VIOLENCE—A DISEASE WITH A CURE?

If we apply the medical model to the problems of intentional injury among young people, as Sims does in labeling urban trauma a chronic disease,[1] then our instructions are clear: recognize the symptoms, treat them, and act to eliminate the disease.

Diagnosis: The symptoms stare us in the face

Homicide is the leading cause of death among young black men. Most homicides occur among the poor, half of whom are black. We live in a structurally violent society in which there is domination by some individuals and social groups over others, resulting in social and economic exploitation and the failure of large numbers of people to meet their basic needs for material sustenance, creativity, security, self-actualization and meaning in life. The resulting "cycle of poverty" flows from the cradle to the grave and beyond: low birth weight, inferior education, unemployment, poor housing, inadequate nutrition, disease and premature death by violence, leaving behind another generation born to these same circumstances. According to federal guidelines, a family of three with an income less than $9,000 per year is poor; in 1989, half of all African American children met these criteria.

Instead of rebellion outward, rebellion is directed inward, and anger is channeled into destruction of self and neighborhood, with many young black men taking what they can get by any means necessary. The "attitude" goes like this:

- . . . . .it's called *respect.* Since I can't be recognized by the wider society, I refuse to be ignored by my own.
- . . . . .it's called *love.* If I can't get it from my parents or the rest of society, I'll get it from my peers.
- . . . . .it's called *leaving my mark.* If I can't be a doctor or a lawyer or a scientist or whatever I wanted to be, then I'll be whatever is left. And I'll be the best at that. They'll know I was here by the babies I leave behind. They'll know I was here by the death and destruction I leave behind. I'd rather go out in a blaze of glory than a puff of smoke.

All of mankind shares the desire for respect, love, and achievement. When these desires are thwarted by the conditions of life in the inner city, man adapts and survives as best he can, and develops an "attitude" in reaction to loss and deprivation. That attitude puts the individual at further risk, and there is now an extensive literature describing the young black man as an endangered species.[25]

Treatment: The tasks are clear

Despite the complexity of the issues, there has been considerable progress and there is potential for much

more. There are many types of community programs available to youth (YMCA, Boys Clubs, young fathers' groups, 100 Black Men, Violence Prevention Projects, etc.) And they do good work. Adult black men who have "made it" are returning to their communities to invest time and expertise and become role models, mentors, and educators—the source of dreams, aspirations, and empowerment. Community programs can provide real education—the process in which a person learns to actively manifest who he is and wants to be, not what someone else wants him to be, and learns the qualities that are necessary for his survival.

The cure: Eradicating the root causes of violence—racial, economic and political inequality

William Oliver suggests that institutional racism—systematic deprivation of equal access to opportunity—has prevented substantial numbers of African American males from achieving manhood through legitimate means.[22] Mincy, from a social science perspective, concurs: "To decrease the substantial developmental risks many young Black men face due to high rates of poverty, non-marriage and dysfunction among their parents and neighbors, these risk markers must be substantially reduced."[25] If we wish, as a nation, to end the problem of youth violence, we must make a commitment to (1) facilitate economic growth within inner city communities; (2) develop educational programs that validate an Afrocentric world view; and (3) provide access to jobs, housing, and health care.[26]

In addition, there is a need to deal with immediate causes of youth violence—to crack down, for example, on gun manufacturers, dealers, and owners. Manufacturers, dealers, and owners should assume liability from injuries caused by guns they produce, sell, or own. Assault weapons should remain banned, and mandatory waiting periods before purchasing a gun should be enforced. Gun buy-back programs and metal detectors should be encouraged. ED practitioners, who see the consequences of violence firsthand, have real experience to share with the public and can speak out at all

CONVERSATION WITH YOUTH VICTIM OF ASSAULT
An Example that Really Happened: Dialogue with a 16-year-old man with a Head Laceration

MD: How are you feeling?

Patient: Not too good. . . .

MD: How did you get hit?

Patient: This guy had a fight with my brother last week; today he hit me with a baseball bat and I never saw it coming!

MD: Are you thinking about getting even?

Patient: Yes! I don't care if I spend 10 years in jail. At least I'll be satisfied!

MD: You're right to be angry, but I'm concerned about what could happen to you. How would it feel to be away from your family that long? I see a lot of victims of violence—20% of those who survive a stabbing or shooting are dead in 5 years, and 40% more wind up back in a trauma center. An argument among acquaintances with a weapon, alcohol or drugs is a deadly combination. . . .

Patient: I know. I was stabbed 6 years ago, and you can still see my wound and where they put in the chest tube.

MD: How ready are you to prevent this from happening again?

Patient: Well, I sure don't want to ever be back here again. Before I was stabbed, I was in a gang and I carried a gun. Since then I've tried to stay home and avoid things . . . until today. I've been out of trouble for 6 years now.

MD: It isn't easy to avoid these troubles when they're an everyday thing. You didn't see it coming today. But there *are* some things you can do to stay safe. You can avoid situations or walk away from an argument. It sounds like you've been trying to do that. . . . Or you could "chill out"—go visit some relatives in another part of the country. Did you ever see the movie *Sugar Hill* with Wesley Snipes?

Patient: Nods yes.

MD: Remember how he finally got out of the gang, drugs, and violence and went south with his girlfriend to start a family? But it wasn't until he got shot in the back and paralyzed. . . . It isn't easy.

Patient: I saw that movie. It did make me think. Just last month two friends of mine were here at the hospital—one was stabbed and one was shot. I *have* been thinking about getting out of here.

MD: We have a youth violence counselor here at the hospital—would you like his number?

Patient: Thanks, Doc. I'll take the number, and I'll think of visiting South Carolina. I have family there, and I've had enough of this.

---

levels as advocates for their patients and for positive policy change.

CONCLUSION

As Greenberg and Schneider reiterate in *Violence in American Cities: Young Black Males is the Answer, but What is the Question?*,[27] researchers, activists, and ED practitioners have focused on the public health issues of violence as a problem of young black men. Progress in eradicating violence will only be possible when we can all learn to widen the spotlight to include not just victims and perpetrators of violence, but the social and economic forces that marginalize (concentrate, ghettoize, segregate) people into neighborhoods that lack jobs, adequate housing, political power, and a chance at the American Dream.[28] There is tremendous resilience among people forced to live under these conditions. Violence-prevention projects can and will work, if they are supported by investment in our urban communities. We either pay the price of community development now, or pay an escalating price for many lifetimes in the consequences of youth violence.

NOTES

1. World Health Organization. *World Health Statistical Annuals.* Geneva: WHO, 1988.

2. Sims DW, Bivens BA, Obeid FN, Horst HM, Sorensen VJ, Fath JJ. Urban trauma: A chronic recurrent disease. *J Trauma* 1989; 29:940–6.

3. CDC. Deaths resulting from firearm and motor vehicle related injuries—United States 1988–1991. *MMWR* 1994; 43:3.

4. U.S. Department of Justice. *FBI Uniform Crime Report, 1960 & 1992.* Washington D.C.: Bureau of Justice Statistics, 1992.

5. Prothrow-Stith D. *Deadly Consequences.* New York, HarperCollins, 1991.

6. Weapon Injury Report, Massachusetts Department of Health, June 1993.

7. Rosenberg ML, Mercy JA. Assaultive violence. In Rosenberg ML & Fenley MA (eds). *Violence in America: A public health approach.* New York: Oxford University Press, 1991.

8. Bureau of the Census. *Money Income of Households, Families and Persons in the U.S.: 1991* (Tables B6 and B11). Washington D.C.: Bureau of Labor, 1992.

9. *U.S. News & World Report,* August 2, 1993.

10. Fingerhut LA. *Firearm Mortality among Children, Youth and Young Adults 1–34 Years of Age, Trends and Current Status U.S. 1985–1990,* No. 231. Washington DC:NCHS, 1993.

11. Bureau of Alcohol, Tobacco & Firearms, *Compliance Operation Fact Book,* Washington D.C., BATF, Office of Compliance Operations.

12. Callahan EM & Rivara FP. (1992). Urban High School Youth & Handguns. *JAMA* 1992; 267:3038–41.

13. Federal Bureau of Investigation (1993) *Crime in the United States. Uniform Crime Reports, 1992,* Washington, D.C. U.S. Department of Justice, 1993.

14. Fingerhut LA, Ingram DD, and Feldman JJ. Firearm & non-firearm homicide among persons 15 to 19 years of age. *JAMA* 1992; 267:3048–53.

15. Fingerhut LA, Ingram DD, & Feldman JJ. Firearm homicide among black teenage males in metropolitan countries. *JAMA* 1992; 267:3054–8.

16. Gil D. *Preventing Violence while Perpetuating Social Injustice: Mission Impossible.* Boston: Brandeis University, 1995.

17. Brown RM. *Strain of Violence: Historical studies of American Violence and vigilantism.* New York: Oxford University Press, 1975.

18. Bulham HA, *Frantz Fanon & the Psychology of Oppression.* New York: Plenum Press, 1985, p. 156.

19. DuRant RH, Cadenhead BA, Pendergast RA, Slowens G, Linder C. Factors Associated with the Use of Violence among Urban Black Adolescents. *AJPH* 1994; 84:612–7.

20. *Time,* February 7, 1994, pp. 48–59.

21. Issacs MR. *Violence: The Impact of Community Violence on African-American Children and Families.* Arlington, VA: National Center for Education in Maternal and Child Health, 1992, p. 55.

22. Oliver W. *The Violent Social World of Black Men.* Boston: Lexington Books, 1994, p. 57.

23. National Center for Injury Prevention and Control. *The Prevention of Youth Violence: A Framework for Community Action.* Atlanta, GA: Centers for Disease Control and Prevention, 1993, p. 55.

24. Ibid, p. 15.

25. Mincy RB (ed). *Nurturing young Black males.* Washington DC: Urban Institute Press, 1992.

26. Myers LJ. *Understanding an Afrocentric world view: Introduction to an Optimal Psychology.* Dubuque, Iowa: Kendall Hunt, 1992.

27. Greenberg M, Schneider D. Violence in American cities: Young black males is the answer, but what was the question? *Soc Sci Med* 1994; 39:179–87.

28. Hutson HR, Noglin DN, Hart J, Spears K. The epidemic of gang-related homicides in Los Angeles County from 1979 through 1994. *JAMA* 1995; 274:1031–6.

10

Battered Women

BARBARA HERBERT
JUDITH BERNSTEIN

CONTENTS

- Definitions of battering
- Epidemiology
- JCAHO and professional organization mandates
- Detection
- Interviewing skills
- Interventions
- Guidelines and protocols

CHAPTER SUMMARY

Domestic violence is recognized as a public health emergency by the Centers for Disease Control and Prevention,[1] the American Medical Association,[2] the American College of Emergency Physicians,[3] the American Public Health Association,[4] the American College of Obstetrics and Gynecology,[5] and other national and local medical groups. Furthermore, The Joint Commission for Accreditation of Health Care Organizations' 1992 Mandate requires EDs to develop and implement policies and procedures for the identification, evaluation, treatment, and referral of battered women.[6] Great strides in awareness have been made since the 1970s, when wife battering was a misdemeanor in most states, yet the same assault against a stranger was classified as a felony. Battered women's shelters—protected, secure, and often se-

cret environments that offer temporary refuge for women experiencing violence—emerged as a result of the activism of the feminist movement, reacting against the millenia-old conceptualization of women as chattel, property to be abused at will.

In the clinical or medical setting, battering includes the exercise of emotional intimidation, nonconsensual sexual behavior, or physical injury by a competent adult or adolescent, which is utilized to maintain coercive behavior in an intimate relationship with another competent adult or adolescent. Legal definitions commonly include acts that attempt or actually cause physical harm, acts that place the affected individual in fear of physical harm, and acts that, by virtue of force, threat, or duress, compel nonconsensual sexual relationships.[7]

Violence against women is cross-cultural and pervasive. It is estimated that one of every three women seen in emergency departments, one of every four women seen by the obstetrician-gynecologist, and one of every seven women seen in general practice have been victims of domestic violence.[8] Studies conclude that there is regular and repeated violence between spouses in 10 to 20% of marriages,[9] and 95% of the instances consist of women being abused by their husbands or ex-husbands.[10] Each year, 4 million women in the U.S. are battered, 2 million are severely injured, and two to four thousand of these women die.[9] Battering is the single major cause of injury to women—more than rapes, muggings, and automobile accidents combined.[1] One-fifth to one-third of all women who visit an emergency department because of injury may have experienced abuse at some time in their lives.[4,11,12]

Case #1

An unknown white female, approximately 30 years of age, dressed in an attractive business suit, is brought to the ED in full cardiac arrest. She has a #8 endotracheal tube placed in her trachea, and a 16-gauge intravenous needle is rapidly infusing normal saline. She has received epinephrine 1 mg, followed by a 1 mg bolus of atropine. The cardiac monitor demonstrates a bradycardial junctional rhythm at 30 beats per minute.

The woman's husband arrives and shares the following information: she is 27 years old, employed as an attorney, and has a distant history of childhood cardiac disease treated in another state by an unknown physician. He reports that she is generally in good health and has been feeling fine throughout dinner at a local restaurant, where he had received an award for civic service. He is a corporate leader in town, and is an advisory board member for the hospital development fund. Shortly after they returned home, he reports, his wife had suddenly complained of severe headache, then chest pain, and had fallen, unresponsive, to the floor. He then called the paramedics. He is calm but concerned, and reports that there are no other relatives living nearby.

The patient is transferred from the stretcher, and additional venous access is obtained in the contralateral arm; the saline infusion is increased, and epinephrine and atropine are repeated. She stabilizes into a sinus rhythm with a rate of 137 beats per minute. There is a thready carotid pulse. A brachial blood pressure of 60/palpation is recorded by doppler, but within 5 minutes it has fallen below measurable threshold.

Q: Should the emergency physician maintain an index of suspicion for every patient? What about families like these—steadily employed people of good reputation who have no obvious indicators for substance abuse or violence?

Studies have identified multiple barriers to the detection of battering, including the physician's sense of powerlessness, close identification with the patient, fear of offending a patient, lack of knowledge and training, privacy beliefs, and time constraints.[13–15] For these reasons, JCAHO and the major professional organizations suggest routine assessment of all fe-

male victims.[6] Battering affects all women, as evidenced by a study of lesbian women that reported a 17% lifetime prevalence.[16]

Case Continuation

Within 5 minutes of initial stabilization, the brachial blood pressure has fallen below the measurable threshold. Dopamine, in a 3µ/kg/min infusion is begun and a BP of 80/palpation is obtained. Breath sounds are heard bilaterally in the anterior chest and are somewhat diminished.

The patient's course continues to be tenuous. She now requires 10µ/kg/min of dopamine to maintain a palpable BP. Ventilator settings are RR of 12, tidal volume of 800cc and 100% oxygen saturation; positive pressure (PEEP) is added for adequate ventilation. As a nurse attempts to palpate the right carotid artery for pulse, she notes a faint ecchymosis extending posterolaterally toward the cervical spine; the trachea appears to be deviated slightly left of midline. On repeat auscultation at the lateral chest wall, breath sounds are significantly diminished on the left, and a faint crackle of subcutaneous emphysema is appreciated.

Q: What factors emerged during the course of patient care that should have raised a suspicion of trauma or domestic abuse?

A young woman who appears to be in excellent health has collapsed for no apparent reason. Despite appropriate treatment, she cannot be stabilized, and deteriorates rapidly. Her husband has no explanation, and appears concerned but detached.

The call to 911 came in at 10:35 P.M., and EMTs arrived at the scene at 10:41 P.M. ED arrival was at 10:56 P.M., but it was not until 11:15 P.M. that symptoms of a potential trauma were noted. Visual inspection by EMTs might have revealed bruising and evidence of free air, and thus permitted much earlier detection. Over an hour has now passed since the medical team's first contact with the patient.

Case Continuation

A tension pneumothorax was suspected because of diminished breath sounds, subcutaneous air, and medi-

astinum shift. A left thoracostomy is performed immediately with placement of a #36 tube, and a hemo-pneumothorax is drained of 600 cc of blood. Radiography demonstrates four posterior rib fractures. The nasogastric tube is curled in the left base of the lung. There are no diaphragmatic markings on the left side. The patient is transported to the operating room for abdominal exploration and repair of her ruptured diaphragm.

On repeat questioning, her husband appears baffled and concerned. When the ED physician continues to push for a more detailed history, he becomes belligerent and leaves the family room to phone a member of the hospital Board of Trustees.

Appropriate diagnosis and treatment are very difficult in the ED setting, especially when the patient presents in a critically ill condition unable to give a history. Because physical violence is only one of many repressive tactics used for pathological control of the victim by the perpetrator, severely battered women are often socially isolated and distant from home and relatives. The battering partner is frequently the only person present to provide history, and is the sole witness to the event. The batterer may be overbearing and overprotective, but is as likely to be calm, articulate, and apparently helpful. A history from this second type of partner may confuse the diagnostic picture. Thorough evaluation of *all* patients and frequent reassessment must remain the standard of care, and acute intentional injury by a partner must be included in the differential diagnosis. In this case, trauma was not identified until the pressure of mechanical ventilation, together with the ball valve effect of a punctured left lung, forced enough of the air out of the lung to visibly distort the patient's external anatomy.

Case #2

A 33-year-old woman presents to the ED at 3:00 a.m. with a complaint of blisters on both feet from wearing sneakers without socks and requests a note for work. She has a past history of alcohol abuse but states that she has been sober for the last 6 months. She denies any other health problems. Vital signs are normal. She is alert and in no apparent distress. On examination, she has a 1 × 1 cm nonulcerated Achilles blister on each foot. There is no evidence of infection.

Q: What about this case suggests that there is more involved here than "inappropriate" use of the ED?

Whenever the seriousness of the complaint and the patient's affect do not dovetail, suspect abuse. A pattern of multiple, minor complaints may be either a mask for abuse or the somatic expression of the misery of victimization. Bombadier, an internist before entering emergency medicine, describes a patient who visited him repeatedly over 12 years with undiagnosable complaints he joked about as "itchy teeth." It was only when she subsequently appeared on his ED shift as a trauma patient that he was able to determine that she had been systematically abused—physically, economically, and emotionally—during this entire period of "hypochondria." "In general," he says, "these patients do not volunteer information about the violence to which they are subject at home. The physician must first suspect it, and then ask about it. This assumes an appreciation on our part of the scope of domestic violence within every level of our society and a degree of comfort in handling the problem when it is uncovered."[8]

Case Continuation

The physician sat down with the patient and said that he was puzzled about why she had chosen this particular time to come into the ED for this problem. He asked if she was having any special problems that day. In response, she poured out her story. Her boyfriend had been abusing her over a 2-year period and had beaten her up last weekend when he was drinking. Today he had started drinking again with a buddy, and the two of them had gotten verbally abusive. Then the friend left, and she was afraid to be alone with her boyfriend until he sobered up. She ran out of the house without her purse and had been walking the streets afraid to go home. The patient accepted referral to a battered women's program for counseling, and the ED staff arranged for a taxi to take the patient to her mother's house where she would be safe for the night.

Q: What is the role of alcohol in family violence?

Studies demonstrate that cultures like the United States in which there are mixed messages about alcohol have a higher rate of female homicide and violence against women than either countries that regulate or countries that integrate alcohol consumption.[17] Someone under the influence of alcohol may not perceive the risks of violence that would be apparent to a sober person; in addition, drinking modifies the rules of behavior and lowers the standards of accountability. Alcohol is present in more than one-half of all domestic violence incidents.[18] Moreover, the fact that this patient had a history of previous alcohol abuse also puts her at higher risk. The discharge plan for this patient contained two very important factors, a plan for safety and a plan for counseling, but lacked the third element, a specific support system for her efforts to remain sober.

Case #3

A 19-year-old Hispanic woman was brought in by ambulance after neighbors called police to report screams. She had been held captive in the house for 2 days by her husband, during which time she was repeatedly slapped, pushed, and kicked. Her husband had started abusing her while she was pregnant, she said, but none of the previous episodes had been so severe. Her two children, a 4-year-old and a 4-week-old, were left behind in the house with her husband when she was taken to the hospital by ambulance.

On examination, the patient had boot tread marks on her right arm, raised red welts on her back, a scalp laceration, and finger marks on her neck. There was also right orbital bruising and swelling. X-rays were negative for fracture. The laceration was repaired and her wounds were dressed. When the policeman was asked to photograph her, he said, "What for . . . she'll just go back to him," and proceeded to tell jokes to the ED staff while photographing the patient's injuries.

She decided not to press charges. The ED staff worked with her to accept referral to a battered women's program and plan a safe discharge; she called her parents, who came to get her, and she went home with her mother while her father and brother left to go get her children from her house. She was tearful, worried about her children and afraid her husband might harm her family when threatened with removal of his children. Before she left, the psychiatric nurse sat down with her, gave her a brochure describing a program oriented to the needs of the Latina community, evaluated her for suicide risk, gave her a card with numbers to call any time she wanted to talk, and encouraged her to seek help.

Q: What other issues might the ED staff have considered?

The staff of this ED made several good decisions for counseling, culturally appropriate referral, and safe discharge. The situation also presented opportunities, however, for education of the policeman who made inappropriate jokes, and of the paramedics, who left a 4-year-old and a baby with an enraged parent. Arrangements need to be made for medical evaluation of these children, since abuse of women by their partners is often an indicator of concomitant child abuse.[19] Young women, particularly those under 20 years of age, appear to be more vulnerable to battering than those in their middle years. Married women are least likely to report domestic violence, while separated women are the most likely to be severely physically assaulted.[1] There is also an increase in incidents during and immediately after pregnancy, and the consequences of psychological stress may adversely affect pregnancy outcomes even in the absence of physical assault.[18]

Women of every age, religious affiliation, racial and ethnic origin, economic or geographic circumstance, and sexual orientation, however, experience violence from intimate partners,[20] but some factors increase the risks. African American women, for example, are more likely to report abuse and seek medical care for sequelae of battering, and several studies show that poverty is associated with a higher prevalence of abuse.[21]

Accurate information on dating violence is just beginning to be assembled, and information for older women is sketchy, partly because domestic violence is often misclassified as elder abuse.[19] Disabled women[18] and recent immigrants[22] appear to experience a high degree of intimate partner violence. These risk factors must be kept in mind for all ED patients, since estimates suggest that one-third of women utilizing emergency services will have been injured in the last year.[4]

IDENTIFICATION AND INTERVENTION PROTOCOLS

Women injured by battering are often more severely injured and more likely to be injured in the head, neck and thorax, and abdomen than women presenting with other mechanisms of accidental injury.[23] In one study surveying 218 domestic violence victims, 28% required hospital admission, 13% required major surgery, and one-third of cases involved a weapon. Forty percent of the victims had previously sought medical care for sequelae associated with abuse.[24]

Standard evaluation technique assumes that any woman injured in more than three separate anatomic areas who was not involved in a motor vehicle crash has been abused until proven otherwise. All women who have experienced traumatic injury should be specifically asked about intentional injury. There should be meticulous documentation in the chart.[25] Where possible, photographs should be appended to the chart.[26]

Implementation of protocols has been shown to improve identification rates.[4,27] The Family Violence Prevention Fund recommends that the possibility of spousal abuse should be investigated thoroughly if (1) there are unexplained delays in seeking treatment; (2) injuries are consistent with battering; (3) pain or seriousness are minimized, and the patient is unusually calm about traumatic injury; (4) injuries do not match the explanation; (5) history or examination reveal old, untreated injuries; (6) there are bruises in many stages of healing or untreated fractures; (7) the patient is pregnant and bruised or in vaginal pain; (8) the patient or the patient's partner has a history of drug or alcohol abuse.

Interviewing techniques that have been suggested include (1) create a safe space; (2) if children are present, make sure that they are safe; (3) interview in private; (4) assure confidentiality; (5) ask direct questions,—that is, "Did someone beat you?" since many women feel relief when asked directly, without prejudice or judgement; (6) ask about rape and sexual abuse; (7) take a complete medical history; (8) understand that passivity may be a survival technique; (9) be patient when your help appears to be rejected—her ability to trust has been badly undermined ; (10) be direct about the risks—the pattern of escalation, the risk to children, the risk to her of suicide; (11) be aware of your own biases as they surface during the interview—remember that she is the best judge of her own experience, and what is necessary to survive.

There are specific guidelines for treatment as well. Document all injuries, using a body map, photographs, and narrative. Allow the patient to retain as much control as possible, and make sure she agrees to each procedure. Do not touch her without her permission; remember that control over her body is what she loses each time she is battered. Remember that mood or perception-altering drugs may compromise her ability to defend herself, if she chooses to return to the abusive situation. Consider admitting her if possible, or keeping her in the ED overnight until she can arrange placement in a shelter in the morning.

Some very simple interventions can help keep her safe. Keep her separated from her abuser if he has accompanied her to your site. Discuss safe discharge, transportation to safety, and the need for legal consult. If she decides to go back to the house, talk with her about an escape plan—money, extra keys, and a person to call for help. Provide culturally appropriate referrals, and access to a private telephone so she can call supportive relatives or friends, and make contact with the hotline or shelter to which you have referred her. Network with local resources, and develop cooperative protocols for follow-up, so she doesn't fall through the cracks when she leaves your site. Encourage her to return any time that she needs medical assistance.

The national health objective for the year 2000 states that 90% of hospital EDs should have protocols in place for routinely identifying, treating, and referring victims of spouse abuse.[28] At present, most emergency departments are far from this goal. A survey was conducted of 414 California hospitals. Although 93% of these institutions had referral lists, only 7% of these were comprehensive. Only 34% reported having brochures about domestic violence readily available, and less than half had any type of written guidelines for domestic abuse. Figure 10-1 provides an example of a pocket guide that was developed as part of a guidelines project.

Emergency medicine practitioners have a responsibility for secondary prevention as well as treatment of physical injuries. The American College of Emergency Physicians (ACEP) has responded to the call of the PHS, JCAHO and advocacy organizations with a campaign to "Blow the Whistle on Violence." Thousands of high-pitched whistles have been distributed to women and lives have been saved. According to Colin Rorie, ACEP's Executive Director, "Anything we can do to get the message out that violence is unacceptable and preventable is one more step toward making violence a thing of the past."

A pocket card, describing the main points to remember about domestic violence, has been developed by the Domestic Violence Program at San Francisco General Hospital and is reprinted here with permission from the program:

Figure 10-1 Pocket Guide to Domestic Violence

DOMESTIC VIOLENCE GUIDE

Domestic violence is a pattern of assaultive and coercive behaviors, including physical, sexual, and psychological attacks, that adults or adolescents use against their intimate partners. Without intervention the violence usually escalates in both frequency and severity, resulting in repeat visits to the healthcare system.

SCREEN ALL PATIENTS FOR A HISTORY OF DOMESTIC VIOLENCE WITH ANY OF THE FOLLOWING:
HISTORY SUGGESTING DOMESTIC VIOLENCE
- Traumatic injury or sexual assault
- Suicide attempt or overdose
- Physical symptoms related to stress
- Vague or nonspecific complaints
- Problems or injuries during pregnancy
- History inconsistent with injury
- Delay in seeking medical care
- Repeat visits

BEHAVIORAL CLUES
- Evasive or reluctant to speak in front of partner
- Overly protective or controlling partner

PHYSICAL CLUES
- All physical injuries
- Unexplained multiple or old injuries

ASK ABOUT DOMESTIC VIOLENCE
- Talk to the patient alone in a safe, private environment

- Use direct, simple questions, such as:
  - Did someone cause these injuries?
  - Who?
  - Are you in a relationship with a person who physically hurts or threatens you?

TAKE A DOMESTIC VIOLENCE HISTORY:
- Past history of domestic violence or sexual assault
- History of abuse to children

SEND IMPORTANT MESSAGES TO THE PATIENT:
- She is not alone
- It is not her fault
- Help is available

ASSESS SAFETY:
- Is it safe to go home?
- Can the patient stay with family or friends?
- Does she need access to a shelter?
- Does she want police intervention?

MAKE REFERRALS:
- Involve social worker if available
- Provide list: shelters, resources, hotline numbers

DOCUMENT FINDINGS:
- Use patient's own words about injury and abuse
- Document injuries clearly, using a body map
- Take Polaroid photographs of injuries

SOURCE: Reprinted with permission of the Domestic Violence Program 1995 at San Francisco General Hospital.

NOTES

1. Flitcraft A, Stark E. Spouse abuse. In M. Rosenberg and M. Fenley (eds.). *Violence in America.* New York: Oxford University Press, 1991.
2. Council on Scientific Affairs, American Medical Association. Violence against women: Relevance for medical practitioners. *JAMA* 1992; 267:3134–89.
3. Varvaro FF. Treatment of the battered woman: Effective response of the Emergency Department. *Am Coll Emerg Phys Newsletter* 1989; 11:8–13.
4. McCleer SV, Anwar R. A study of battered women presenting in an emergency department. *Am J Pub Health* 1989; 79:65–6.

5. Randall T. ACOG renews domestic violence campaign, calls for changes in medical school curricula. *JAMA* 1992; 267:3131.

6. JCAHO. *Accreditation manual for hospitals.* Oakbrook Terrace IL: Joint Commission, 1991.

7. Harshbarger S. *The abuse prevention act in family violence: The health professional's role in assessment and intervention.* Boston: Office of the Attorney General, 1995.

8. Bombadier G. Domestic violence: A public health emergency. *Insights in Risk Management* 1995; 2:5–9.

9. Gelles RJ, Straus MA. *Intimate violence: The definitive study of the causes and consequences of abuse in the American family.* New York: Simon & Schuster, 1988.

10. National Crime Survey. *Family violence report.* Washington DC: Bureau of Justice Statistics, 1984.

11. Novello AC, Rosenberg M, Saltzman L. From the Surgeon-General, U.S. Public Health Service. *JAMA* 1992; 267:3132.

12. Stark E, Flitcraft AE. Spouse abuse. In *The surgeon general's workshop on violence and public health: Source book.* Atlanta, CDC, 1985.

13. Sugg NK, Inui T. Primary care physicians' response to violence. *JAMA* 1992; 267:3157–60.

14. Council on Ethical and Judicial Affairs. Physicians and domestic violence, ethical considerations. *JAMA* 1992; 267:3190–3.

15. Jecker NS. Privacy beliefs and the violent family: Extending the ethical argument for physician intervention. *JAMA* 1993; 267:776–80.

16. Loulan J. *Lesbian passion.* San Francisco: Spinsters, 1987.

17. Parker R. The effects of context on alcohol and violence. *Alcohol World* 1993; 17:117–22.

18. Hotaling GT, Sugarman DB. An analysis of risk markers in husband to wife violence: The current state of knowledge. *Violence Victims* 1986; 1:101–24.

19. McKibben L, DeVos B, Newberger E. Victimization of mothers of abused children: A controlled study. *Pediatrics* 1989; 84:531–5.

20. Straus M, Gelles R, Steinmentz SK. *Behind closed doors: A survey of family violence in America.* NY: Doubleday, 1980.

21. Walker L. *The battered woman syndrome.* New York: Springer, 1984.

22. Hogeland C, Rosen K. *A needs assessment of undocumented women.* San Francisco: Immigrant Women's Task Force of the Coalition for Imigrant and Refugee Rights and Services, 1990.

23. Stark E, Flitcraft A, Zuckerman D. *Wife abuse in the medical setting: An introduction for health personnel,* Monograph no. 7. Washington DC: Office of Domestic Violence, 1981.

24. Berrios D, Grady D. Domestic violence: Risk factors and outcomes. *West J Med* 1991; 155: 133–5.

25. Haack D. *Suggested protocols for victims of spousal and elder abuse.* Denver: Colorado Department of Health, 1992.

26. Schiffrin E, Waldran C. *Identifying and treating battered adult and adolescent women and their children: A guide for health care providers.* Boston: Department of Public Health, 1991.

27. Tilden VP, Sheperd P. Increasing the rate of identification of battered women in an Emergency Department: Use of a nursing protocol. *Nurs Res Health* 1987; 10:209–15.

28. PHS. *Healthy people 2000.* Washington DC: U.S. DHHS(PHS)91-50212, 1991.

29. MMWR. Emergency Department response to domestic violence: California 1992. *JAMA* 1993; 270: 1296–8.

11

Rape and Sexual Violence: The Adult and Adolescent Female Victim

DAVID L. LEVINE
LAURA E. KAUFMAN

CONTENTS

- Prevalence/risk
- Rape trauma syndrome
- Sexual assault protocols
- ED intervention
- Screening for the unknown victim
- STDs
- Training
- Research
- Prevention

CHAPTER SUMMARY

While the specific legal definition varies from state to state, sexual assault can generally be defined as forced sexual contact without consent. Sexual assault is not a crime of passion, but rather an act of violence using sex as the weapon. Emergency medical providers have often viewed sexual assault as largely a criminal matter. Thus many emergency departments have focused on the details of evidence collection and/or the victim's presenting physical injuries while neglecting the victim's mental health needs. In addition, many sexual assault victims leave the ED having received little or no information regarding possible future mental or physical health issues connected to the assault. Many sexual assault victims seek care in the nation's emergency departments for symptoms related to sexual violence, but because they are not asked the right questions or are afraid they will not be believed, they never disclose their victimization. This chapter explores the important role emergency medical providers play in aiding the sexual assault victim and preventing sexual violence in general. It argues for the establishment of standard protocols and staff/medical student training procedures to help insure that sexual assault victims are identified and given appropriate care. Patient education strategies are recommended to encourage more victim reporting and to reduce future violence. The emergency medical provider's role is presented as an important part of the criminal justice process, and an avenue for physicians, nurses, and EMTs to help *prevent* future sexual violence. Finally, the following pages suggest further research to uncover the best methods of intervention/prevention in sexual assault cases and call for emergency medicine professionals to participate in relevant initiatives to improve community-wide systems of care for adult sexual assault victims. Given that over 90% of all sexual assault victims are female,[1] and given the differing responses and needs of child victims, this chapter will focus on adolescent and adult female victims of sexual violence. In addition, because the vast majority of sex offenders are male, the offenders discussed herein are assumed to be men.

Case #1

AR is a 17-year-old G0 P0 white female brought into the emergency department at midnight. Her mother accompanies her. In triage, the patient states she was raped at a party, by a male classmate, approximately 2 hours ago. ED staff assure AR she is safe in the hospital. AR complains of vaginal pain and bilateral thigh and arm abrasions. AR's mother requests a physical exam and any evidence collection necessary to prosecute the assailant. AR also agrees to the exam. When given the option by the triage nurse, AR and her mother choose to have a victim advocate called. The ED staff also calls a report of the sexual assault in to the city police. AR and her mother are taken to a quiet, private room. The advocate arrives, and the mother steps out of the exam room to get a cup of coffee. Physician history is taken after the mother leaves. The history reveals that AR was sexually assaulted by her current boyfriend (the mother did not know AR was dating) at the boyfriend's house. AR was "making out" with her boyfriend, which included consensual oral intercourse. AR firmly stated "no" to attempts at vaginal intercourse before she was pinned by her boyfriend and forced to have vaginal intercourse. The boyfriend did not wear a condom and ejaculated in the vagina. There was no oral ejaculation. There was no use of foreign objects or mechanical restraints. AR ran home when her boyfriend fell asleep. AR does not wish her mother to know about her relationship with the assailant. AR did not change clothes, douche, or defecate prior to arrival. She did try to wash herself off and did urinate.

AR is not taking any medications. Her tetanus immunization is up to date, and she has no allergies. There is no past history of sexually transmitted diseases or GYN problems. There was no use of alcohol or drugs. She does smoke one pack of cigarettes a day. AR has been sexually active in the past.

The physical exam reveals normal vital signs. AR is withdrawn and quiet but laughs at unusual times. Her clothes appear intact. Multiple abrasions and contusion to both shoulders and forearms are noted. Both thighs also appear bruised. The pelvic exam reveals small uptake of toluidine blue, illustrating a small laceration to the vaginal mucosa. No other injuries are noted. Appropriate specimen collection and labs are performed while informing the patient of all steps prior to performance.

AR receives local care to her wounds, antibiotic prophyllaxis for STD, and a "morning-after" pill to prevent pregnancy. The victim advocate and health care providers encourage her to tell the complete story to her mother and help her to do so when her mother returns. AR is scheduled for medical follow-up in 1 week and referred to the rape crisis center for crisis counseling.

Case #2

RT is a 45-year-old G1P1 divorced African American female who presents to the emergency department at 3:00 a.m. with a chief complaint of inability to sleep, feeling like being strangled in her sleep, and shortness of breath. She denies any chest pain, abdominal pain, nausea, vomiting, or neurological deficits. She has not had any fevers, chills, shakes, sweats, or URI symptoms. She notes she has had trouble sleeping for about a year, but the choking and shortness of breath sensation is new. She has not taken any medicine or sought medical intervention for the sleeping problem. There is no history of psychiatric problems. The patient does not have the choking feeling now, and is able to swallow without difficulty. RT's only cardiac risk factor is that she smokes one pack of cigarettes per day. She denies any trauma. She denies leg pain or swelling. She does not drink alcohol or use drugs.

The physical exam reveals an anxious, thin female in no apparent distress. She is without a fever and vital signs are normal. Her pulse oximetry is 99% on room air. Physical exam is completely normal including a normal throat, neck, pulmonary, cardiac, and extremity exam. She has no evidence of a DVT. Her EKG, chest x-ray, and blood gas are normal.

The physician's impression is anxiety disorder. She sends the patient home with outpatient psych follow-up. RT returns 2 hours later, hyperventilating, and notes she is scared to be at home alone. The same physician quickly assesses the patient and orders a psychiatry consult. After a lengthy interview, the patient reveals she was sexually assaulted 2 years ago today by a stranger. She states she has never told anyone because she felt it was her fault, and she worried no one would believe her.

DEFINITION OF THE PROBLEM

Prevalence/Risk Factors

The term rape suggests the following common media image: A woman walks alone through a dark alley. Suddenly, she is confronted by a strange man. After a struggle, he forces her, at knife or gunpoint, to engage in vaginal sexual intercourse against her will.

Research suggests that the reality of sexual violence in the United States is, in fact, quite different. First, sexual assault is not merely limited to forced vaginal penetration with a penis. Sexual assault occurs along a continuum which runs from unwanted touching and fondling of sex organs to forced vaginal, anal, and oral penetration. The weapon of choice in sex crimes is often a penis, but sexual assault can also involve penetration with the fingers or objects such as broomsticks, soda bottles, the butts of guns or knives.

Second, stereotypical assumptions that paint the rapist as a menacing stranger have led us to overlook the most common settings for rape and to vastly undercount the extent of sexual violence. Sexual assault is *not* generally a crime among strangers. Numerous studies have found that as many as 78 to 82% of women are raped by someone they know.[2–4] The assailant can be a spouse, boyfriend, family member, co-worker, friend, or neighbor. Someone with whom the victim is less intimately acquainted, such as the plumber or the boy who bags her groceries each week, can also be the offender.

The emergency medical provider who is unwilling to consider the prevalence of sexual violence among intimates and acquaintances will fail to identify many sexual assault victims and miss an opportunity to provide proper treatment. One study found, for instance, that more than one-half of rape victims over age 30 had been sexually assaulted by an intimate partner.[5] Among women suffering physical abuse by a partner, 33 to 46% also report being sexually assaulted by that partner.[6] Rape by acquaintances, sometimes called "date rape," is similarly very common. A 1993 study of sexual victimization of 401 undergraduate women found that 26% (106 women) had been sexually assaulted by a romantic or other acquaintance at some time after the age of fifteen.[7] Over the past 15 years, there has been a marked increase in reported incidents of rape of women and girls by nonmarried intimate partners.[8]

Age is another significant predictor of sexual violence. Research suggests that adolescent girls and young women face particularly high rates of sexual assault. Women are most likely to be raped in their adolescent and late teen years.[9] The 1992 National Women's Study, outlined in *Rape in America*, found that almost one in three (32%) of all sexual assaults are committed against girls aged 11 to 17. Another 22% of total rape victims fell between 18 and 24 years of age at the time of the assault. Seven percent of rape victims were 25 to 29 years old, and only 6% of all rapes occurred after the victim was 29 years or older.[3] Women 50 and older were found to comprise 2.2% of

all rape victims reporting a sexual assault in a recent study of Dallas County, Texas.[10]

It is also important to note that, over a lifetime, many women suffer multiple sexual assaults. The National Women's Study concluded that 56% of women were raped only once in their lifetimes, while 39% experienced more than one rape and 5% were unsure how many times they had been raped.[3] Adult survivors of childhood sexual abuse are at particularly high risk for experiencing further sexual violence as adult women. A random-sample study found that 17% of women who were not victims of child sexual assault experienced sexual violence as adults, while 33 to 68% of those who experienced childhood sexual abuse were raped as adults.[11]

Accurately determining the general prevalence of rape is extremely difficult. Estimates drawn from law enforcement authorities are limited by restrictive legal definitions of sexual violence which often exclude marital and acquaintance violence and which vary from state to state. Studies exploring reporting to the police find that anywhere from only one in ten rape victims[2] to only one in six[3] disclose their sexual assault to the police. Random surveys regarding the extent of sexual violence among women have been equally inconclusive. Prevalence rates in studies completed over the past two decades have found that from 2 to 25% of American women have been raped.[12] The varying methods of study and consequent varied results have led sexual assault researcher Mary P. Koss to conclude that "confident assertions regarding the true scope of rape remain premature." Nonetheless, Koss points to the study *Rape in America*, which finds that one in every eight women has been raped in her lifetime, as one of the more exhaustive studies and still finds it too conservative in estimating the extent of rape.[5] It *is* safe to argue that sexual violence is a significant public health problem deserving of careful treatment, research and prevention.

Rape Trauma Syndrome

The emergency medicine professional treating a rape victim can expect her to exhibit some combination of physical and mental symptoms called *rape trauma syndrome*. First described by Burgess and Holstrom in 1974, it is now generally accepted as a special category of posttraumatic stress disorder (PTSD) as defined in DSM-IV. A study has shown that 31% of rape victims develop rape-related PTSD.[3]

There are various models of rape trauma syndrome which describe from two to five phases. The three-phase model will be described below. Each survivor is different, and all victims do not naturally progress through all phases. Victims may also experience more than one phase at a time.

The initial phase, or the acute phase, begins immediately after the assault and lasts from days to weeks. During this period, victims exhibit emotional shock, disbelief, and despair. Moscarello describes a classic triad of symptoms following the traumatic event which include (1) haunting and intrusive recollections, (2) numbing of feelings, and (3) generalized hypersensitivity to environmental stimuli.[13] A patient's outward response may vary from emotional instability to well-controlled behavior. She may be crying one minute and laughing the next. Her mood swings may seem inappropriate to family, police, or medical providers. Embarrassment, self-blame, and feelings of powerlessness are common. Since control over her body has been ripped away from her during the assault, a victim may have trouble exercising the control to make the simplest decisions. She may all of a sudden be unable to decide what to wear or whether or not to brush her teeth. Finally, victims can suffer from somatic symptoms such as nausea, abdominal pain, and headaches, as well as from eating and sleep disorders.

The second phase, coined the outward adjustment or recoil phase, begins several days to weeks after the assault and may last from months to years. Some victims never move beyond this phase. During this period, the victim focuses on returning to her preassault pattern of living and works hard to have everything "get back to normal." Therefore, it is common for victims to deny the significance of the rape. During this phase, there is a tendency to miss follow-up appointments with medical, legal, and community providers. Symptoms of anxiety or depression emerge, although the victim may ignore these and contend that everything is fine. Studies show that 30 to 50% of rape victims experience at least one major depressive episode.[3,13] Psychosomatic complaints such as extreme fatigue, abdominal pain, nausea, headaches, musculoskeletal pains, and insomnia are common. During this stage, victims seeking medical care often do not report that they were sexually assaulted. The recoil phase can last as long as the victim

is able to suppress or deny that she was raped or to ignore the feelings associated with the assault.

The final phase of rape trauma syndrome is called resolution and reorganization. It usually occurs months to years post-assault. This is the period where a victim faces her feelings about the rape and seeks to incorporate the experience into her life history. This phase may be triggered when the victim experiences something that reminds her of the assault, or her depression may become so substantial that she is willing to confront her feelings. Physical, psychological, social, and sexual difficulties may occur as the victim reexplores the assault and her feelings associated with it.

Social support has been found to be the most important factor correlated with recovery from rape.[14] The reaction of family and friends is variable, but the most common response is silence.[15] The victim is discouraged from talking about the assault, and there is no acknowledgment of how the assault affects her life. It is common for victims to lose the support of those closest to them. For instance, between 50 to 80% of women lose their boyfriend or husband after a rape.[16] The efficacy of different treatment modalities varies tremendously, but group therapy with other survivors has been found to be very successful.[16] Group therapy tends to decrease the isolation of the victim while providing clear and unambiguous support.

Recovery is a long process, and some victims never recover. Resnick et al. found most victims were able to function within their family in 1 month, function in social situations in 2 months, and function at work in 8 months. Despite these findings, Resnick also notes that anxiety remained 1 year after the rape.[17] Burgess and Holstrom interviewed rape victims 4 years after the assault and found that none of the victims felt their lives were back to normal.[18]

Sexual Assault and Medical Utilization

Given the possibility that as few as 1 in 10 sexual assaults are reported to police, it is not surprising to learn that the National Victim Center's study found only 17% of all rape victims sought a medical exam. The same study concluded that 60% of rape victims seeking a medical exam did so within 24 hours of the assault.[3] This might lead to the conclusion that the vast majority of rape victims never seek care from the ED. However, the research that does explore post-assault physician visits by rape victims and several studies that consider the rate at which domestic violence victims are detected by emergency departments suggests that emergency medical providers may actually be seeing numerous victims who seek medical care without disclosing their history of sexual victimization.

Existing studies of medical usage by sexual assault victims focus on visits to physicians in general and do not single out emergency physicians for particular attention. A 1991 study of female patients in a health maintenance organization found that rape victims increased their visits to all physicians by 56% in the year following the crime. Prior to the crime, victims averaged 4.4 and 4.1 physician visits annually. In the year after the sexual assault, they averaged 6.4 and 7.3 physician visits.[19] A second study in 1994 showed similar patterns in medical utilization by rape victims, with significant increases in physician visits noted as early as 4 months post-assault.[20]

Studies regarding ED detection of domestic violence show that appropriate staff training and targeted screening questions increase identification of domestic violence significantly. A continuous quality improvement model in a busy public emergency department increased detection of domestic violence in women presenting with trauma by twofold.[21] A more intensive mandated interview protocol increased detection of domestic violence from 5.6% to 30%.[22]

More research is needed as to whether the low detection rate discovered in domestic violence cases also applies to sexual assault. Nonetheless, given the substantial increase in medical usage by rape victims following their assault, the high rates of nondetection of domestic abuse in emergency departments, and the frequency of female sexual assault, emergency medical personnel should strongly consider the possibility that adolescent and adult females visiting the ED may be rape survivors. This should be considered regardless of whether the woman makes herself a "known" victim by disclosing that she has been assaulted, or whether the fact that she is a rape survivor is initially "unknown."

THE EMERGENCY MEDICAL PROVIDER'S ROLE IN TREATING AND PREVENTING SEXUAL VIOLENCE

Whether rape victims present as such or not, the nation's emergency departments are handling a large caseload of sexual assault. Emergency medical providers play a vital role in assuring that sexual assault victims receive proper care both in the ED and in subsequent follow-up. However, the role of the emergency medicine professional does not stop there; he or she is also a critical link in the chain of efforts being utilized to *prevent* sexual violence. By routinely screening female patients for sexual violence, sharing violence prevention information with patients, and ensuring that medical exams in rape cases are carried out so as to best preserve crucial evidentiary material, the emergency medical provider will go a long way towards preventing future sexual assaults. Finally, emergency medical professionals can expand research into rape prevalence, treatment, and prevention and can work even more closely with others in the community trying to treat and prevent sexual violence.

Sexual Assault Protocol for the Known Victim

Proper care of the rape victim who discloses a recent assault requires both an understanding of the treatment steps which must be followed as well as an appreciation of the victim's state of mind. Although emergency medical providers are part of the criminal justice process in the case of sexual assault, it is *not* the job of emergency medicine professionals to judge the actions or account of the victim. Physicians, nurses, and EMTs provide medical care and should leave criminal analyses up to judges and juries.

Public understanding of the horrors of rape and the needs of its victims has increased greatly over the past two decades. Nonetheless, stereotypical and judgmental views of sexual assault victims are still common. Many continue to believe that women lie about being raped or that a woman engaging in high-risk behavior who is then raped deserved to be a crime victim. Rape victims are painfully aware of the way others may see them. The National Victim

Center study found that 69% of rape victims are worried that people will think the assault was their fault. Victims are also concerned about others learning they were raped: 71% fear their families discovering they were assaulted, and 68% worry about those outside their family learning of the attack.[3] As discussed above, rape survivors may also suffer from some combination of shame, heightened fear, and a sense that they have lost control over their lives.

The ED is often the first official "system" to which the victim reports her assault. If she is met with judgmental attitudes or insensitive treatment by emergency medical staff, she may be reluctant to share her story with personnel in the criminal justice system. This is a problem for both the individual victim and society as whole. Many rapists are repeat offenders. If insensitive treatment discourages a victim from pursuing the difficult course of reporting her rape to police, her offender will remain free to victimize others in the community. Therefore, not only is victim-sensitive care the appropriate treatment for medical personnel to provide, it also serves to help prevent future assaults. The following protocol is designed considering both the victim's state of mind and the medical interventions necessary to promote a victim's health.

Prehospital Intervention

All patients should have a primary and secondary survey to assess for life threatening injuries. Standard prehospital protocols should be followed for any life-threatening injury detected. If stable, the victim should be reassured she will be safe in the ambulance. To protect evidence, the victim should be discouraged from changing clothes, eating, drinking, taking any medications, gargling, brushing teeth, urinating, defecating, douching, or showering. Throughout succeeding interviews with ED personnel and law enforcement officials, the victim may have to retell the events of what happened multiple times. Therefore, history of the assault should be kept to a minimum and should be directed only to assess potential life-threatening injuries.

Paramedics or EMTs need to take care not to disturb evidence at the rape site or on the patient.

Unless necessary, the genitalia should not be examined or packed as this may be traumatic for the victim and may destroy evidence. If the victim consents or local policy requires, police should be contacted. The patient should be promptly transported to either a designated hospital for handling sexual assault or a hospital of the victim's choice, if stable. Involving the victim in decision making throughout contact will help her begin to regain a sense of control over her life and help to start the healing process.

Emergency Department Intervention

When any patient presents, life-threatening injuries and unstable vital signs should be assessed. Five percent of rape victims have major nongenital physical injuries.[23] When the patient is stabilized, evidence collection and full psychological support should be implemented.

The patient's name and reason for visit should be confidential. The patient should be placed in a quiet, private room, out of the mainstream area but accessible to department personnel. Ideally, the room should have the facilities to perform a pelvic exam so the patient does not have to be moved multiple times. Staff should regularly assure the patient of her safety. In addition, staff must not be judgmental about the behavior of the victim, her clothing, or her explanation of the assault. A designated nursing provider and physician, who are trained in the sexual assault protocol and aware of the multiple emotional manifestations that might occur, should be assigned to the patient. A community or in-hospital advocate should be called if the patient consents. The number of providers should be kept to a minimum.

The victim must give written consent prior to any exam, test, or treatment. It is important to let the victim guide the process in order to restore as much control as possible to the victim. Hospital security should be alerted to the possibility of the assailant presenting to the emergency department. Police also should be contacted if the patient consents or if local policy requires.

History. The purpose of the history is twofold. First, the history guides the provider about any medical conditions that could affect the victim's treatment. Second, the history provides details of the assault that will guide the exam. In eliciting the history, the provider should avoid using questions starting with "why" since it may be interpreted as judgmental and feed into the victim's self-blame.

A complete history should be obtained even if the victim does not wish to file charges. The history of the event will include the time and place of the assault, race, and number of assailants, and a brief description of the assault including whether there was oral, vaginal, or rectal penetration and/or ejaculation. Use of force, threats of force, use of restraints, use of foreign bodies, use of foams, jellies, or lubricants should be elicited. It is important to assess what the victim has done since the assault such as changed clothes, douched, bathed, urinated, defecated, ate, or used a tampon. The gynecological history should include use of birth control pills, history of missed pills, last menstrual period, gravity, parity, history of surgeries, and history of sexually transmitted diseases. Last voluntary intercourse within the previous week should be assessed as sperm may be motile in the cervix up to 5 days and in the vagina for 6 to 12 hours. Only facts pertinent to the case should be asked and recorded. The history should also include all physical complaints and the patient's tetanus immunization status. Use of alcohol and drugs in the time period around the assault as well as a psychological history should be assessed as this may have impaired the victim's ability to consent to intercourse. The history should be obtained in a nonjudgmental fashion. The patient should be allowed to pause and proceed at a comfortable pace.

Physical Exam. Detection of injuries is critical for both proper medical care for the victim and for successful legal prosecution. Although up to 70% of rape victims reported no physical injuries, 4 to 5% of victims sustained serious physical injury, and 24% sustained minor physical injury.[3,24] Other studies report injury rates as high as 50%.[25] Evidence of trauma is significantly associated with successful prosecution. Specific injuries associated with successful prosecution include multiple contusions, abrasions, human bites, lacerations of the perineum, lacerations or puncture wounds to the extremities, burns, and depressed skull fractures with severe head injury.[25]

Even if the victim is unsure about reporting to the police, a sexual assault evidence kit should be collected. It should be emphasized that the collection of evidence does not add time to the physical exam. If performed by a male physician, the physical exam should be chaperoned by a female. If the victim consents, a photograph of her prior to undressing should be taken. Prior to disrobing, the general appearance of clothes including staining, tears, mud, leaves, sand, and other foreign material should be noted. A Woods lamp may be used to detect seminal stains on the clothes. The patient should disrobe and place all clothes in a paper bag. Underwear should be put in a separate bag. Paper bags are used instead of plastic since plastic bags cause mold to develop on semen stains and bacteria count to increase on blood stains. If possible, the clothing should only be handled by the victim. Eighty percent of the population secrete blood group antigens in their saliva, perspiration, and semen and the helper may contaminate potential evidence. As the clothing will not be returned arrangements should be made to obtain replacement clothes for the victim.

A complete physical should be done with emphasis on the following items. The whole body should be searched for abrasions, lacerations, bites, scratches, foreign bodies, and areas of ecchymoses. Dried semen may be found on the patient's skin. The most common areas of injury besides the vagina are the mouth, throat, wrists, breasts, and thigh. Oral cavity injuries include a torn frenulum, broken teeth, abrasions, and lacerations. Bite marks on the genitalia and breast are common.[26] Lacerations must be visualized closely to ensure they are not stab wounds.

Forensic collection includes fingernail scrapings which are taken with a fingernail file and placed collectively in a test tube or envelope. Head hair specimens are collected by combing the hair and placing the combings in an envelope. Hair specimens will be compared to pubic hair specimens and also examined for the offender's hair. If there was oral penetration, the spaces between the teeth should be swabbed for the presence of acid phosphatase and sperm, and a throat culture for gonorrhea collected.

The gynecological exam may be the most traumatic aspect of the victim's exam since it may remind her of the assault. Explanation of procedures is necessary. Allow the patient to guide the exam. Pubic hair should be combed and collected per local protocol. Genital trauma is common even in asymptomatic victims. Up to one-third of pelvic injuries were asymptomatic, although none required medical intervention. The vulva should be examined for signs of trauma. Eight percent of patients have vulvar trauma.[27] The speculum should be lubricated only with water. Toluidine blue dye can be used to identify small pelvic lacerations from traumatic intercourse. The dye is best applied to the vaginal mucosa at the introitus. Special attention should be given to the hymen as this is one of the most common places for trauma. Lacerations of the vaginal wall are more common in younger patients near the introitus. More sexually experienced patients have lacerations higher up. Small abrasions or telangiectasia in the posterior fourchette and distal vagina can be seen by colposcopy or local application of toluidine blue.[28,29] Secretions pooled in the posterior fornix should be aspirated and placed in a sterile container to be examined for sperm and acid phosphatase. If there are no secretions in the posterior fornix, it should be wiped with a cotton tip swab and swabbed onto two slides for sperm and acid phosphatase examination. Gonorrhea and chlamydia cultures should be obtained. It has been found that 1% of all victims have moderate to severe genital injuries requiring surgical intervention.[25,30] A rectal exam should be performed if there was penetration or attempted penetration. Lacerations, fissures, and bleeding should be noted. Gonorrhea and chlamydia cultures should be obtained from the rectum.

The postmenopausal woman presents with similar frequency of trauma but a significantly different pattern of injury. Genital trauma in the postmenopausal woman is more severe with a significantly increased proportion of women requiring surgery. Genital edema, abrasions, and lacerations are more common. Frequency of extragenital trauma is significantly increased in younger patients, especially to the head and neck regions. Trunk and extremity trauma is common to both groups.[10]

Baseline labs that should be drawn include syphilis serology, hepatitis B, blood type, and pregnancy. An HIV baseline should also be collected if the patient gives consent after appropriate counseling.

Treatment. Pregnancy is a serious consequence of sexual assault. The estimated risk of pregnancy is 2 to 4% for women who were not using contraceptives at the time of the assault. All victims should be coun-

seled concerning pregnancy testing and options for termination. The victim should give informed consent to testing and pregnancy prophylaxis if implemented. Hormonal therapy within 72 hours of the assault with 100 µg of ethinyl estradiol at the time of exam and repeated in 12 hours decreases the risk of pregnancy 60 to 90%.[31] For assaults between 72 hours and 7 days, an OB/GYN consult should be obtained for possible use of an intrauterine device (IUD) if the pregnancy is not desired. For hospitals that do not provide services of pregnancy prophylaxis, the patient must be referred to a facility that will provide services if desired. Tetanus immunization should be given if the patient is not already protected. Prophylaxis for sexually transmitted diseases and HIV is discussed in the special consideration section below.

Follow-up. All plans should be in writing. Psychological follow up should be in 1 to 2 weeks. Medical follow up should be in 2 to 4 weeks unless medically indicated sooner. All patients should be given a 24-hour crisis phone number. Many communities have a rape crisis center, and these programs are excellent resources. A safe place for the patient to go should be arranged if the offender has not been placed under arrest. The patient should be encouraged to express her feelings. She should be told briefly about rape trauma syndrome and warned that she may experience sudden changes in mood.

Screening for the Unknown Victim of Sexual Assault

Many sexual assault victims go undetected in the emergency department or by their primary care provider. Victims told their doctors in only 67% of rape cases that they had been sexually assaulted.[3] Most commonly victims will reveal a history of sexual assault only in response to a direct physician inquiry.[16] In fact, when physicians are trained to take a patient's sexual history as part of a routine history and physical, significant previously undisclosed past traumatic sexual experiences are uncovered.[29] There is a misperception that patients will be offended if routinely asked about sexual violence. It has been shown that patients at both private and public hospitals favor routine physical and sexual abuse inquiry. Patients believe physicians can help with problems. Patients surveyed also stated that they would answer physicians truthfully if asked about abuse.[32]

Some common symptoms that may indicate a history of sexual assault victim include rapid or pounding heartbeat, headaches, nausea, back pain, skin disorders, menstrual symptoms, sudden weight change, sleeping disorders and persistent abdominal pain. Sometimes symptoms may be trauma specific. For example, a patient forced to have oral sex may suffer from a gagging sensation or a patient who was choked may exhibit trouble breathing.

In order to carry out primary prevention by detecting unknown rape victims, all female patients presenting for medical care should be screened for sexual violence. Questioning should be routinely incorporated into the history and physical. When inquiring about sexual assault, behaviorally specific questions that elicit information about the threat of injury as well as different types of criminal assault should be used. Nonlegal terms will best counteract respondents' stereotypes about the nature of the violence committed.[33] It has been shown that using the term rape in questioning compared to behaviorally specific questions decreased the detection rate from 20 to 2.6%.[17] Typical questions may include "Has anyone made you have sex by using force or threatening to harm you?" or "Has someone either touched you in a sexual manner anywhere on your body, touched your genitals or breasts, or engaged in oral, vaginal, or anal sex against your will?"

If a patient discloses being raped within the last 72 hours, implement the protocol discussed above. If the assault occurred more than 72 hours ago, the patient should still be examined for physical injuries and should be given appropriate medical and mental health follow-up instructions.

Special Considerations: Sexual Assault and Drug Use

The association of drug and alcohol use with sexual assault is very strong. There is a high incidence of previous sexual abuse among chemically dependent women: estimates run as high as 46% for rape and 28 to 40% for incest within the chemically dependent population compared to a rate of 20 to 25% for rape and incest in the general population.[34] Studies show that as many as 75% of women in treatment for

substance abuse have been victims of sexual violence.[31]

Sexual abuse has been associated with high risk behavior including initiating drug use by age 15, pressure by a male partner to use drugs during pregnancy, and engaging in sex in exchange for drugs. Victims of sexual abuse were 2.9 times more likely to engage in sex for drugs than those not sexually abused.[31] Rape in America found that rape victims were 5.3 times more likely to have used prescription drugs nonmedically than nonvictims. It also found that rape victims were 3.4 times more likely to use marijuana, 6 times more likely to use cocaine, and 10.1 times more likely to use hard drugs other than cocaine compared to women who were not raped.[3]

Rape-related PTSD is an additional risk factor for drug use. Rape victims with PTSD were 5.3 times more likely to have two or more major alcohol related problems and 3.7 times more likely to have two or more serious drug related problems than rape victims without PTSD. Compared with noncrime victims those with PTSD are 13.4 times more likely to have two or more alcohol related problems and 26 times more likely to have two or more drug related problems.[3]

Special Considerations: Sexually Transmitted Diseases

Poor medical follow-up of victims, differing baseline prevalence of STDs in various regions of the US, and the difficulty in differentiating preexisting STDs from those acquired during the assault, make it hard to accurately determine the risk of acquiring sexually transmitted diseases during a rape. The most common infections are trichomonas, bacterial vaginosis, and chlamydia. The CDC estimates the risk of an adult rape victim acquiring gonorrhea as 6 to 12%. The risk of chlamydia is 4 to 17% while the risk of syphilis is 0.5 to 3%.[35] Another study showed the risk of acquiring gonorrhea was 4%, chlamydia 2%, syphilis 0%, and trichomonas 12%.[36]

The CDC recommends prophylaxis because follow-up can be difficult and patients may be reassured if offered treatment or prophylaxis for possible infections. The recommendations include ceftriaxone 125mg IM in a single dose plus metronidazole 2g orally as a single dose, plus doxycycline 100 mg orally two times a day for 7 days.[37] The CDC has expanded alternatives for general outpatient treatment of chlamydia and gonorrhea, but has not expanded them for rape victims. Standard alternatives if the patient is allergic to the above apply.

When giving information, it should be provided in a nondirective manner using open-ended questions and discussion. It is recommended that baseline post-assault testing be done anonymously as the assailant may have access to health records and previous HIV infection may be used against the victim. Follow-up testing should begin within 6 weeks of the assault. The vast majority of individuals infected with HIV have detectable antibodies within 3 to 6 months.[36] There is no clear data establishing the efficacy of prompt institution of zidovidine (AZT) prophylaxis.[37]

THE NEED FOR MORE EXTENSIVE TRAINING

Clear and constructive protocols are not enough in guaranteeing better identification, treatment and prevention of sexual violence. As discussed previously, recognition of sexual assault by clinicians is poor. Patient care for those who either disclose their rape or are later identified as victims is suboptimal, especially in regards to information on pregnancy and sexually transmitted diseases, including HIV. Appropriate follow-up for medical issues and counseling is also lacking. Patients are not consistently being given information about STD testing or risks of exposure. Rape in America reports that 39% of victims did not receive information about testing for exposure. In a subgroup analysis of more recent patients, 33% of patients did not receive appropriate information. Despite the significant risk of pregnancy, 60% of rape victims reported that they were not advised about pregnancy testing or how to prevent pregnancy. Finally, even with the increased awareness of HIV, only 50% of rape victims, surveyed in the last 5 years, were given information about HIV.[3]

Both the Surgeon General's Workshop on Violence and Public Health and the Attorney General's Task Force on Family Violence recommend that the medical school curriculum include teaching about violence against women.[38,39] Currently, only 53% of medical school curricula include teaching about domestic violence.[40] A recent national survey of emergency medicine residencies showed only 45% included sexual assault education as part of orientation for new residents. Sixty two percent offered less than one hour of education on evidence collection and 66% included less than one hour on psychosocial sequelae surrounding the assault. Less than 4 hours of any additional training was offered during subsequent years of residency in 63% of the programs.[41]

Education has been shown to increase detection and appropriate treatment for another form of violence against women, domestic violence. A continuous quality improvement model in a busy public emergency department increased detection of domestic violence in women presenting with trauma by twofold.[21] A more intensive mandated interview protocol increased detection of domestic violence from 5.6% to 30%.[22] Figure 11-1 provides an example of such a protocol.

Training on detection and appropriate treatment and referral is necessary for all medical students as well as for all residents in emergency medicine, internal medicine, family practice, obstetrics and gynecology, and psychiatry. Education is also needed for nurses, attending physicians, prehospital providers, physician assistants, nurse practitioners, social workers, and psychologists. Formal education should include both initial training and continuing medical education.

RESEARCH, PREVENTION EDUCATION, and COMMUNITY INVOLVEMENT

Much needs to be done to improve services for victims of sexual violence. Detection is paramount to being able to provide appropriate care. Routine triage questions and routine history and physical questions need to be incorporated into exams of all patients. The addition of chart prompts may be useful especially with more voice dictation modalities and the push for computerized records. Continuous quality improvement can be used to follow compliance with charting more complete sexual histories. Education for all levels of providers is necessary and model curricula need to be developed which emphasize detection, appropriate treatment for pregnancy, STDs including HIV, and rape trauma syndrome. Accreditation of hospitals should be contingent on

Figure 11-1 Flow Diagram for Better Identification of Sexual Assault

Triage: Known Rape Victim?

YES	NO
↓	↓
Follow protocol herein	Assess and evaluate for ED visit

↓

Ask all female patients standard screening questions, e.g., Has anyone made you have sex by using force or threatening to harm you?

↓   ↓

YES   NO

↓   ↓   ↓

≤72 hours   > 72 hours   Share sexual assault prevention education wtih patient

↓   ↓

Follow rape exam protocol herein   Assess patient for physical injuries and for rape trauma syndrome, and refer to follow-up recommended in protocol herein

appropriate implementation of protocols with appropriate and continuous education.

Public education about crimes against women is necessary. Discussion of age-appropriate issues should begin in grade school. Primary prevention programs should be implemented in settings such as prenatal care visits, well-child care visits, and adolescent clinics. Secondary prevention can be implemented with high-risk groups such as alcohol and drug abstinence groups. The emergency medicine provider should take advantage of opportunities to discuss with male patients that it is wrong to force anyone to engage in sexual acts against her or his will. Female patients should be counseled that no one has the right to force one to perform sex acts against one's will and also told of resources available if they are feeling pressured.

Better networking and cooperation is necessary between medical providers, community advocates, and members of the criminal justice system. Many initiatives are created in one sector without communication to other parts of the system. In many communities, there is already a well-developed community-based system of rape crisis centers. These programs offer some combination of crisis intervention, long-term individual and group counseling, medical accompaniment, and legal advocacy. If not already doing so, emergency providers should work closely with these community-based providers to offer a complete continuum of care for sexual assault survivors. Staff from these programs can be a valuable resource for physician, medical student, nursing, and nursing student training. In addition, rape crisis center staff can also provide invaluable support to a victim whose case is in the criminal justice system.

Emergency medicine providers do provide testimony in sexual assault cases and may want to work closely with local prosecutors to familiarize themselves with the criminal justice system. Working in concert with the criminal justice system in certain jurisdictions, the emergency medicine physician has been in the forefront of developing and reevaluating standardized evidence collection kits. This should continue to be encouraged.

CONCLUSION

Emergency medical providers play a key role in providing quality treatment to sexual assault victims and preventing future assaults. It is vital that all providers work to understand the extent of rape in our society and seek to identify those victims who do not initially disclose a history of victimization. With a combination of protocols, training, public education, public policy participation and community coalition-building, emergency medicine professionals can provide a strong line of defense against the growing epidemic of sexual violence in our country.

NOTES

1. Jamieson KM, Flanagan TJ. *Sourcebook of Criminal Justice Statistics—1988.* Washington, DC: U.S. Department of Justice, Bureau of Justice Statistics, 1989.
2. Russell DEH. *Sexual Exploitation.* Beverly Hills, CA: Sage Publications, 1984.
3. National Victim Center and Crime Victims Research and Treatment Center. *Rape in America: A Report to the Nation.* Arlington, VA: National Victim Center, 1992.
4. Ullman SE, Siegel JM. Victim-offender relationship and sexual assault. *Violence and Victims* 1993; 8: 121–34.
5. Stark E, Flitcraft A, Zuckerman D, Grey A, Robinson J, Frazier W. *Wife Abuse in the Medical Setting: An Introduction for Health Personnel.* Washington DC: Office of Domestic Violence, 1981.
6. Frieze IH, Browne A. Violence in marriage. In Ohlin L, Tonry M (eds.). *Family Violence: Crime and Justice, A Review of Research.* Chicago: University of Chicago Press, 1989; pp. 163–218.
7. Santello MD, Leitenberg H. Sexual aggression by an acquaintance: Methods of coping and later psychological adjustment. *Violence and Victims* 1993; 8:91–104.
8. Council on Scientific Affairs, American Medical Association. Violence against women: Relevance for medical practitioners. *JAMA* 1992; 267:3184–9.
9. Bureau of Justice Statistics. *Criminal Victimization in the United States, 1982.* Washington, DC: U.S. Department of Justice, 1984.
10. Ramin SM, Satin AJ, Stone IC, Wendel GD. Sexual assault in postmenopausal women. *Obstetrics and Gynecology* 1992; 80:860–4.
11. Russell DEH. *The Secret Trauma: Incest in the Lives of Girls and Women.* New York: Basic Books, 1986.
12. Koss MP. Detecting the scope of rape: A review of prevalence research methods. *J Interpersonal Violence* 1993; 8:198–222.
13. Moscarello R. Psychological management of victims of sexual assault. *Can J Psychiatry* 1990; 35:25–30.
14. Gise L, Paddison P. Rape, sexual abuse, and its victims. *Psychiatr Clin N America* 1988; 11:629–48.
15. Heinrich L. Care of the female rape victim. *Nurse Practitioner* 1987; 12:9–27.
16. Dunn SFM, Gilchrist VJ. Sexual assault. *Primary Care.* 1993; 20:359–73.
17. Resnick PA, Calhoun KS, Atkeson BM, Ellis EM. Social adjustment in victims of sexual assault. *J Consult Clin Psychol.* 1981; 49:705–12.
18. Burgess AW, Holmstrom LL. Adaptive strategies and recovery from rape. *Am J Psychiatry* 1979; 136:1278–82.
19. Koss MP, Koss PG, Woodruff WJ. Deleterious effects of criminal victimization on women's health and medical utilization. *Arch Intern Med* 1991; 151:342–7.
20. Kimerling R, Calhoun KS. Somatic symptoms, social support, and treatment seeking among sexual assault victims. *J of Consult Clin Psychol* 1994; 62:333–40.
21. Levine DL, Herbert B. CQ1 promotes integration of battered women's protocol. Abstract No. 204, APHA: San Francisco, 1993.
22. McLeer SV, Anwar R. A study of battered women presenting in an emergency department. *Am J Public Health* 1989; 79:65–66.
23. Marchbank PA, Lui KJ, Mercy JA. Risk of injury from resisting rape. *Am J Epidemiol* 1990; 132:540–9.
24. Dupre AR, Hampton HL, Morrison H, Meeks GR. Sexual assault. *OB Gyn Surv* 1993; 45:640–8.
25. Rambow B, Adkinson C, Frost TH, Peterson GF. Female sexual assault: Medical and legal implications. *Ann Emerg Med* 1992; 21:727–31.
26. Deming JE, Mittleman RE, Wetli CV. Forensic science aspects of fatal sexual assaults on women. *J Forensic Sci* 1983; 28:572–6.
27. Schiff AF. A statistical evaluation of rape. *J Forensic Sci* 1973; 2:339.
28. Lauber AA, Souma ML. Use of toluidine blue for documentation of traumatic intercourse. *Obstet Gynecol* 1982; 60:644–8.
29. McCauley J, Guzinski G, Welch R, et al. Toluidine blue in the corroboration of rape in the adult victim. *Am J Emerg Med* 1987; 5:105–8.
30. Geist RF. Sexually related trauma. *Emerg Med Clin N America* 1988; 6:439–66.

31. Yuzpe AA, Smith RP, Rademaker AW. A multicenter clinical investigation employing ethinyl estradiol combined with dl-norgestrel as postcoital contraceptive agent. *Fertil Steril* 1982; 37:508–13.

32. Friedman LS, Samet JH, Roberts MS, Hudlin M, Hans P. Inquiry about victimization experiences: A survey of patient preferences and physician practices. *Arch Inter Med* 1992; 152:1186–90.

33. Resnick HS, Kilpatrick DG, Dansky BS, Saunders BE, Best CL. Prevalence of civilian trauma and posttraumatic stress disorder in a representative national sample of women. *J Consult Clin Psychol* 1993; 61: 984–91.

34. Paone D, Chavkin W, Willets I, Friedmann P, Jarlais, DD. The impact of sexual abuse: Implications for drug treatment. *J of Women's Health* 1992; 1:149–53.

35. Schwarcz SK, Whittington WL. Sexual assault and sexually transmitted diseases: Detection and management in adults and children. *Rev Infect Dis* 1990; 12S6:S682–S690.

36. Jenny C, Hooton TM, Brown A. Sexually transmitted diseases in victims of rape. *NEJM* 1990; 332:713–16.

37. Centers for Disease Control and Prevention. 1993 Sexually Transmitted Diseases Treatment Guidelines. *MMWR* 1993; 42:1–102.

38. U.S. Department of Justice. *Surgeon General's Workshop on Violence and Public Health.* Washington, DC: U.S. Department of Health and Human Services, Public Health Service, 1986.

39. U.S. Department of Justice. *Attorney General's Task Force on Family Violence: Final Report.* Washington, DC: U.S. Department of Justice, 1984.

40. Centers for Disease Control. Education about adult domestic violence in U.S. and Canadian medical schools: 1987–1988. *MMWR* 1989; 38:17–19.

41. Levine DL, D'Onofrio G, Herbert B. The need for structured EM curriculum and management of domestic violence and sexual assault. *Acad Emerg Med* 1995; 2:412.

12

Elder Abuse and Neglect

JEFFREY S. JONES

CONTENTS

CHAPTER SUMMARY

Though the plight of battered spouses and the problem of abused children have been well recognized, another form of domestic violence, elder abuse and neglect, has recently gained the attention of American society. As the number of elderly persons in the United States continues to increase, elder maltreatment (including physical and sexual assault, neglect, abandonment, exploitation, psychological abuse, and violation of personal rights) is being recognized as a major health problem, affecting hundreds of thousands of vulnerable people across all classes of society.

Emergency practitioners are in a unique position to have an impact on maltreatment of elders and can make a major contribution in the early identification of abused or neglected victims. Awareness of the scope of the problem and its manifestations is essential to an effective response. The components of such an awareness include (1) thorough evaluation and accurate detection; (2) knowledge of applicable state legislation; (3) proper interventional procedures; and (4) coordination with available community support services.

The following case illustrates these points and serves as a focus for discussion of the epidemiology, definitions, and classification of elder abuse and neglect. The accompanying protocol provides a framework to aid the emergency department (ED) clinician in the crucial first steps of identification, assessment, and documentation of abusive and high-risk families. The chapter concludes with recommendations for interventional strategies, focusing on providing safe, acceptable alternatives for the elderly victim.

Case #1

Emma Tyson is a 76-year-old blind white female who is brought to the emergency department by ambulance, suffering from a fractured right hip. Concerned neighbors contacted the police when they discovered the patient's caregiver, an alcoholic, had been away from the home for several days. Mrs. Tyson is a widow and has lived with her son for approximately 4 years. The patient is unable to provide additional information because of weakness and dehydration.

Q: How do emergency physicians decide which elderly patients may be victims of abuse or neglect?

The AMA recommends that physicians now routinely ask every patient questions related to elder abuse and neglect.[1] This recommendation is reasonable, given the prevalence of the problem and the tendency for "asymptomatic" family violence to go unrecognized. Even if the patient has a cognitive impairment, it is reasonable to ask about mistreatment. Dementia does not necessarily prevent the elderly patient from describing recent events at home. If the patient cannot answer questions about abuse, the ED physician should seek out an appropriate respondent who is not likely to be a perpetrator.

As with battered women, it is essential that part of the history be obtained while the patient is alone. Excusing the caretaker during the examination will provide privacy. Confidentiality of the interview should be stressed. Developing a level of trust to allow the patient to disclose abuse or neglect is essential. Questions that may be seen as threatening should be deferred until later in the interview.

Medically ill patients, like Mrs. Tyson, constitute the largest portion of abused elderly presenting to the ED.[2,3] Therefore, besides querying patients about the circumstances surrounding their injuries and asking psychiatric patients about their domestic situation, practitioners should explore medical complaints as a screening device for domestic violence. While giving attention to the presenting complaint, the health care provider should include specific questions about the nature of the abusive situation. Many abuse victims could be identified simply by asking patients direct questions such as

> "Are you receiving enough care at home?"
>
> "Has anyone ever scolded or threatened you?"
>
> "Are you afraid of anyone in your family?"
>
> "Has anyone at home ever hurt you?"

Questioning the patient about recent daily routine and activities may reveal a history consistent with abuse, confinement, isolation, environmental exposure, lack of needed appliances (e.g., walker, dentures) or supervision, or other types of neglect. A brief social history may reveal alcohol or drug abuse in the home or other instances of increased caregiver stress. Medical records might indicate previous suspicious injuries or evidence of neglect. Furthermore, an examination of medication bottles and review of the medication history may reveal noncompliance or inappropriate dosing, suggesting neglect or medication abuse.

Q: Why is the diagnosis of elder abuse or neglect often difficult to make in the Emergency Department?

Two major barriers must be overcome in order to diagnose and evaluate cases of elder mistreatment accurately. First, emergency care providers must be aware that the problem exists and that, in the face of present economic and demographic conditions, its prevalence may be increasing. Second, the detection of elder abuse and neglect requires a high index of suspicion. Many of these cases involve only subtle signs, such as poor hygiene or dehydration, and have a great potential to pass undetected.[2]

Multiple factors cause both the elderly victim and family to conceal or minimize the abuse or neglect. The patient may not realize that he or she is a victim of abuse, or, because of dependence upon a caregiver, may fear what may happen to him or her if maltreatment is reported. The abused may also feel at fault for the situation and therefore not pursue any recourse. Furthermore, unlike victims of child abuse or spouse abuse, the elderly are often homebound and hidden from public scrutiny. They often do not come into contact with anyone other than their caregivers because of their lack of mobility. Older women experiencing spousal abuse may be particularly vulnerable, both economically and emotionally, and fear abandonment if their problem surfaces. Furthermore, the domestic violence programs to which a younger woman might turn generally do not have either safe housing or programs oriented toward the needs of older women, especially the very old.

Abusers may accompany the victim to the ED and be reluctant to leave the victim alone with health care workers.[4] When this reluctance is caused by a fear that the maltreatment will be discovered, it is often masked in inappropriate affection or comments that the elder "just doesn't understand." Clinicians should arrange to interview and examine the patient alone, even when the family objects. Every clinical setting should have guidelines that describe the type of information necessary for detecting and reporting cases of elder abuse and neglect. Providers are more likely to inquire about an elderly patient's bruises if they are trained in detecting mistreatment and familiar with the protocol for identifying and reporting suspected victims. Although several excellent protocols are available,[1,2,5–7] few have been subjected to reliability and validity tests.

Q: What additional information might be obtained from prehospital personnel?

Gatekeeper programs are a recommended approach to identifying elderly people at risk for abuse, domestic violence, and neglect.[8] Gatekeepers are people (e.g., postal or utility workers) who have regular contact with the elderly in their homes and could identify those who may need help. A group ideally suited to this case-finding role is prehospital health care providers. The elderly are frequent users of EMS services. Strange and colleagues[9] estimated that of the 11.3 million patients arriving at EDs by ambulance in 1990, 4.1 million (36%) were geriatric patients.

As initial responders to calls for medical assistance, EMS providers can observe the home situation and record problems that they believe warrant further investigation. Indications of neglect include (1) the lack of necessary appliances, such as walkers and bedside commodes; (2) the lack of necessities such as heat, food, and water; (3) unsafe conditions in the home; and (4) caregiver illness. Proper medical care for chronic health problems may have been withheld, or the patient may appear over- or undermedicated (Table 12-1). A recent survey demonstrated that prehospital personnel, despite a lack of training or continuing education, *are* identifying elderly victims of abuse.[10] However, only 27% of these suspected cases are reported. The most common reasons given for not reporting are listed in Table 12-2.

Case Continuation

Clinical assessment in the ED revealed the following information: Mrs. Tyson was found by EMS personnel lying on the floor in her own excrement, probably for days. The home was filthy, and the heat was turned off despite winter temperatures. The patient's primary caregiver was her son, an unemployed teacher with a history of al-

Table 12-1 Clues to Possible Elder Abuse or Neglect Observable by Prehospital Personnel[2,4]

Delay in seeking medical care for illness or injury

Injury inconsistent with history provided

Conflicting reports of injury from patient and caregiver

EMS contacted by someone other than caregiver

History of similar episodes or of other suspicious injuries in the past

Alcohol use, drug abuse, and/or mental illness among family members

Soft tissue injuries (especially burns) in various stages of healing

Malnutrition and/or dehydration

Poor personal hygiene (soiled linens or clothing)

Inappropriate clothing for season

Temperature not properly adjusted for the season

Filthy living quarters

Placed in restraints when no one is in the house

Under- overmedicated

Lack of necessary appliances (dentures, walker, hearing aid)

coholism. He had been away from the home for at least 3 days. Mrs. Tyson could not describe how she fell.

Physical examination revealed tenderness and swelling about the right hip. She also had several large infected decubitus ulcers and signs of dehydration and malnutrition.

Q: When interviewing the primary caregiver (when available), what questions should be addressed?

In assessing the primary caregiver, the ED physician should inquire about lifestyle, family structure, and caregiving skills. Determining whether or not the family understands the patient's medical condition and the necessity of care and medication is crucial to deciding whether inadvertent or willful neglect is involved. Other factors in the caregiver's history that might be factored into such a judgement include excessive use of alcohol or drugs, mental illness in the

Table 12-2 Frequent Reasons for Not Reporting Elder Maltreatment[10]

Unsure which authorities take reports of elder abuse

Unaware of mandatory reporting laws

Concerned about the lack of anonymity

Assume that other professionals (police) will report suspicious cases

Unclear about legal definitions of abuse/neglect

Abuse involved only minor injuries

Do not want to get legally involved

Did not recognize the abuse at the time

Patient denial

Patient's own responsibility to report abuse

Limited knowledge of available community services

Table 12-3 Interview with Possible Perpetrator[7,11]

Introductions—Establish trust and support
"Tell me what you want us to know about your mother."

Determine level of caregiving skills
"What is her medical condition? What medicine does she take?"
"How involved are you with mother's everyday activities and care?"

Identify areas of stress—Financial problems, health impairment, or mental illness
"Please describe a typical day for yourself"
"What responsibilities do you have outside the home?"

Support system
"How do you cope with having to care for your mother all the time?"
"Do you have family support or respite care?"

Future plans—Explore alternatives to the present situation
"Are you prepared to care for your mother should her health decline?"

Corroborate report—Discuss present situation with caregiver
"Is there a reason for waiting this long to seek medical care for your mother?"
"You know those bruises on your mother's arms? How do you suppose she got them?"

residence, alienation, social isolation, poor self-image, and behavior that reveals unmet dependency needs or senility.

The caregiver may resist an interview with the health care provider, but if a protocol is introduced as a standard part of the exam and read to the caregiver by the interviewer, the response may be less defensive, and the individual is less likely to feel unjustly accused of wrongdoing. Harborview Medical Center in Seattle has developed a written script for interviews with potential perpetrators of elder abuse or neglect.[7] The interview is designed to provide a picture of the family situation, stresses, and available resources (Table 12-3).

Q: What are the physical indicators that may alert a physician to elder abuse?

Physical indicators have been described as "observable conditions of the aged person that range from signs of physical neglect to obvious physical injury."[11] Because an adequate history of mistreatment is frequently not obtainable from the older patient, one of the most important aspects of case detection is understanding the physical indicators (Table 12-4). Emergency care providers need to be aware of these signs because of the potential urgency of treating a patient's injury and the necessity of gathering hard

evidence to legitimize and facilitate further interventional steps. The classic symptoms of child abuse do not always pertain to elder abuse cases. For example, improper skin hygiene or bruises in infants indicate abuse; in the case of the elderly, diagnosis must be more circumspect. Because of decreased skin elasticity, minor trauma may result in significant ecchymosis, falsely implying abuse.

Physical injury is the most obvious type of abuse and any ED protocol should call for the documentation of any bruises or burns. Undress the patient completely and look for unusual patterns that might reflect the use of an instrument (i.e., electrical cord, belt buckle), human bite marks, or confinement with ropes or chains. Injuries that appear in different stages of resolution must have multiple explanations to account for them. A knowledge of the stages of

Table 12-4 Common Clinical Signs of Elder Maltreatment

Inappropriate or soiled clothing

Injury that has not received proper care

Malnutrition or dehydration

Decubitus ulcers

Lacerations, abrasions, bruises in various stages of healing

Unusual soft tissue injuries (bite marks, scratches)

Traumatic alopecia or scalp hematomas

Eye injuries or broken teeth

Burns (cigarette, immersion burns)

Evidence of improper restraints (rope marks)

Multiple fractures (spiral fractures, various stages of healing)

Evidence of sexual assault (bruises or bleeding of genitalia)

Sexually transmitted disease

Evidence of improper administration of medication

Emotional status (fearful or agitated, overly quiet and passive, depressed)

healing can contribute to an assessment of the likelihood of intentional injury. The time elapsed since the injury can be estimated by assessing contusions according to the following parameters:

Color of Lesion	Approximate Time Elapsed
Swollen, tender	0–2 days
Red-blue	0–5 days
Green-yellow	5–7 days
Yellow-brown	10 days
Normal tint	3 weeks

Thermal injuries, both burns and cold injuries, can also be suspicious because of their shape and location. The injury may take the shape of common hot objects, such as curling irons, cigarette tips, and heating grills. Scald burns often fit one of three patterns: (1) evidence of immersion without splash marks, and/or a burn that is uniform in depth with a vivid demarcation between burned and unburned tissue; (2) a burn that spares flexed surfaces, since the antecubital fossa is spared when the elbow is im-

mersed into the water; and (3) a burn of the buttocks and genitals from sitting in scalding water.[4]

The presence of a neurologic deficit or abnormal mental status may be due to an unreported head injury. Head injuries, lacerations and abrasions to the face, and trauma to the eyes are frequently encountered in elder abuse and should be treated with a high index of suspicion.[12] Hair loss with ecchymoses at the roots suggests hair being pulled. Eye evaluation may disclose subconjunctival or vitreous hemorrhage, orbital fractures, traumatic cataracts, or visual field deficits. Posttraumatic dentition, mandibular or maxillary fractures, oral burns, and poor dental hygiene should be subject to a more detailed investigation. The neck may also reveal evidence of choking, particularly when linear marks are noted, and tracheal patency must be confirmed.

Ambulation must be observed when possible; painful or unusual gait may reflect signs of sexual assault or occult injuries. As with children, multiple fractures should be investigated as potential abuse. Osteoporosis, falls, metastatic disease, and renal osteodystrophy should be differentiated in these patients from those with traumatic bone fractures.[13] Bilateral injuries to the upper extremities may indicate shaking or an attempt to ward off the abuser. Blunt abdominal trauma may present with Grey Turner's or Cullen's sign, the former characterized by blue-green ecchymosis in the flank 2 to 3 days after trauma, and the latter by blue periumbilical discoloration. Both types of stigmata are indicative of extravasation of intraabdominal hemolyzed blood.

Observe the interaction between the older patient and caregiver. The patient may become fearful or demonstrate a sudden change in behavior when the caregiver is present. The elder may be reluctant to speak for himself or herself, especially while the abuser is present. Overt antagonism may be evident.[12] The caregiver may appear contrite and overly concerned, or be domineering or show a lack of appropriate concern. Either the victim or abuser may have overt clinical signs (irritability, crying, silence) indicative of depression or social withdrawal.[13]

Q: What physical findings are consistent with neglect?

Physical neglect should be suspected if the physical examination shows the aged patient is malnourished, dehydrated, or has wasting of subcutaneous tissue. These problems are common among frail and immobile elderly, however, and are therefore difficult to associate with abuse by the caretaker. Nail care may be a sensitive barometer in evaluating hygiene negligence. Except in debilitated patients, decubitus ulcers are usually preventable and their presence suggests neglect. Improper care of medical problems, untreated injuries, poor hygiene, and inappropriate dress for the weather require care to discriminate, if possible, the effects of poverty from those of neglect.[2] Either case necessitates involvement of social services.

Q: What laboratory data might be necessary in the assessment of suspected cases of elder maltreatment?

Laboratory data are needed in the evaluation of the chief complaint, as well as for the assessment of cases of suspected elder mistreatment. The workup may include metabolic screening for nutritional, electrolyte, or endocrine abnormalities; hematologic, and coagulation studies to assess abnormal bruising or bleeding tendencies; a urinalysis to rule out urinary system trauma; and a toxicologic or drug-level screen to determine over- or undermedication. The laboratory evaluation of the elderly patient suspected of having been sexually abused may include serology and cultures for sexually transmitted disease. Collection of evidence should follow standards for suspected rape.

Radiologic studies appropriate for the short-term management of the older patient must be obtained. X-rays can be invaluable in identifying previously undetected fractures and may indicate the "age" of the trauma. All elders with suspected abuse plus any patient with documented radiologic injuries should have survey films taken. Special signs to look for include periosteal thickening and transverse or oblique fractures of the midshafts of long bones and fingers. A computerized tomography (CT) scan may be necessary if there has been a major change in neurologic status or head trauma.

Case Continuation

Initial treatment in the ED included oxygen supplementation, intravenous hydration, antibiotics, tetanus im- *munization, and local wound care. Diagnostic radiographs revealed an acute fracture of the right femoral neck as well as multiple healing rib fractures of varying ages.*

Mrs. Tyson was subsequently admitted to the hospital for 15 days. On hospital discharge, she refused protective services and returned home with her son. Arrangements were made for a visiting nurse to check on Mrs. Tyson every other day for 2 weeks. The son was given information on various alcohol treatment programs in the community.

Q: What can be done if elderly patients refuse protective services?

The older adult has the right to refuse protective services and may elect to return home with his or her family.[14] Unless a court issues a finding of incompetence and appoints a temporary guardian, elders are assumed to be able to judge their own needs. This differs from child abuse, in which the government assumes the right to intervene, if necessary, without regard to the parents. Upon discharge from the ED, the health care provider should attempt to modify the home situation by involving other family members to unburden the stressed caregiver, contact the appropriate reporting agency, and ensure involvement of social service authorities to guarantee a timely follow-up home visit (i.e., visiting nurse, social worker).[4] The key to getting help for nonconsenting elders is to gain the elder's trust and/or be able to work with the family and significant others in the elder's life. In some cases, providers may be able to reach the elder by asking a person close to the patient to explain the need for services. In all cases, victims should be counseled that violence may escalate, and that the physician is a potential source of help.

Q: What community resources should be mobilized?

Once it has been determined whether or not the elder is capable of and willing to take action, a range of intervention alternatives may be considered. Among the community social services that should be available are: case management, home health services, alternative housing, legal intervention, police protection and cooperation, and counseling (for the abused and the abuser). Although the family is often the source of the abuse, it is still potentially the most nurturing source of long-term care for the elderly person.[15] Efforts should be directed toward assisting the stressed caregiver to cope with the role and to prevent the occurrence of situations that might lead to abuse. Drug and alcohol programs may help those caregivers dependent on such substances. If additional skilled help is required for the care of the victim, this can be arranged with the local visiting nurses association or home health service of the hospital. Emergency care providers must take the responsibility of educating themselves about various local community social and health services available (Table 12-5). In some cases, it may be clear as to what steps need to be taken in order to halt the abuse or prevent further abuse from occurring. In other cases it may be necessary to convene a team comprising various disciplines to brainstorm possible solutions and facilitate decision making.[1] The patient's primary care physician can participate in ongoing management or at least provide follow-up after a referral has been made and serve as a monitor who can reactivate assistance if the situation is deteriorating.

Table 12-5 High-Risk Situations Conducive to Mistreatment

Alcohol or drug abuse, and/or mental illness among family members

Physical, functional, or cognitive problems in caregiver that may prevent them from providing proper care

Elderly persons whose primary caregiver is under severe external stress (loss of job, personal illness, divorce)

Families with a history of domestic violence (spouse, child abuse)

Caregiver demonstrates poor impulse control

Caregiver is forced by circumstances to care for elder who is unwanted

Caregiver is unemployed, without sufficient funds, or dependent on the elder for housing and money

Increasing care needs because of progressive or unstable conditions, such as Alzheimer's disease, parkinsonism, or severe stroke that exceeds the caretaker's ability to cope

Elderly victim exhibits problematic behavior: incontinence, shouting, paranoia

GENERAL DISCUSSION

Prevalence

"How many elders in the United States have been abused or neglected?" is one of the questions most frequently asked about elder abuse. Unfortunately, even after more than a decade of elder abuse research, the exact answer is unknown. Among the early attempts to estimate the prevalence of elder abuse and neglect, Block and Sinnott found 40/1,000 in Maryland,[16] and Gioglio and Blakemore reported 15/1,000 in New Jersey.[17] The Maryland survey gave rise to the widely cited figure of 4% of elderly people who suffer abuse. However, because the response rate was so low and the final sample so small, the authors concluded that the findings were essentially invalid.

The most complete study to date is the Pillemer and Finkelhor prevalence study,[18] which was based on a random, stratified sample of all community dwelling persons 65 years and over in the metropoli-

tan Boston area. Over 2,000 persons were contacted, either by telephone or in person, and asked about their experience with three types of mistreatment. The survey found that 3.5% of elderly Boston residents had been mistreated, by physical abuse (2%), verbal aggression (1.1%), and neglect (0.4%). The investigators also demonstrated that spouse abuse was more prevalent (58%) than abuse by adult children (24%) and that economic status or age was not related to the risk of abuse. Among virtually all studies, women are reportably abused or neglected more often than men. In the Boston survey, however, men reported more abuse but appeared to suffer less serious injuries and less emotional stress. This hypothesis may account for the larger proportion of women than men among the victims reported to protective service agencies.

Elizabeth Podnieks and colleagues[19] repeated the Boston study as a national prevalence study in Canada a few years later, with two major changes. Financial exploitation was added as a category of mistreatment, and the in-home interviews for those who were unable to respond on the telephone were eliminated. The survey, which reached 2,086 elderly persons living in private dwellings, reported that approximately 4% of the elderly population experienced some serious form of maltreatment at the hands of a spouse, relative, or significant other. The most common form was financial exploitation (2.5%), then verbal aggression (1%), followed by physical violence (0.6%) and neglect (0.4%). Exclusion of persons unable to answer a phone survey may account for the low number of physical violence cases compared to the Boston results. Lower physical violence rates also are not unexpected, since similar findings have been noted when other Canadian and United States violence and crime statistics are compared.

If the Canadian prevalence rate for financial exploitation is added to the U.S. data, then the total rate for the four types of mistreatment (physical, psychological, financial, and neglect) would be about 5.7%. While the exact number of cases may not be known, it seems reasonable to say that, at the very minimum, 5 out of 1,000 older persons are mistreated. A central problem in obtaining national incidence data is the absence of uniform legal statutes, reporting requirements, definitions, and methods of record-keeping. Basing its projections on data compiled from a nationwide survey of elder abuse reports, the National Aging Resource Center on Elder Abuse (NARCEA) estimated that nearly 1.57 million older people were abused in 1991.[20] This estimate was arrived at by determining the substantiated number of abuse cases nationwide (112,415 people) and multiplying that number by 14, the number arrived at by Pillemer and Finkelhor[18] based on their estimate that only 1 out of 14 cases of elder abuse is reported.

Underlying the growing concern about elder abuse and neglect is the realization that this problem is just in its "infancy." By the year 2000, the number of Americans aged 65 to 75 is expected to increase by 23% and the number of those aged 75 and older by 40%.[21] This increased population will have longer life expectancies and will therefore require personal care for longer periods of time. In addition, the increasing geographical mobility and growing number of two-income families are trends that significantly reduce the number of caregivers available for the care of older adults. These factors suggest that the problem of elder mistreatment will increase.

Definitions

From the very beginning of scientific investigation into the nature and causes of elder abuse, definitions have been a major issue.[22] Lack of agreement on the precise meaning of "elder abuse" has made it impossible to compare research findings from early studies. Even greater variability is evident in state protective service laws. Without federal legislation for elder abuse, each state has established its own definitions, clinical criteria and reporting systems. In the extreme, this can mean 50 variations on a theme. Some states do not use the word *abuse* and an act may be defined as abuse in one state but not in another. Neglect is defined even more broadly, with some state laws focusing on intent and others on consequences. Difficulties in compiling national incidence data and in transferring specific model programs between states are only some of the problems that stem from the lack of common elder abuse definitions.[23] The American Medical Association has described elder abuse and neglect as "actions or the omission of actions that result in harm or threatened harm to the health or welfare of the elderly."[1] At least 33 different types of elder abuse (from endangerment to passive neglect) have been described in various studies, but all can be condensed into five primary categories: physical abuse, neglect, psychological abuse, violation of personal rights, and financial abuse.[2]

Physical abuse.   Physical abuse or battery involves acts of violence that may result in pain, injury, impairment, or disease.[1] This includes beatings, deliberate burns, sexual assault, force feeding, and unreasonable physical restraint. Emergency physicians should suspect physical abuse when the older patient presents with unexplained injuries, delays in seeking care for an injury, or the history provided by the patient or caregiver is inconsistent with the medical findings (see Tables 12-3 and 12-4). In one prevalence study, 63% of the victims described being pushed, shoved, or grabbed; 45% had something thrown at them; 42% were slapped; and 10% were bitten or kicked.[24]

Neglect.   This category of elderly abuse seems far more common than deliberate injury. Neglect of the elderly raises difficult questions about who exactly the responsible caregiver is, what his or her precise responsibilities are to the neglected person, and whether the neglect was intentional or unintentional. Examples include withholding personal care, medical therapy, or mechanical aids (e.g., walker, dentures) that enable an older adult to thrive in the community. Nonambulatory patients may be left unattended for long periods, resulting in vermin infestation and decubitus ulcers.

Victims of neglect tend to be in poorer health than victims of psychological or physical abuse. As such, abuse by neglect is found more frequently in debilitated elderly patients and is more common than physical abuse in nursing home residents. Persons in good health are often able to do something about the deprivation, whereas the bedridden cannot. The study by Kimsey and colleagues cites anecdotal evidence expanding these observations.[25]

Self-inflicted neglect presents ethical problems because older adults, unlike children, can choose their own lifestyle. Therefore, self-neglect may stem from an older person's decision not to accept funds, services, or medical care.[13] The right to self-determination is relinquished only if and when the older adult is legally declared incapable or incompetent. Self-neglect will probably continue to be the type of abuse most often detected and the most challenging for emergency care providers to treat.

Psychological abuse. Emotional or mental mistreatment occurs on a more subtle level but is not necessarily less damaging than physical abuse. Infantilization; derogation; social isolation; and threats of institutionalization, abandonment, and homicide fall under this category. Fear may be provoked when family members, who are aware of their power over the aged, use subtle or obvious pressures and threats to force the elderly to conform. Distinguishing this abusive behavior from hostile or resentful communication can be difficult.[4]

Psychological abuse is difficult to measure, especially if the victim is suffering from mental impairment. Behavioral signs include passivity, withdrawal, depression, or agitation. The elder may act confused, disoriented, and fearful; or show signs of infantile behavior in the presence of the caregiver. At times, questions asked of the elder will be deferred to the caregiver, or when a stressful topic is broached, the elder may suddenly change the subject.

Violation of personal rights. This type of abuse occurs when caretakers or providers ignore the older person's inalienable or legal rights and capacity to make decisions for himself or herself.[1] Typical examples of this behavior include the refusal to grant the older adult privacy, denying self-determination or decision making regarding personal issues, or forcible eviction and/or placement in a nursing home.

Financial abuse. Financial abuse, or exploitation, usually occurs in one of two forms.[26] It may be the misuse of the elderly person's funds by another person, usually a caregiver or close relative, or a caregiver may withhold medical attention or refrain from making necessary expenditures for the elderly person's benefit. Money saved to provide for retirement needs may be used by the family for other purposes, sometimes with the result of depriving the aged person of basic needs. Financial abuse should be suspected if the patient is suffering from substandard care in the home despite adequate financial resources, medical bills are not being paid, or if the patient seems confused or unaware of his or her financial situation. Older adults are particularly susceptible to this type of mistreatment, yet it may be the most difficult to identify.[1]

The majority of victims suffer from more than one type of mistreatment. Not only does one incident lead to another, but the occurrence of one form of abuse or neglect appears to provoke other forms.[26]

Etiology and Social Context

During the past 20 years, investigators have turned their attention towards identifying risk factors for elder mistreatment both for older adults and their caregivers. These risk factors are based on etiologic theories or explanations for the occurrence of elder abuse and neglect. Unfortunately, these theories are generally based on small retrospective studies and nonrepresentative samples. Nevertheless, awareness of such factors, and the theories underlying them, may help health care professionals understand, recognize, and prevent situations in which elder mistreatment may occur.

Perhaps the easiest theory of all to understand is that of the psychopathology of the abuser.[14] According to this theory, abusers have personality traits or character disorders that cause them to be abusive. A provider who is mentally retarded, has a psychiatric disorder, or is a substance abuser may not have the capacity to make appropriate judgments regarding the older person's needs.

A related explanation underlying elder mistreatment is that of transgenerational violence, which asserts that violence is a learned behavior in some families. In a Detroit study of 77 cases of elder abuse, 10.4% of the documented cases showed clear evidence of mutual abuse between family members.[27] In this vicious cycle, family members alternatively reinforce the abusive behavior of one another.

A third theory emphasizes stress as an important factor in elder mistreatment. Many duties and responsibilities that are associated with providing care for elderly persons may place overwhelming demands on providers. They may have to give up previous lifestyles, social relationships, and possibly jobs to be home to care for the older adult. These stressors may cause the abuser to lash out in anger or slowly transfer personal enmities to an elder scapegoat.[26] The abused may have behavioral problems (i.e., nighttime shouting) that contribute to stress at home.[2]

Theories of impairment and consequent dependency underlie much of the analysis of child abuse.[15] The inability of the elderly person to do some activities of daily living leads to dependency and consequent vulnerability to abuse and neglect by a caregiver. It has been suggested that as these needs increase, the burden and the stress level of caregivers increase.[13] In one sample of 240 elderly clients referred for intensive home supports because of significant unmet needs, 17% were reported to have been abused or severely neglected.[28] Evolving changes in the delivery of health care have increased pressure for shorter hospital stays and may result in early discharges of elderly patients. It is important to consider whether early discharge adds to home caregiver stress and contributes to elder abuse, since these patients may require extensive care at home and, therefore, be at high risk for abuse.[14]

Other authorities point out that the caregiver may be dependent, especially economically, on the older adult.[1] This dependency may lead to resentment and, when combined with caregiver stress, may predispose to violence. Other potential causes for abuse and neglect include: a lack of knowledge (or misinformation) by caregivers, ageism, greed, social isolation of the victim, and lack of community support.

Most of the etiologic theories used to explain elder mistreatment can also be applied to formal caregivers (such as nursing home personnel). Although abuse and neglect in institutional settings cannot be ignored, the vast majority of elder care is given by family members living in the same household. Seventy percent of the population more than 60 years of age reside with family members; 25% live on their own in the community; and only 5% reside in institutions.[29] With these statistics in mind, no one should be surprised to learn that most abusers are the relatives of the older person—that is, a spouse, a child, a grandchild, or a sibling. Approximately 60% of the abusers (or neglecters) are spouses of victims, and about 24% are adult children.[18] In a review of the literature, Hudson and Johnson conclude that the "pioneering studies have uncovered an important fact about elder abuse and neglect—they are primarily family affairs."[30]

High-risk situations conducive to elder mistreatment are summarized in Table 12-5. Further study remains to be done to identify with precision the highest-risk groups and to identify marker conditions for elder mistreatment.

Documentation

Thorough, well-documented medical records provide concrete evidence and may prove to be crucial to the outcome of any legal case. Documentation should include the following historical factors and clinical findings:[1,2]

- Chief complaint and description of the abusive event or neglectful situation using the patient's own words whenever possible. If patient, caregiver, or other informants (EMS, police) give different histories, document what is said by each.

- Past medical history. Include other current problems, severe cognitive and/or physical impairment requiring extended care, history of previous abuse or neglect, repetitive admissions because of injuries or poor health.

- Relevant social history. Include recent household crises or conflicts; determine the patient's dependence on the caregiver.
- A detailed description of injuries with possible causes and explanations given. Take color photographs whenever possible or record the location and nature of the injuries on a body chart or drawing.
- Results of all pertinent laboratory and other diagnostic procedures.
- An opinion on whether the injuries were adequately explained.
- If the police are called, the name of the investigating officer and any actions taken.

Informed consent should be obtained with regard to several aspects of the evaluation including taking photographs and the release of medical records to authorities.

Crisis Intervention

If an emergency health care provider suspects elder mistreatment, proper intervention will depend on the type of mistreatment, its severity, the victim's desire to remain at home, and the caregiver's interest in improving the home environment. Immediate action is needed in cases where the magnitude of abuse and neglect may lead to permanent physical or mental damage. Hospitalization is warranted in these high-risk situations and is more likely to be accepted by the elder and family as treatment for a specific problem (i.e., dehydration, decubiti) rather than as protection from further harm.[2] Hospitalization then provides adequate time and opportunity to define the actual care needs of the patient and arrange for necessary services.

If the patient is in no immediate danger, crisis intervention should be guided by choosing the alternatives that least restrict the patient's independence and decision-making responsibilities (Figure 12-1). Reporting suspected abuse to state authorities, either in accordance with legislative requirements or voluntarily, enlists the assistance of Adult Protective Services, whose professional staff members have expertise in this area. Geriatric assessment clinics, which conduct multidisciplinary evaluations that are typically focused on the patient and caregiver, are also appropriate for this purpose if they are available.

These specialists may have important referral information for patients or family members—support groups and other services in the community that focus on aging parents, home care, substance abuse, family violence, and financial and legal planning. Perhaps most important, physicians need to become familiar with long-term care and in-home health service options in their communities.

For patients who no longer retain decision-making capacity, the court may need to appoint a conservator or guardian to make decisions about finances, living arrangements, and care. Typically, the state Adult Protective Services agency participates with the patient's clinician in these proceedings.

Legal Considerations

All emergency care providers should become familiar with applicable elder mistreatment laws and the procedure for referring a suspected case. An Alabama survey revealed that a majority of emergency department personnel did not understand the state's mandatory reporting law.[31] In most states, there is a designated agency—generally, the local adult protective services unit of the state department of social services—but in some areas, it may be a private agency. Providers may be unaware of the mandatory reporting laws that have been enacted in 46 states and the District of Columbia, most within the past 8 years.[32] Only four states (Colorado, New York, Wisconsin, and Illinois) have voluntary reporting laws; that is, they state abuse "may be reported" instead of mandating that it "shall be reported." In every law, the physician is either named specifically as a reporter or included with others as "any person with knowledge of, or who reasonably suspects abuse." At least 30 state statutes contain penalties for the failure to report, which range from fines of up to $1,000 to a maximum of 6 months' imprisonment.

The issue of mandatory reporting of elder abuse and neglect is still being debated by practitioners in the field. While mandatory reporting has proven to be a valuable tool in child abuse, some authorities maintain that it deters elderly persons from seeking needed medical care and other assistance. Although these laws vary from state to state, they typically provide no funds that would allow for meaningful intervention in abuse or neglect situations.[23] While the states spend an average of $22 per child for pro-

Figure 12-1 Case Management of Abused or Neglected Elderly Patients[1,15]

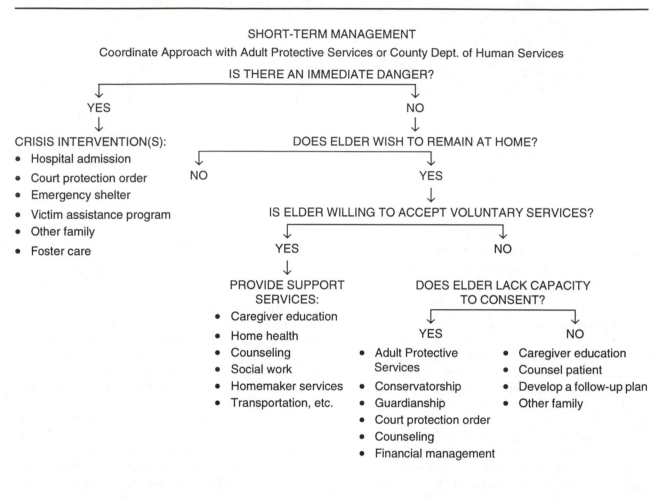

SHORT-TERM MANAGEMENT

Coordinate Approach with Adult Protective Services or County Dept. of Human Services

IS THERE AN IMMEDIATE DANGER?

YES

NO

CRISIS INTERVENTION(S):
- Hospital admission
- Court protection order
- Emergency shelter
- Victim assistance program
- Other family
- Foster care

DOES ELDER WISH TO REMAIN AT HOME?

NO

YES

IS ELDER WILLING TO ACCEPT VOLUNTARY SERVICES?

YES

NO

PROVIDE SUPPORT SERVICES:
- Caregiver education
- Home health
- Counseling
- Social work
- Homemaker services
- Transportation, etc.

DOES ELDER LACK CAPACITY TO CONSENT?

YES

NO

- Adult Protective Services
- Conservatorship
- Guardianship
- Court protection order
- Counseling
- Financial management

- Caregiver education
- Counsel patient
- Develop a follow-up plan
- Other family

tective services, only $2.90 is spent for each elderly person.[14] Laws that mandate reporting but do not provide adequate resources or protective services may actually inflict harm by creating false expectations.

For physicians and other health care providers who are protected by privileged communication statutes, mandatory reporting of abuse and neglect presents another dilemma. It may be necessary to violate the law or to break the trust of a patient and possibly jeopardize a therapeutic relationship.[26] The AMA suggests that the provider should explain to the patient that he or she is obligated to report suspected mistreatment and strive to maintain a positive provider-patient relationship, keeping in mind the

medical need for intervention.[1] The goal is not to punish the individual or family but to stop the abuse or neglect and to assure access to help in the form of outside resources. All states protect the health care provider from civil or criminal liability for the content of the report.[26] Most of these laws have added that the provider must have acted "in good faith" or performed their duties with "reasonable competence."

On the other side of the issue is the question of whether a provider may be liable for not reporting suspected elder abuse or neglect. No tort as yet addresses this liability issue. However, based on the provider's documented legal responsibility concerning child abuse, there is a good chance that providers can be held responsible for subsequent abuse if the elderly person's ability to escape the situation is questionable.[23,26]

Most states have resource hotlines that both physicians and patients can call with questions about maltreatment of the elderly. Clinicians should consult state government directories under the listing "Adult Protective Services" or "Department of Aging" or contact the National Center on Elder Abuse (c/o American Public Welfare Association, 810 First St. NE, Suite 500, Washington, DC 20002).

NOTES

1. Aravanis SC, Adelman RD, Breckman R et al. *Diagnostic and Treatment Guidelines on Elder Abuse and Neglect.* Chicago: American Medical Association, 1992.
2. Jones J, Dougherty J, Schelble D. Emergency department protocol for the diagnosis and evaluation of geriatric abuse. *Ann Emerg Med* 1988; 17:1006–15.
3. Goldberg WG, Tomlanovich MC. Domestic violence victims in the emergency department: New findings. *JAMA* 1984; 251:3259–64.
4. Stewart C, Stewart C, Jones J, Weissberg M. Confronting the grim realities of elder abuse and neglect. *Emerg Med Reports* 1991; 12:179–86.
5. Aravanis SC, Adelman RD, Breckman R et al. *Diagnostic and Treatment Guidelines on Elder Abuse and Neglect.* Chicago: American Medical Association, 1992.
6. *Elder Mistreatment Guidelines for Health Care Professionals: Detection, Assessment, and Intervention.* New York: Mount Sinai/Victim Services Agency Elder Abuse Project, 1988.
7. *Elder Abuse Diagnostic and Intervention Protocol.* Seattle, Harborview Medical Center, 1990.
8. Gerson LW, Schelble DT, Wilson JE. Using paramedics to identify at-risk elderly. *Ann Emerg Med* 1992; 21:688–91.
9. Strange GR, Chen EH, Sanders AB. Use of emergency departments by elderly patients: Projections from a multicenter data base. *Ann Emerg Med* 1992; 21:819–24.
10. Jones J, Walker G, Krohmer J. To report or not to report: Emergency services response to elder abuse. *Prehosp Disaster Med* 1995; in press.
11. Sengstock MC, O'Brien JG, Goldynia AM, Trainer T, deSpelder TG, Lienhart KW. *Elder Abuse Assessment and Management for the Primary Care Physician.* East Lansing, MI: Office of Medical Education, Research and Development, Michigan State University, 1990, pp. 51–6.
12. Rathbone-McCuan E, Voyles B. Case detection of abused elderly parents. *Am J Psychiatry* 1982; 139:189–92.
13. Benton D, Marshall C. Elder abuse. *Clin Geriatr Med* 1991; 7:831–45.
14. Council on Scientific Affairs: Elder abuse and neglect. *JAMA* 1987; 257:966–71.
15. O'Malley TA, Everitt DE, O'Malley HC, et al. Identifying and preventing family-mediated abuse and neglect of elderly persons. *Ann Intern Med* 1983; 98:998–1005.
16. Block MR, Sinnott JD. *The Battered Elder Syndrome: An Exploratory Study.* College Park, MD: Center on Aging, University of Maryland, 1979.
17. Gioglio GR, Blakemore P. *Elder Abuse in New Jersey: The knowledge and experience of abuse among older New Jerseyans.* Trenton: Department of Human Services, 1983.
18. Pillemer K, Finkelhor D. The prevalence of elder abuse: A random sample survey. *Gerontol* 1988; 28:51–7.
19. Podnieks E, Pillemer K, Nicholson JP, Shillington T, Frizzell A. *National Survey on Abuse of the Elderly in Canada: Final Report.* Toronto: Ryerson Technical Institute, 1990.
20. Tatara T. *Summaries of the statistical data on elder abuse in domestic settings for FY90 and FY91.* Washington, DC: National Aging Resource Center on Elder Abuse, 1993.
21. Sanders AB. Care of the elderly in emergency departments: Where do we stand? *Ann Emerg Med* 1992; 21:792–5.
22. Wolf RS. Elder abuse: Ten years later. *J Am Geriatr Soc* 1988; 36:758–62.
23. Brewer RA, Jones JS. Reporting elder abuse: Limitations of statutes. *Ann Emerg Med* 1989; 18:1217–21.
24. Kosberg JI. Preventing elder abuse: Identification of high-risk factors prior to placement decisions. *Gerontologist* 1988; 28:43–50.
25. Kimsey LR, AR, Bragg DF. Abuse of the elderly—the hidden agenda. I. The caretakers and the categories of abuse. *J Am Geriatr Soc* 1981; 29:465–72.
26. Palincsar J, Cobb DC. The physician's role in detecting and reporting elder abuse. *J Leg Med* 1982; 3:413–41.
27. Sengstock M, Liang J. *Identifying and Characterizing Elder Abuse, Final Report Submitted to the NRTA-AARP Andrus Foundation.* Detroit: Institute of Gerontology, Wayne State University, 1982.
28. Shaughnessy PW, Kramer AM. The increased needs of patients in nursing homes and patients receiving home health care. *N Engl J Med* 1990; 322:21–7.
29. Movsas TZ, Movsas B. Abuse versus neglect: A model to understand the causes of and treatment

strategies for mistreatment of older persons. *Issues Law & Medicine* 1990; 6:163–73.

30. Hudson MF, Johnson TF. Elder neglect and abuse: A review of the literature. *Ann Rev Gerontol Geriatr* 1986; 6:81–134.

31. Clark-Daniels DR, Baumhover L. Abuse and neglect of the elderly: Are emergency department personnel aware of mandatory reporting laws? *Ann Emerg Med* 1990; 19:970–7.

13

Emergency Department Staff as Victims

ERIC S. FREEDLAND
MICHAEL TARMEY
MARK DAVIS
KENNETH SAVAGE
KATHLEEN HIGGINS

CONTENTS

- ED violence, a crisis for providers
- Coping with patient and provider anger
- Factors contributing to ED violence
- Strategies for avoiding and containing violence
- Safety training
- Communications skills
- Restraint protocols
- Critical incident debriefing

CHAPTER SUMMARY

Violence in America is a public health emergency; more than 1.6 million individuals in the U.S. are victims of assault each year, and many of them are treated in the ED.[1] Verbal and physical abuse toward the emergency department health care provider presents a crisis in our profession and a threat to our well-being. Significant numbers of medical staff injuries and even deaths have been described as the result of violent acts in the ED. A recent study confirms that violence and the threat to personal safety are major concerns of EM residents, many of whom did not believe that their hospital or residency program provided adequate security.[2]

This chapter presents an overview of the problem of violence against ED health care providers. Two case studies examine the challenges of abusive confrontation and the responses elicited from both provider and patient. Inappropriate responses are critiqued, and a model of optimal conflict resolution presented. The public health implications and the present lack of adequate training in dealing with the potential for violence are both discussed. A case is made for approaching every patient with *universal precautions:* a heightened awareness for potential violence, a safe approach, a plan, and skill in verbal and physical assessment techniques. Adoption of universal precautions will result in protection for both practitioner and patient.

Case #1:

At 3:00 a.m. on a busy Saturday morning, Dr. Jones is asked by the triage nurse to deescalate the following situation. Mr. Martino is a 40-year-old owner of a construction company who is complaining of severe low back pain, which has been getting progressively worse. He is unable to sleep or get comfortable. Mr. Martino has been waiting for 3 hours in the ED waiting room, pacing back and forth. He is tired of waiting, in severe pain, and demands to speak with whoever is in charge.

Mr. M (shouting): Are you the doctor in charge?

Dr. J (impatiently): Yes, I am, what's the problem?

Mr. M: I've been waiting over 3 hours!

Dr. J (loudly): Could you please lower your voice? We are very busy! Can't you see how busy it's been, and how sick some of the other patients are?

Mr. M (angrily): Well, I am in great pain! Can't you see how I'm hunched over? I can barely walk. If I can't get my problem taken care of by you people, then I am going somewhere else. I have insurance.

Dr. J (annoyed): We'll get to you as soon as we can!

Mr. M (walking toward the door): Well, I'm leaving and going somewhere else if you can't do anything for me now!

Dr. J (impatiently): Well, you're welcome to go somewhere else.

Mr. M: I'm outta here! (He leaves.)

Q: Does this patient have a need for emergency department care?

Emergency medicine serves everyone regardless of social or financial status. When the patient self-defines as an emergency, ED staff must then provide necessary evaluation, treatment, appropriate reassurance, and optimal disposition. Patients evaluate symptoms based on subjective, or "feeling," data that include a much larger perspective of emotional, physical, and social needs than the provider is accustomed to evaluating from his professional, objective, or fact-based perspective. When there is conflict between these two worldviews, one position does *not* devalue the other. An illness may not be life-threatening in the eyes of the practitioner, but it is still person-threatening. When these impasses occur, there is a need to deepen the level of patient-practitioner communication.

Q: Why is it important to pursue nonemergency complaints in the ED setting?

In the specialty of emergency medicine, it is the patient who determines that an emergency exists. Some complaints may seem trivial to an observer and might be handled as well or better by a primary care provider in a less acute setting. However, even a seemingly rather benign complaint can mask a serious underlying disorder. In the case of a patient with back pain, one must rule out potentially life-threatening and debilitating conditions such as multiple

myeloma, metastatic disease, herniated disc with cord compression, osteomyelitis, discitis, urinary tract infection, renal stone, or a ruptured abdominal aortic aneurysm.

Certainly a confrontational discussion with this patient is inadequate to elicit the emergent nature of the problem. The complaint of severe pain must lead to further clinical evaluation and appropriate treatment of the pain. An angry patient may be agitated or have serious psychosocial issues such as cocaine use that should be evaluated with great care. An illustration of this is the landmark Libby Zion case,[3] in which a young woman's fatal medical condition was initially, mistakenly, determined to be an agitated state and a behavioral issue.

Q: How appropriate is this patient's anger?

When we consider the appropriateness of a patient's expressed anger, we must consider that all anger is appropriate. It is an honest emotion. A patient who has waited in pain without evaluation or treatment has the right to the legitimate emotion of anger. How he chooses to express that anger is open to discussion and negotiation, and, if all else fails, restraint may be necessary. Unequivocally, the patient does *not* have the right to assault a health care provider.

Q: What about the provider's anger?

By the same token, it is acceptable for the provider to feel anger when confronted in a hostile manner but not to behave in kind and provoke the patient. We too, are entitled to our legitimate emotions. Emotions are partly determined by our thoughts; if we can exercise control over our thoughts, then we can, to a large degree, control our emotions. The ideal strategy, which is not always easy to master, is to not personalize the attack but rather to recognize it as a suffering patient's expression of pain. A better response to this patient would have been:

Case Continuation

The next day, when Dr. Jones has caught up on his sleep, he is able to handle the same situation much better. In this next confrontation, he attempts to legitimize the patient's anger in a calming tone of voice, saying "I can see why you are angry. Waiting 3 hours while you are in such pain is unreasonable. I'm sorry. Let's see how we can make this right." He turns to the nurse and says, "Let's see this patient right away, even if it is out of turn, if possible. He seems to need reassurance, and maybe there's more to his problem than it appears."

Q: What might have prevented the first situation from getting out of hand?

Confronting the patient with anger will usually serve to escalate the situation. One can choose to practice personal detachment and to suspend the ego. The hostile interaction might have been prevented altogether if a patient advocate, in the form of a nurse or other staff member, served as a liaison and constantly updated waiting patients and family regarding the length of wait and reasons for the delay. A simple display of rapport, empathy, and understanding of the patient's suffering can prevent or defuse an escalating hostile situation and protect all parties.

Q: What are the rights of ED providers and what procedures can be introduced to enhance safety?

The emergency department health care provider, in accordance with OSHA and JCAHO mandates, has the right to work in a safe environment.[4] To ensure this, we must take a proactive approach in establishing procedures and policies. All ED personnel must receive education and training in self-protection, recognition, and management of violence. Well-trained, experienced security personnel, stationed on site, are preferable. These officers must have considerable skill in verbal deescalation and physical restraint techniques. Security audits should occur routinely, and consideration should be given to such physical measures as strategically located emergency alert systems, controlled and monitored access, metal detectors, and bullet-proof, glassed-in triage stations.[5]

Case #2

Mr. Russell is a 25-year-old white male who is obviously agitated, but cooperative, and admits to chronic and recent IV cocaine use. He presents with a fever of 102.4°F, shaking chills, and drenching sweats. The physician is quite occupied with a serious trauma in the

next room, but, in passing, sticks his head into the cubicle and gives the nurse, Ms. Lasser, a rapid order to start an IV. Neither he nor the nurse have introduced themselves. The nurse goes out to get the necessary equipment, and she is gone quite a while because of competing demands. She comes back with the tray, puts on gloves, sits down at the bedside, and grabs Mr. Russell's right arm. He does not understand what she is doing, perceives her hold on his arm as a physical threat, pulls his arm away and attempts to punch her.

Q: Could this assault have been avoided?

Possibly, but not necessarily. Clearly both providers are at fault for not introducing themselves, attempting to obtain rapport, and explaining their actions. Both the history of substance abuse and the anxiety and confusion that accompany a serious infection predispose to miscommunication and a potential for violence that should have been recognizable before the event occurred. But the assault might have been attempted even if both providers had acted in exemplary fashion.

Q: When the patient's behavior is inappropriate and there is a potential for violence, what can be done to permit necessary care to be provided without compromising the safety of the ED providers?

This second patient clearly represents a true emergency. An IV drug user with a fever could have a number of life-threatening ailments, including endocarditis, sepsis, infected pulmonary embolism, pneumonia, or tuberculosis. A reasonable judgment can be made that this patient's assaultive behavior is inappropriate from the provider's point of view, although it may seem very appropriate from this ill patient's perspective. The provider must not consider this as simply "part of the job" and accept being a victim of assault.

Precautions can be taken to avoid being a victim in much the same manner as gloves are used to protect from blood or saliva-borne pathogens. These include planning to approach the patient so as to be out of reach of potential weapons (teeth, fists, elbows, knees, and feet). Once a patient is out of control and

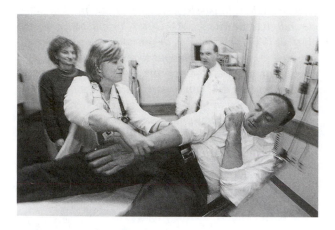

physically assaultive, verbal intervention is not usually effective.

Q: What is the best way to block an attack that happens when an IV is being started?

When an IV is being started with two hands on the patient's upper extremity, if the opposite fist is projected toward you, an initial defense would be to push the IV arm across the patient's body toward his face. This will block the oncoming blow while redirecting his momentum. An even more effective technique would be to push the patient's straightened IV arm toward his shoulder, as illustrated in the photograph, directing his energy back toward the bed and forcing him to lay back. At this point, a trained team should be called to restrain the patient. While employing such defensive techniques, the provider must reposition his or her body out of the way of an attack. Such techniques and strategies must be learned and practiced beforehand, much in the same way as we have had to consciously train ourselves to use *universal precautions* against HIV disease.

DISCUSSION

Contributors to ED Violence

There are many reasons for the increase in violence in the ED. Violence is more prevalent in the community at large. There are liberal gun control laws, and an increase in weapon carrying. Drug and alcohol use

have also increased, and there was a 12% surge in drug-related ED cases during the first two quarters of 1991 alone.[6] The ED sees more homeless people with mental disorders, and there are more psychiatric patients brought into the ED by police, partly because since 1955, the total number of state psychiatric hospitals has been reduced by 80%.[7] Today, only 900,000 of the 1.7 to 4 million Americans with severe mental illness reside in institutions. Narcotics and cash are known to be present in the ED, and the doors are open to all, 24 hours per day. There is physical crowding, long waits in a congested area, and poor communication between providers and visitors or family in the waiting area. Communication problems between ill patients and care providers contributes to ED violence, along with anxiety-provoking conditions and moderately uncomfortable ambient temperatures, although extremely hot temperatures may actually decrease aggression and lead to flight rather than fight. Family disputes and marital or lover's quarrels frequently escalate into ED violence, and gang-related activities and crack use are more widespread.[8,9] Grief-stricken relatives who have just been told that their loved one had died have been known to assault the messenger. People who have had some of their control taken away (i.e., clothes removed) and the sick or hurting patient who feels ignored in a busy ED, are also likely candidates for violence.[10]

Under these conditions, every patient or visitor has the potential to be violent. This includes the frail, elderly man who suddenly becomes agitated and scratches the provider with his long nails because his phenytoin level has become too high, or the intoxicated, docile young woman who begins to sober up and then becomes violent toward the medical worker who reminds her of an abusive parent. The assailant is often someone other than the patient,—for example, the parent who witnesses her child having a painful chest tube placed and attacks the emergency medicine resident, or the young man who has just been informed of his fiancee's unexpected death and who throws a chair at the informant.[11]

Force or physical and chemical restraints should be employed only when reasonably necessary and when used carefully and for the patient's benefit. The basics of safety in the management of acutely violent patients include (1) know when verbal deescalation techniques are appropriate, (2) have adequate manpower who are trained to subdue a patient, (3) be familiar with physical restraint techniques, and (4) dress appropriately if participating in physical restraint maneuvers.

The key to avoiding medical malpractice is to establish and document that the actions taken are indeed reasonable and necessary for the protection of the patient and provider. Meticulous documentation is the best defense. Compliance with filing incident reports is important for assessing the extent of the problem accurately and for determining the efficacy of instituted measures.[12]

Etiologic Factors of ED Violence

Violent patients are not a homogeneous group. Clinicians must therefore evaluate the underlying cause of violence on a case-by-case basis. Recognizing and understanding etiologic factors may aid in evaluation, treatment, and prevention of violence, because these violence-provoking conditions may be reversible. Common etiologic factors include a wide range of medical systemic disorders; primary CNS/organic brain disorders; psychoactive substance use; and delusional and other psychiatric disorders. Developmental factors include a history of child abuse and exposure to domestic violence. Psychosocial risk factors include an inability to tolerate stress, poor personal insight, and a tendency to react by blaming others. Social isolation—lack of friends and support systems—also contribute to violent tendencies.[13]

Violent behavior has been correlated with age (young teens to thirties), sex (male), and socioeconomic status (low), but not with race when the study was controlled for socioeconomic status.[14] Persons from an environment in which violence is common may also be more likely to be violent themselves. Triggers in violence-prone persons include a recent loss, such as a romantic disappointment, death, or unemployment. The most reliable predictor of violent behavior is a history of violent behavior.

Implications for Emergency Medicine

During the period between 1980 and 1989, homicide was the leading cause of occupational death from injury for women, and the third leading cause for all

workers.[15] In the 1990s, there has been an increase in injuries to hospital workers involving violence occurring in every area of the health care arena.[16] Recent data indicates that violent situations occur in 5% of calls in a metropolitan city-county EMS system servicing over 500,000 people in Nashville, Tennessee.[17] Injuries to prehospital providers inflicted by violent patients over the previous year were reported by 67% of respondents of a 1993 published survey. Weapons were evident in 12% of violent encounters.[18]

In a survey of 47 pediatric ED directors, with 94% responding, more than three-fourths reported one or more verbal threats per week and one or more physical attacks per year. Reported physcial attacks occurred between 0 and 12 times per year, with a mean of 2. The majority reported that their staff members practice with at least occasional fear (55%).[19] In a recent survey of emergency medicine residents and recent graduates in California, 62% of respondents worry about their own safety while working in the ED, and 50% believe that their hospital residency programs do not provide adequate security in the ED. Data from a 1988 survey of large teaching facilities reported frequent verbal threats (≥1/day in 32% of facilities), display of weapons as a threat (≥1/month in 18%), and battery of medical or nursing staff (≥1/month in 43%).[2] Emergency medicine staff work in a battleground.

Failure to Report Incidents of Violence

Verbal and physical assaults toward ED health care providers exact a high toll in the form of physical injury, lost time, emotional distress, decreased morale, lack of self-esteem, a negative attitude toward the job and patients, burnout, posttraumatic stress disorder, and attrition. Yet, the problem remains underreported and underdocumented.[12]

The reasons for the lack of reporting include denial. It is distressing to confront the reality of our own vulnerability to violence, and easier to avoid the issues. Analogies have been drawn between health care providers and victims of domestic abuse.[20,21] The practitioner who assumes that verbal and physical abuse are part of the job, or that violence is deserved, or that complaining is a sign of weakness is acting out a pattern suggestive of the responses of battered women. Fourteen percent of male physicians and 31% of female physicians in one study had themselves been victims of abuse at some point in their own lives.[19] In one study, 25% of nurses had a personal history of domestic violence, which is higher than the general population of women.[22] These factors may well contribute to a syndrome in which one hesitates to report abuse in the workplace. It is curious to compare the absence of guidelines for such situations, with the detailed protocols and near-universal compliance for reporting accidental needle sticks and the risk of HIV exposure that exist today.[23] In reality, the health risk to the ED practioner from physical violence may be even greater than that posed by HIV exposure.

A provider typically enters a helping profession with altruistic goals. To be assaulted by the very individual whom you are attempting to help shatters the image of the patient in need seeking help from the provider and being grateful for the services that he or she provides. The provider is also brutally forced to confront his or her own vulnerability which may have been kept carefully and conveniently denied. These discontinuities make it difficult to confront the issue directly.

Training

Despite the urging of the Joint Commission on Accreditation of Hospitals Organization (JCAHO), the Emergency Nurses Association (ENA), and the American College of Emergency Physicians (ACEP) for health care workers to be versed in self-protection and the management of violence,[24–26] only a minority of ED staff have received such training. According to Lavoie,[27] only 40% of emergency department directors responding to a national survey reported that their ED nurses received formal training in the recognition and management of violent patients; yet 16% stated that there have been one or more litigious actions in the last 5 years involving restraint of violent patients in the ED. Confrontations with security officers and health care providers can result in disability and workers' compensation for staff and in injuries to patients. These negative outcomes often occur in the process of attempting to restrain the patient who is a danger to himself and others. Removal of restraints is an even higher-risk activity.

Universal Precautions

Precaution is not paranoia. We treat known AIDS patients, and every patient as potentially having HIV, yet we display respect and treat them with dignity as we take precautions. Physicians are taught to examine patients from the right side of the bed, and in fact, many physicians feel awkward if they approach in any other way. Practitioners should develop the habit of approaching each patient with safety in mind. This means out of reach of human weapons. Recently a resident was suddenly and unexpectedly kicked in the chest while talking with a patient. Had she practiced the habit of maintaining a protected distance and angle, she would not have been assaulted. An effective program for managing violent patients limits liability as well as minimizes injury to all parties. Self-protection and the management of violence should be a part of competency requirements along with CPR and ACLS.

Live Safe Medical, Inc. is an example of a program for training health care providers in universal precautions, self-protection, and management of violence in the workplace that includes assessment of physical plant security and workshops on medicolegal considerations, verbal self-protection and deescalation techniques, physical self-protection and escapes, and restraint and control techniques. The Live Safe Medical program provides participants with a quickly learned yet functional method of self-protection that emphasizes avoidance and minimizing confrontation, and, when necessary, subduing and restraining the patient safely. The program addresses not only the physical aspects of self-defense but the often-neglected psychological ramifications of violence. This is an integrated approach of didactics and actual practice of escape and defensive techniques. These techniques do not depend on exceptional physical conditioning or coordination. They focus on the psychological and emotional mind sets of the attacker and defender. In addition to a comprehensive training program, a collaborative, proactive approach allows input from physicians, nurses, medical workers, and security staff to ensure an optimally safe environment. In addition, ongoing positive peer support, immediate debriefing, and psychological, economic, and legal advice should be provided.

NONPHYSICAL INTERVENTIONS

Develop More Than One Strategy

There is no single nonphysical approach to a violent patient that will be effective in all cases, nor is there consensus in the literature. Each violent situation must be managed individually. What works in one setting may have devastating consequences in others. It is unusual for a psychotic or delerious patient to respond favorably to verbal interventions. Some patients may need to be treated with a serene, outwardly calm approach, while others require a structured environment.

Monitor Feelings

The violent patient commonly elicits strong, emotional responses. Fear felt by the provider may be a clue to the patient's potential for violence and should be followed by protective measures. It is important that fear and anger not color objectivity or lead to retaliation. Provocative individuals, either family members or uniformed security guards, should be asked to leave. If the latter are the only security staff, they should remain nearby.

Making Emotions Work for, Not against You

We appraise each thing that we experience in the world in terms of involvement, relationship, and interaction, not objective distancing. The Live Safe Medical program uses a streamlined collection of practical defensive tactics culled from Ninpo Taijutsu, a Japanese martial tradition more than 800 years old. Emotions can be made to work for you if a balanced, integrated strategy is employed. Feelings can guide you to a response that is right for you in a given situation—provided you are able to access your own feelings and mindset as well as those of the attacker.

Heighten Your Awareness

Pay attention to clues of impending violence and communicate this to your co-workers, so no unsuspecting staff member walks into danger. Keep waiting time to a minimum for potentially violent patients. Certain staff members who know the patient from other ED encounters may have a calming effect; others with an antagonistic relationship should be kept away. The most experienced personnel should deal with the situation—with appropriate back-up and a prepared show of force. Also, make sure there is a clear path for the patient to escape, and make sure you have a way out of a possible physical confrontation at all times.

Talking with the Agitated, Threatening Patient

Although it is difficult to verbally deescalate the seriously agitated or already violent patient, certain patients who are beginning to escalate might be amenable to various deescalation techniques. Again, remember to be flexible and individualize. The following are some *general* guidelines.

- Remain calm, appear in control.
- Show concern and respect.
- Speak calmly, using an increasingly slow cadence. You might want to speak more quickly with a rapidly talking anxious patient and then slowly bring down the cadence as you talk him down to a calmer pace.
- Avoid using angry glares, clenched fists, or rigid body language against a challenging patient. A relaxed body, level voice, and eyes that exude confidence may go a long way toward deescalating a situation.
- Give choices such as where the patient can sit. Three choices instead of two provides a less confrontational atmosphere; e.g., "You can either sit in the chair or be restrained." This implies that one of the answers is correct and the other wrong. A better approach might be to state, "You can sit in the chair, lie on the stretcher, or be restrained." This appears to provide less of an ultimatum.

- Speak softly in a nonprovocative, nonjudgmental manner and begin by commenting in a neutral, concrete tone about the obvious; e.g., "You seem upset."
- Attempt to develop rapport prior to addressing the issue of violence. The violent patient may feel helpless, terrified of losing control, or frightened by the intensity of his or her own emotion. Acknowledge these feelings.
- Offer food or drink—safely. Avoid hot drinks or potential weapons.
- When asking about violence, be direct and honest.
- Assure the patient that you will do what you can to help him or her stay in control of violent impulses. Set limits firmly but try not to threaten or display anger.
- Guard against allowing your fear or anger to lead to punitive measures.
- Limit setting can involve talk, sedation, or physical restraints.
- Avoid emotional, provocative, or judgmental commands or comments; e.g., "Act like an adult." These could escalate violent behavior.
- Pay attention to patient's personal space—there should be adequate space between the clinician and the patient, and, ideally, both should be sitting. Display respect for the patient.
- Do not tower over him or stand in front of him with an aggressive posture; e.g., hands on hips or folded or pointing a finger. Avoid appearing intimidating.
- Avoid intense direct eye contact. This could appear challenging.
- When the patient speaks, listen empathically, and uncritically. Avoid early interruptions.
- Try to elicit the patient's view of the situation and what led up to the violent situation.
- Subtly and gently try to correct patient's misperceptions, if there is no evidence of paranoia. Point out the correctness of perceptions you agree with; e.g., "You are right. The wait to be seen is too long," and ally yourself, as in "I'd be angry, too, if I had to wait so long."
- Other strategies include the ice-breaker, "How can I help you?" or "Help me to help you" or "Tell me what needs to happen now to make the situation right."
- Do not make promises you cannot keep.

- Give paranoid patients who are threatening violence plenty of physical space and try to ally yourself in an attempt to face the problem together. Do not, at this time, point out the patient's delusional behavior. Be aware that the patient may incorporate you into his or her delusional system, increasing risk for assault.[28]

The Interviewing Environment

Decide whether those who accompany the patient are a stabilizing or destabilizing force and act accordingly in recruiting or dismissing them. The safety of the physical setting should be considered. At the bedside, be sure that potential weapons are out of reach (IV poles, walkers, canes). In isolation rooms, furniture should be too heavy to move or throw. However, a light chair for the examiner to sit in could be used for defensive purposes in cases of attack, particularly against sharp weapons. Avoid loose objects such as ashtrays. Be sure that there is an easy exit route for you. Sit between the patient and the exit. If both of you are sitting, place the chairs at 45 degrees to each other. A "panic button" is desirable so that help could be summoned, if needed. An isolation room should not be cramped, especially if the agitated patient has a need to pace.[28]

Attention to Dress

When interviewing violent or explosive patients, remove eyeglasses, jewelry, neckties and scarves, and stethoscope. Patients should be rigorously searched prior to isolation, and pens, jewelry, matches, and lighters removed.[29]

Signs and Symptoms of Imminent Violence

Some signs that a patient may become violent are

- A gut feeling of fear or feeling threatened experienced by the healthcare provider.
- Speech that is loud, threatening, pressured, and profane.
- Increased muscle tension—for example, sitting forward on the edge of a chair and gripping the arms, tightened lips, gnashing of the teeth, or clenching of the fists.

- Hyperactivity, such as pacing, diaphoresis, slamming doors, or knocking over furniture.
- Individuals with certain kinds of tattoos are at greater risk of violent behavior. Having three or more certain types of tattoos is often associated with a history of incarceration, often for a violent crime. "Misfit," "Unlucky," "Born to Lose," "Death Before Dishonor," and so on may be associated with antisocial behavior.[30,10]

Display of weapons. Expose as few staff as possible when a gun or knife is displayed. Keep a calm appearance, and encourage the patient to talk and build rapport. Do not intimidate, confront, or insult. Encourage the patient to talk. You can make an observation, such as, "Oh, I see you have a gun," or, "You seem upset." Suggest that the patient put the gun down. Do not reach for the gun. Abandon any thoughts of being a hero! If the patient is unwilling to surrender a weapon or plans to leave the ED, ideally, let security or the police deal with it. Plan ahead, especially for hostage situations.[31,28]

Hostages. Hostages should maintain a low profile and avoid physical and verbal interaction, intimidating or argumentative behavior, and heroism. Don't panic or become hysterical, nor should you display extreme helplessness or passive behavior. Try to maintain a calm, controlled demeanor. Do not make suggestions. The first 15 to 45 minutes are the most dangerous. Follow instructions. Treat the captor like royalty. Be observant. Think twice about trying to escape. If rescue comes, be prepared to drop instantly to the floor for your protection.[32,28]

PHYSICAL INTERVENTIONS

Restraints

Contraindications.

- Use for punishment; i.e., for seeking retribution for an act when no danger exists to the patient or others.
- Inability to properly monitor patient for aspiration and circulatory compromise every 15 minutes.

Adverse effects.

- Circulatory obstruction, if too tight.
- Aspiration, if patient positioned precariously.
- Positional asphyxia.
- Sudden death, secondary to stress response triggering fatal dysrhythmia.[33,34]

Indications.

- After other means of controlling violent behavior have been considered or tried.
- To prevent imminent harm to the patient.
- To prevent imminent harm to others.
- To prevent serious disruption to the treatment environment.

Techniques.

- Restraint equipment should be stored carefully and be readily accessible.
- Ideally, there should be at least five team members, one assigned to each limb and a team leader controlling the patient's head. Each team member should wear gloves. If the patient is female, at least one member of the team should be a woman. The most experienced member should be designated team leader.
- Explain to the patient in a nonthreatening way what his or her options are at this point. Consider other methods; e.g., verbal intervention or chemical sedation alone. Once the decision to restrain the patient is made, further discussion or negotiation is inappropriate and possibly dangerous.
- Give the patient a few seconds to comply. At times a patient who is out of control and recognizes this will comply. The patient often fears losing control and may feel relieved when restrained.
- Maintain the patient's dignity at all times.
- If the patient refuses to cooperate, divide the team into two and approach the patient from opposite sides.
- Use the least amount of force required. The team should hold the patient at the head, elbows, and knees and should carry him to a stretcher or secure him to the one he is in with four-point leather restraints. Two-point restraints permit the patient to fall from the stretcher.
- Restrain in a supine position or, if there is any risk for aspiration, in the prone position.

- Search the patient for weapons and drugs.
- Examine every 15 minutes and reposition once an hour to prevent pressure sores.[28,5,32]
- Monitor vital signs and O_2 saturation.

Removing Restraints.

Caveat: Communication among staff is crucial! Coordinate the decision regarding the removal of restraints with the nursing, medical, and psychiatry staff. Problems arise when a physician who has not had continuing contact with the patient is seduced and manipulated into removing restraints without the knowledge of and consultation with the nursing staff. Michael Stultz, director of security services, Stanford University Medical Center, states that, . . . "more security and other hospital staff are injured after a nurse or physician makes a bargain with a restrained patient and releases him or her on condition of good behavior than are hurt during the original restraint. This is particularly true in a teaching hospital, where large numbers of new residents come through the ED for training. Injury incidents frequently occur when a physician has released a patient without consulting with nursing or security personnel on the advisability of such an action. On seven occasions during the past year, security personnel have had to restrain an ER patient four to six times during a single ER visit at Stanford. On four of these occasions, security personnel have been bitten, punched, or scratched."[35]

Medicolegal considerations.

- In 1982, the U.S. Supreme Court, after ruling in *Youngberg* v. *Romeo,* deferred to professional judgment the management of violent people.
- Most restraints are initiated by nursing staff. JCAHO regulations specify that within 1 hour of seclusion or restraint, an order (telephone or written) by a physician is needed.[30]

Chemical Restraints

If the patient is combative, IM administration of medications is the most practical option. Initially, Haloperidol, 5 to 10 mg IM,[36] or Droperidol, 5 mg IM may be used followed by Haloperidol, 5 mg or Droperidol,[37] 5 mg every 30 minutes. Lorazepam (1 to 4 mg)[38] or Midazolam 2 to 5 mg IM,[39] may also be used. Once IV access is established, titration of sedation can be achieved with benzodiazepines or butyrophenones. The sedated patient must have continuous pulse oximetry and cardiac monitoring with frequent vital signs recorded. Ideally, a sitter or medical aide should be one-to-one with the patient at all times. In addition to oversedation, butyrophenones can exert an anticholinergic and alpha-blocking effect as well as extrapyramidal reactions—for example, twisting of the neck and tongue, and oculogyric crisis. These effects can be treated with diphenhydramine or cogentin. In head trauma patients, or patients in whom a potential CNS insult is suspected, controlled intubation with neuromuscular blockers may be indicated. Once a patient is controlled, organic etiologies must be addressed in a timely fashion—for example, hypoxia by oxygen saturation, hypoglycemia by rapid fingerstick test, CNS insult by CT scan, and so on. A history and physical exam as possible must be done as well as selective laboratory tests.

CRITICAL INCIDENT STRESS DEBRIEFING (CISD)

After an episode of violence, the team should be allowed to debrief and decompress. The devastating effects of violence and mayhem in the ED have been cited as a major cause of burnout among health care providers.[40] In a busy ED, there may not be adequate time available at a given moment, but even a brief 2-to-3-minute debriefing that recognizes the events, their effects, and the feelings that they elicit may prove a wise investment for future well-being. When deemed appropriate, a more in-depth critical incident stress debriefing (CISD) can be conducted away from the ED environment.[41] Emotional aftershocks can occur, and the ED worker may experience delayed effects days, weeks, or months later. The incidence of posttraumatic stress disorder (PTSD) is significant among healthcare workers. Similarities have been found between hospital staff victims of violence, victims of street crimes, and victims of disasters. Even closer similarities have been found between hospital staff and police, fire, and rescue personnel who are victims of violence or other traumatic experiences.[42] Clinicians are not immune. In one study, clinicians reported reactive symptoms at a higher rate than nonclinicians. In some studies, a relatively small number of providers were found to be repeatedly attacked. The possibility should be explored that staff who are repeatedly attacked may have a management style or behavior that is subtly, if not overtly, adversarial, or otherwise makes them a target.[43]

CONCLUSION

Violence against ED health care providers by patients and visitors is a significant public health issue. The assailant can be a patient, family member, or visitor. Such incidents are underreported and underdocumented. The reasons for this are complex. Physical injury, lost time, emotional distress, decreased morale, burnout, attrition, and PTSD are serious potential consequences. Skills in approaching patients safely and managing assaults should be considered part of *universal precautions*. An effective program for managing violent patients limits liability as well as minimizes injury to all parties. Positive peer support is critical to ensuring the wellness of the ED staff.

NOTES

1. Lundberg G, Young R, Flanagin A, Koop C. Violence: A compendium from *JAMA, American Medical News,* and the specialty journals of the American Medical Association (Foreword). Chicago: American Medical Association, 1992, no. OP350092.
2. Anglin D, Kyriacou DN, Hutson HR. Residents' perspectives on violence and personal safety in the emergency department. *Ann Emerg Med* 1994; 23:1082–4.
3. Spritz N. Oversight of physicians' conduct by state licensing agencies, Lessons from New York's Libby Zion case. *Ann Int Med* 1991; 115(3):219–22.
4. OSHA General Duty Clause (29USC 1900(a)(1); covered by the Occupational Safety and Health Act of 1970.
5. Taigman M. Self-protection for health care employees. Joint Commission on Accreditation of Healthcare Organizations (JCAHO). *Plant, Technology & Safety Management Series: Security in Health Care Facilities.* Chicago, IL: Joint Commission, 1991.
6. Drug Abuse Warning Network (DAWN). National Institute on Drug Abuse (NIDA). 1991, cited in: *Dealing With Hospital Violence: Volume I: Emergency Rooms.* Port Washington, NY: International Association for Healthcare Security & Safety (IAHSS), Rusting Publications, 1992.
7. Lamb H. Is it time for a moratorium on deinstitutionalization? (Editorial). *Hosp Community Psychiatry* 1992; 43:669.
8. International Association for Healthcare Security & Safety (IAHSS). *Dealing With Hospital Violence: Volume I: Emergency Rooms,* Port Washington, NY: Rusting Publications, 1992.
9. Lindley D. The many faces of violence in U.S. and Canadian hospitals. *Journal of Healthcare Protection Management* 1993; 10:33–41.
10. Taliaferro EH. Coping with the Violent Patient. *Emerg Med* 1992; 155–6, 161–4.
11. Freedland E. Personal observation. 1995.
12. Foust D, Rhee KJ. The incident of battery in an urban emergency department. *Ann Emerg Med* 1993; 22:583–5.
13. Tardiff K. The current state of psychiatry in the treatment of violent patients. *Arch Gen Psychiatry* 1992; 49:493–9.
14. Swanson J, Holzer C, Ganju V, Jono R. Violence and psychiatric disorder in the community: Evidence from the Epidemiologic Cachment Area surveys. *Hosp Community Psychiatry* 1990; 41:761–70.
15. NIOSH. *Homicide in U.S. Workplaces: A Strategy for Prevention and Research.* Morgantown, WV: U.S. Department of Health and Human Services, Public Health Service, Centers for Disease Control, National Institute for Occupational Safety and Health, DHHS (NIOSH) Publication no. 92-103; 1992.
16. NIOSH. *Fatal Injuries to Workers in the United States, 1980–1989: A Decade of Surveillance; National Profile.* Cincinnati, OH: U.S. Department of Health and Human Services, Public Health Service, Centers for Disease Control and Prevention, National Institute for Occupational Safety and Health, DHHS (NIOSH) Publication no. 93-108; 1993.
17. Fowlie E, Eustis T, Wright S, Wrenn K, Slovis C. Prospective field study of violence in EMS (abstract). *Ann Emerg Med* 1994; 23:620.
18. Tintinalli JE. Violent patients and the prehospital provider. *Ann Emerg Med* 1993; 22:1276–9.
19. McAneney CM, Shaw K. Violence in the pediatric emergency department. *Ann Emerg Med* 1994; 23:1248–51.
20. Worthington K. Taking action against violence in the workplace. *American Nurse* 1993; (June):10–12.
21. Nordberg M. ED Staffs Underreport Assaults by Patients. *Emergency Medical Services* 1993; (June):63–4.
22. Sugg NK, Inui T. Primary care physicians' response to domestic violence: Opening Pandora's box. *JAMA* 1992; 267:3157–60.
23. Cadigan C, Higgins K, Thompson T. *The occupational health knowledge base, assessment and intervention techniques and policies for domestic violence victims in the*

workplace. Master of Science Nursing thesis, Simmons College, 1994.

24. Joint Commission on Accreditation of Healthcare Organizations. Plant and Safety Management (PL. 1.2.2.2). In *Accreditation Manual for Hospitals.* Chicago: Joint Commission, 1993.

25. Emergency Nurses Association position statement: Violence in the emergency setting. *J Emerg Nurs* 1991; 17(6).

26. American College of Emergency Physicians. Protection from physical violence in the emergency department (position paper). *Ann Emerg Med* 1993; 22:1651.

27. Lavoie FW, Carter GL, Berg RL. Emergency Department Violence in United States Teaching Hospitals. *Ann Emerg Med* 1988; 17:419.

28. Tardiff K. *Concise Guide to Assessment & Management of Violent Patients.* Washington, DC: American Psychiatric Press, 1989.

29. Kinkle SL. Violence in the ED: How to stop it before it starts. *Am J Nurs* 1993; (July):22–4.

30. Blumenreich P, Lippmann S, Bacani-Oropilla T. Violent patients: Are you prepared to deal with them? *PostGraduate Med* 1991; 90:201–6.

31. Wasserberger J, Ordog G, Landers S, et al. Weapons in the emergency department. *Top Emerg Med* 1994; 16:6–17.

32. Deagle JH, Franaszek JB, Gavin LJ, et al. *Emergency Department Violence.* American College of Emergency Physicians, Dallas, TX; 1988.

33. Bell MD, Rao VJ, Wetli CV, Rodriguez RN. Positional asphyxiation in adults: A series of 30 cases from the Dade and Broward County Florida medical examiner's offices from 1982–1990. *Am J Forensic Med Pathol* 1992; 13:101–7.

34. Robinson B, Sucholeiki R, Schocken DD. Sudden death and resisted mechanical restraint: A case report. *J Am Geriatr Soc* 1993; 41:424–5.

35. Stultz MS. Emergency room security: commonsense measures. *Journal of Healthcare Protection Management* 1993; 10(1):12–26.

36. Clinton J, Sterner S, Stermachers Z, Ruiz E. Haloperidol for sedation of disruptive emergency patients. *Ann Emerg Med* 1987; 16:319.

37. Thomas HJ, Schwartz E, Petrilli R. Droperidol versus haloperidol for chemical restraint of agitated and combative patients. *Ann Emerg Med* 1992; 21:407–13.

38. Hyman S. The violent patient. In Hyman S, Tesar G (eds.). *Manual of Psychiatric Emergencies.* Boston: Little, Brown,1994.

39. Wright SW, Chudnofsky CR, Dronen SC, et al. Midazolam use in the emergency department. *Am J Emerg Med* 1990; 8:97–100.

40. Taliaferro E. Violence in the emergency department: A very real concern. *Ann Emerg Med* 1988; 166:1248.

41. Ordog G, Wasserberger J, Ordog C, et al. Violence and general security in the emergency department. *Acad Emerg Med* 1995; 2:151–4.

42. Caldwell MF. Incidence of PTSD among staff victims of patient violence. *Hospital and Community Psychiatry* 1992; 43:838–9.

43. Cooper AJ, Mendonca JD. A prospective study of patient assaults on nurses in a provincial psychiatric hospital in Canada. *Acta Psychiatr Scand* 1991; 84:163–6.

14

Ethnicity, Culture, and the Delivery of Health-Care Services

CAROL JACK SCOTT

CONTENTS

- Definitions of culture, race, and ethnicity
- Racism and health care
- Health beliefs and familial folk remedies
- Disease-illness dichotomy and the cultural construction of reality
- Guidelines for culturally sensitive care

CHAPTER SUMMARY

Physicians diagnose and treat *disease* (abnormalities in structure and function of body and system), but patients have symptoms and *suffer illnesses* (experience changes in body states). While physicians think in terms of anatomy and physiology, their patients may be thinking in terms of yin and yang, thick or thin blood, or hot and cold.

This chapter uses three clinical vignettes to illustrate specific knowledge, attitudes, and skills that can be tools for culturally competent health care providers. Cross and Bazron's concepts of cultural competency[1] are presented as a model for cultur-

The author wishes to acknowledge the contribution of Thomas N. Robinson, Jr., Ph.D., Assistant Professor, Department of African Studies, University of Maryland, for his assistance with research for this chapter.

ally competent delivery of emergency department care.

DIVERSITY IN THE ED

Cultural beliefs and attitudes determine behavior, guide decisions, and affect interactions with colleagues, staff, and patients. As the recent Society for Academic Emergency Medicine (SAEM) position paper, "Emergency Medicine and the Health of the Public" (see Chapter 1), points out: "Specific issues may vary among different racial and ethnic minority groups ... each has its own cultural, social, and economic and political characteristics that define their public health needs."

Case #1

It is 7:00 A.M. in the morning, and the following case is presented at change of shift. The resident says, "The patient in room 4 is ready to go home as soon as he is seen by you. He is 72 years old and lives alone. His neighbors brought him in. His chief complaint is 'can't take the stomach pain any more.' He doesn't believe in doctors and hasn't seen one in more than 10 years. He ate an egg for his pain but had no relief. He has normal vital signs, reduced bowel sounds, and no rebound or guarding. His abdomen was not distended but there was a little tenderness to deep palpation. He refused to have his blood drawn or have a rectal exam. He kept talking about his pulse. He hasn't demonstrated any pain since he got here. I think he can go home. There's been no objective evidence for any pathology in the 12 hours he has been here. I can get him a spot in the clinic within the week." Before you can respond, the nurse interrupts to ask if the translator is still going to be needed for this patient, or can he go home?

Q: The resident has summed up this situation as a trivial complaint. What has he missed that might tip him off to the seriousness of this problem?

First, the seriousness of the reported complaint does not correlate with the physical findings, yet this 72-year-old is brought in by his neighbors in the middle of the night. The need for translation alerts you to potential misinterpretation. Based on incomplete data (no rectal exam or white count), the resident has decided that this is not a serious problem, and the patient can be sent home. What has he missed?

The first tip-off is that this gentleman has avoided the medical care system for the last decade or more. If he has permitted himself to be brought in, something must be seriously wrong. His attention to pulse is based on his perception of a radical change in pulse or life force, or *piao*, that portends imminent death.[2] His use of herbal remedies did not improve his abdominal pain, and, unfortunately, delayed his entry to care. He would say that his yin and yang are out of balance. After further evaluation, the ED resident realized that this traditional Chinese-American patient had mesenteric ischemia, a life-threatening condition requiring immediate surgery. This case illustrates that health care providers must be willing to apply knowledge of ethnic health beliefs and practices with due attention to the individuality and specific needs of the patient.

Q: Could knowing this patient's ethnicity and/or culture influence the provision of care?

Competent care requires attention to the lifestyle, culture, ethnicity and spiritual beliefs of patients. We learn from our own cultural and ethnic backgrounds *how* to be healthy, *how* to recognize illness, *how* to be ill, and *how* to live. Estes and Zitzow describe culture, ethnicity, and religious background as *heritage consistency*, or the degree to which a person's lifestyle reflects a traditional way of life.[3]

Culture. Anthropologists and other social scientists generally use the word *culture* to mean the *standards for behavior* that one acquires as a member of a social group. These standards include, "precepts, concepts, beliefs, and values that help individuals to order and thereby give meaning to their experience of both social relationships and the physical world."[4] Fejos describes culture as "the sum total of socially inherited characteristics of a human group that comprises everything which one generation can tell, convey, or hand down to the next; in other words, the nonphysically inherited traits we possess."[5]

Ethnicity. Although the concept of ethnicity has undergone a great deal of rethinking in recent years,[6–9] Schermerhorn defines ethnicity as

> . . . a collectivity within a larger society having real or putative common ancestry, memories of a shared historical past, and a cultural focus on one or more symbolic elements defined as the epitome of their peoplehood.[10]

This definition highlights three important aspects of ethnicity:

1. Ethnicity establishes social ties by reference to common origins.
2. Ethnicity also implies that the people of a particular collectivity or group share at least some learned standards for behavior.
3. Ethnic collectivities or groups participate with one another in a larger social system.

Ethnic categories are sometimes defined by the people themselves, and sometimes by the larger sociocultural system. For example, the single category "Hispanics" includes immigrants from vastly different Spanish speaking countries as well as native-born Americans of Spanish-speaking origin. The symbols and behavioral standards that have served to differentiate ethnic collectivities in one geographic context may thus be collectivized or reinterpreted by a dominant majority.

There are at least 106 ethnic groups and more than 170 Native American groups in the United States, all of which occupy different positions of power. Members of one ethnic group may function as the guardians of the dominant value system, incumbents of governmental offices, and dispensers of rewards, whereas others are systematically excluded.

People from every country in the world now reside in the U.S. Some nations, such as Germany, England, Wales, and Ireland are heavily represented; other nations, such as Japan, the Philippines, and Greece have smaller numbers of people living here. Ethnic groups within this country often believe in and practice their original healthcare system and continue their ancestral or traditional practices.

Religion. The third major component of heritage consistency is religion. Religious teachings help to present a meaningful philosophy and system of practices within a system of social controls having specific values, norms, and ethics. These are related to health in that adherence to a religious code may be conducive to spiritual harmony and health, and illness may be perceived as punishment for the violation of religious codes and morals.

Q: What relationships between specific health and illness measures and ethnicity, culture, and outcomes have been studied?

Disease rates. Ethnic groups have been observed to vary in rates of morbidity and mortality for different diseases. Statistical summaries and comparative studies involving African Americans, Chinese Americans, Jewish, Mexican Americans, Navajos, and Puerto Ricans, for example, all reveal important differences in disease prevalence, morbidity and mortality. These differences may reflect biases in vital statistics;[11–13] unequal access to treatment; genetic predisposition; shared risk factors (largely due to class membership), such as poverty, poor nutrition, or exposure to different pathogenic agents; or ethnically patterned, pathogenic cultural standards or behaviors. Ethnic differences in disease rates serve as an important background against which to view differing health beliefs and behaviors.[14–15]

Health maintenance and home treatment. Comparative studies have shown that ethnic subcultures differ both in their conceptions of well-being and in their health maintenance practices. Individual perceptions of size, weight, and "quality of life" are ethnically influenced. Understanding this is increas-

ingly important as we promote and support prevention and self-care. Ethnic home health practices also involve the use of nonmainstream sources of medicine, and this may help towards understanding why large proportions of illness episodes reach health care providers late, if ever.[16]

Access to care and utilization patterns. Many common barriers to access to care have been identified for minorities.[17–21] Barriers that have been cited include institutional racism; lack of bilingual-bicultural health care providers; financial constraints of community health care facilities; lack of familiarity with the U.S. health care system; provider insensitivity to sociopsychological and cultural characteristics of minority patients; catchment area confinement and lack of transportation; and traditional sociocultural health beliefs and practices. Alternative providers of health care may be used prior to, in conjunction with, or following mainstream services. For example, *Curanderos* and other lay practitioners among Mexican Americans, *espiritistas* and *santiguadores* among Puerto Ricans, singers among the Navajo, herbalists and other curers among Chinese Americans, bonesetters among French Canadians, *remède-mans* among Louisiana Cajuns, and various healers among urban blacks are just a few of the ethnic curers who have recently been described in the literature. For members of many ethnic groups, the range of options available for treating illness thus extends considerably beyond establishment and even "marginal" providers (chiropractors or osteopaths).

Ethnicity influences people's concept of symptoms, disease, and illness. Beliefs in the health effects of *Susto* among Mexican Americans, the evil eye among various circum-Mediterranean groups, Arctic hysteria among Eskimos, *battement de coeur* among Haitian Americans, theories of hot and cold among Hispanics, etiological ideas about God's punishment or possession by the devil among Southern blacks, or *gaz* and blood perturbations among Haitian Americans are all examples of culturally different perceptions of disease causality.

Q: Can *race* and *ethnicity* be used interchangeably?

The concept of *race* historically implied a degree of genetic homogeneity among persons designated by a range of visible characteristics. In contrast, *ethnicity* reflects a broader view of factors that may influence the susceptibility of individuals to etiologic agents and the ways in which individuals may respond to those agents.[22] For example, a newly immigrated Nigerian, a Haitian, and an African American might be considered racially identical—"black"—but they may not share nutritional habits, attitudes, and beliefs about medical care, or even biological inheritance. Anthropologists have long recognized that the racial lines drawn by a society are cultural rather than scientific constructions. Moreover, within the international medical community, racial divisions are not perceived in the same way. What is "black" to someone from the United States, for example, may be "white" to a Brazilian or a Caribbean Islander. The terms *black* and *white* say more about how U.S. society has been structured than about medically relevant, biological realities. Cauldwell recommends that the terms *black* and *white* be dropped from oral and written medical presentation and that more attention be paid to detailed history taking that provides important ethnic and cultural information.[23]

Q: What about racism and health care?

To date, only a small fraction of epidemiologic research in the United States has investigated the effects of racism on health—that is, the health consequences of racial subordination, as opposed to the more traditional public health concern with racial differences in disease. Most of these studies on racism and health have focused on determining whether health outcomes are comparable among members of different racial/ethnic groups at the same socioeconomic level.

Although racism clearly has its damaging economic dimensions, other aspects are also likely to be detrimental to people's health. These include the psychosocial effects of racial discrimination and oppression (e.g., all forms of racial exclusion and subordination), the problems resulting from a lack of access to adequate health care, and the physical and psychosocial consequences of residential and occupational segregation and of incarceration.

Both subtle and overt forms of racism, within and across social classes, can invalidate people's sense of self-worth and lead to internalized oppression. Eth-

nic minorities subjected to bigotry often adopt the oppressor culture's denigrating views and judge both themselves and others in their racial and ethnic group according to these criteria. This self-denigration in turn can potentially compromise available support and resources.[13]

Researchers need to develop and validate new methodologies to elicit the objective and subjective components of discrimination, oppression, and internalized oppression to permit testing these factors' association with risk of poor health. Empirical approaches to quantifying objective evidence of discrimination must be refined in order to assess residential and occupational segregation or pay inequities, for example, and also expanded to assess potentially discriminatory patterns of health care. Specific questionnaires also must be created and validated to assess people's subjective recognition of, attitudes toward, and reactions to unfair treatment, as well as their specific experiences of and responses to racist and class-biased situations.[24]

Case #2

A 25-year-old Mexican American mother of four brings her 22-month-old daughter to the ED, saying "She's sick and I'm scared. She usually is so bad, but now she doesn't even want to have her brother play with her. I think something bad has happened."

Examination reveals a lethargic infant who appears somewhat dehydrated. Temperature is 39°C. Numerous ecchymotic areas are noted on the child's trunk. No source for fever is noted. The mother's level of emotional distress and the finding of bruises prompt a call to Social Services for evaluation of child abuse.

Q: What do clinicians need to know about folk illnesses?

Pachter has highlighted at least five reasons why we should be familiar with folk illness beliefs and their implications for health care delivery.[25] First, people who experience sickness episodes that are perceived as folk illnesses may present for care to a traditional provider. One may expect that in culturally pluralistic settings, people go to "doctors" for "medical" illnesses and to "folk healers" for folk illnesses. In fact, this view is much too simplistic, and the data have proven it incorrect. Individuals may use many sources of care during a single episode of illness. Patients sometimes go to biomedical practitioners for relief of symptoms while simultaneously using a folk therapist to eliminate the cause of the illness.

Second, while many folk remedies are quite effective, others may be potentially hazardous. It is uncommon for folk remedies to cause major adverse effects, but occasional examples have been reported, and the potential for serious harm does exist. Marijuana tea, used to treat asthma by some West Indian patients, is one example of a potentially harmful remedy.

Third, traditional health practices may be misinterpreted by medical practitioners. Folk therapy can produce skin lesions that may be mistaken for signs of abuse. Most widely recognized are the Southeast Asian practices of "coining" (*cao gio*), the Chinese practice of moxibustion, and the Mexican-American and Southeast Asian practice of "cupping." In coining, warm oil is placed on a child's trunk and the area is briskly rubbed with the edge of a coin or spoon, which creates areas of ecchymosis. This practice is thought to relieve fevers.

Fourth, folk illnesses may be cultural interpretations of states of pathophysiology that require medical attention. *Caida de la mollera* is the term used for an infant's sunken fontanelle. In some instances this entity may reflect severe dehydration, and the infant may not receive timely care, because this condition is not associated in traditional beliefs with dehydration, and a healer is called instead to elevate the fontanelle back into place. If folk beliefs and behaviors become an impediment to biomedical care because of delay in medical attention or because of harmful folk treatments, significant morbidity may occur.

And, finally, folk illnesses represent ways of thinking that may be very instructive for health care professionals. A degree of humility may be the best medicine for both patient and physician. We can learn a lot from how our patients understand and treat their illnesses. Let us remember that many of our staple medicines—aspirin and digitalis—are derived from lay approaches to disease. Concepts of hot and cold, or thick or thin blood, may spark ideas for further investigation. At the very least, familiarity with them will provide a jumping off point for communication between patient and physician.

In this case study, cupping was practiced. Although it may have been entirely appropriate to consider abuse in a differential, given the physical lesions, this mother's care for her daughter was misinterpreted. Sensitive questioning—otherwise known as a comprehensive history—would have included the question, "What home remedies have you used to bring down her fever?" Ultimately, the child was found to have a viral syndrome and the mother was found to be an impoverished but caring parent.

Case #3

Mr. Jones is a 58-year-old African American who returns to the emergency department for a wound check. Sutures were placed 7 days ago for a minor accidental laceration. As was noted 7 days ago, his blood pressure was elevated to 250/130. He again was queried about his apparent lack of compliance with his antihypertensive medication. He stated, ". . . I'm okay . . . not like my brother who had a stroke when he was 55 years old . . . I feel as good as I should for my age . . . I can work everyday . . . no aches or pains . . . why do I need to take anything? If it's not broke, don't go fixin' it." The provider left the room. Outside of the treatment bay area, the provider was overheard conversing with a colleague, ". . . they just don't get it . . . why won't they take one little pill a day?"

Q: The provider is making an assumption about this patient—that he is illogical or ignorant. How could he reframe the way he looks at the situation?

This case study illustrates the clash between two worlds. Physician and patient must negotiate a shared understanding in some areas and agree to disagree with respect in others. The physician perceives a disease that manifests itself without symptoms (hypertension), and prescribes medication to be taken now for a future effect (prevention of stroke). The patient is experiencing no symptoms or troubles, and does not wish to take medication if he feels well. In his mind he is disease-free. The temporal connection between medication taken now and future illness has not been made clear to him. The physician values medication as "helpful." The patient views medication as "dangerous"; if he feels well, his blood *can't* be "too thick," and medication might "thin it out" dangerously. Physician and patient have different ideas of causality and different experiences to bolster their approaches. Without direct communication, neither will be able to learn from the other, and there will be no common negotiated treatment plan. Failure of compliance is usually just this kind of failure of communication.[26]

Q. What is a useful approach for resolving these different perceptions of disease and illness?

Neither disease or illness should be regarded as distinct entities. According to Kleinman,[27] both concepts are explanatory models, two aspects of a complex total phenomenon: sickness. What is most important is that these explanatory models help construct "clinical reality." As health professionals, our approach has traditionally been focused on recognition and treatment of disease (curing). The health care system has tended to disregard illness as a legitimate clinical concern. Again, this may be in part responsible for patient noncompliance, and patient and family dissatisfaction with some aspects of the provision of health care.

Kleinman describes the cultural construction of clinical reality as the process whereby for a particular episode of sickness, the patient and provider negotiate to label the patient's needs. The experience of an illness is determined by what illness means to the sick person. Furthermore, illness refers to a specific status and role within a given society. Not only must illness be sanctioned by a physician in order for the sick person to assume the sick role, but it must also be sanctioned by the community or social structure of which the person is a member. There may be major discrepancies in therapeutic values, expectations, and goals.

In case #3, Mr. Jones has not assumed responsibility for having a disease. He has, to date, been asymptomatic. His perception was that he was not likely to acquire any problems from what the doctors described as a disease. He had no perceived benefits from the adoption of a regimen of taking medication. Neither Mr. Jones nor his providers had negotiated a construct of reality from which each perceived that appropriate action would result.

CULTURAL COMPETENCE

Q: What can I do to enhance my ability to provide care, given these facts?

The concepts of heritage consistency and the cases presented here suggest that we all need to consider a new set of competencies. As discussed earlier, *culture* is the integrated pattern of human behavior that includes thought, speech, action . . . the customary beliefs, social forms and material traits of a racial, religious, or social group. *Competence* is the state of being capable. For an individual, *culture competence* is "the state of being capable of functioning effectively in the context of cultural differences." For an organization, it is "a set of congruent practice skills, attitudes, policies, and structures, which come together in a system, agency, or among professionals and enable that system, agency or those professionals to work effectively in the context of cultural differences."[1] Culturally competent professionals create and support multicultural environments. *Multiculturalism* is the state of the environment in which diverse populations not only coexist harmoniously but also thrive, valuing the heritage, cultures, contributions, needs, and potential of all individuals and populations.

Q: How does all of this apply to me? I am a reasonably nonbiased person and I don't see color—is there something else I need to know or do?

Culturally competent individuals and settings acknowledge and incorporate (not tolerate)—at all levels—the salience of culture, the assessment of cross-cultural relations, a vigilance towards the dynamics that result from cultural differences, the importance of expanding cultural knowledge, and adapting to meet culturally unique needs. Fortunately, cultural competency is a developmental process. No matter how comfortable we are, there is always room for growth and improvement.

To understand where one is in the process of becoming more culturally competent, it is useful to think of the possible ways of responding (thinking and behaving) to cultural differences. Imagine a continuum which ranges from cultural proficiency to cultural destructiveness. There are a variety of pos-

Figure 14-1   Cultural Competence Continuum

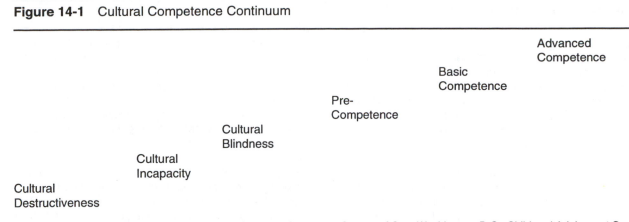

SOURCE: From Cross, Barzon, et al. *Towards a Culturally Competent System of Care.* Washington, D.C.: Child and Adolescent Service System Program Technical Assistance Center, Georgetown University, Child Development Center, 1989.

sibilities between these two extremes. Described below are six points along the continuum and the characteristics that might be exhibited at each position. This developmental continuum allows us all an opportunity for continuous improvement (see Figure 14-1).[1]

Cultural Destructiveness. The most negative end of the cultural competence continuum is represented by attitudes, policies, and practices that are destructive to cultures, and, consequently, to the individuals within the culture. The most extreme example of this orientation are programs that actively participate in the purposeful destruction of a culture. An example of "cultural genocide" is the systematic attempted destruction of Native American culture by the very services set up to "help" Indians—that is, boarding school. Another example is the Exclusion Laws of 1885–1965 that prohibited Asians from bringing spouses to this country. This law was destructive to the Asian family.

Historically, some of our institutions and training programs denied physicians of color access to certain training programs and professional organizations, and patients of color were denied access to nonsegregated care. The medical education of the Negro was considered by Flexner in his landmark report of 1905 (See Figure 14-2). While we do not often see examples this overt today, this history pro-

vides us with a reference point for understanding some of the barriers to adequate health care that people of color currently experience in the American health care system.

Cultural Incapacity. The next position on the continuum is one in which individuals do not intentionally seek to be culturally destructive but rather lack the capacity to function and to allow others to function effectively in settings where colleagues or patients are of diverse cultures. Extreme biases, beliefs in the racial superiority of the dominant group, and assumption of a paternal posture towards "lesser" groups may be present. Individuals and/or settings may not be aware of these biases. Such settings and individuals may support the rights of all persons to have equal opportunity. At this stage of development we are characterized by ignorance and an unrealistic fear of people of other cultures. The characteristics of cultural incapacity include: discriminatory practices, "microinequities," subtle messages to people of differing cultures that they are not valued or welcome, and generally lower expectations of members of certain cultures (colleagues and/or patients).

Cultural Blindness. At the midpoint on the continuum, we express a philosophy of being unbiased—"I

146 *Chapter 14*

Figure 14-2 The Medical Education of the Negro

"The medical care of the negro race will never be wholly left to negro physicians. * Nevertheless, if the negro can be brought to feel a sharp responsibility for the physical integrity of his people, the outlook for their mental and moral improvement will be distinctly brightened. The practice of the negro physician will be limited to his own race, which in its turn will be cared for better by good negro physicians than by poor white ones. But the physical well-being of the negro is not only moment to the negro himself. Ten million of them live in close contact with 60 million whites. Not only does the negro himself suffer from hookworm and tuberculosis; he communicates them to his white neighbors, precisely as the ignorant and unfortunate white contaminates him. Self-protection not less than humanity offers weighty counsel in this matter; self-interest seconds philanthropy. *The negro must be educated not only for his sake, but for ours.* He is, as far as human eye can see, a permanent factor in the nation. He has his rights and due and value as an individual; but he has, besides, the tremendous importance that belongs to a potential source of infection and contagion.

The pioneer work in educating the race to know and to practice fundamental hygienic principles must be done largely by the negro physician and the negro nurse. It is important that they both be sensibly and effectively trained at the level at which their services are now important. *The negro is perhaps more easily 'taken in' than the white; and as his means of extricating himself from a blunder are limited, it is all the more cruel to abuse his ignorance through any sort of pretense.* A well-taught negro sanitarian will be immensely useful; an essentially untrained negro wearing an MD label is dangerous.

Make-believe in the matter of negro medical schools is therefore intolerable. Even good intention helps but little to change their aspect. The negro needs good schools rather than many schools — schools to which the more promising of the race can be sent to receive a substantial education in which hygiene rather than surgery, for example, is strongly accentuated. *If at the same time these men can be imbued with the missionary spirit so that they will look upon the diploma as a commission to serve their people humbly and devotedly, they may play an important part in the sanitation and civilization of the whole nation. Their duty calls them away from large cities to the village and the plantation, upon which light has hardly as yet begun to break.*

Of the seven medical schools for negroes in the United States, five are at this moment in no position to make any contribution of value to the solution of the problem above pointed out. Flint at New Orleans, Leonard at Raleigh, the Knoxville, Memphis, and Louisville schools are ineffectual. They are wasting small sums annually and sending out undisciplined men, whose lack of real training is covered up by the imposing MD degree.

Meharry at Nashville and Howard at Washington are worth developing, and until considerably increased benefactors are available, effort will wisely concentrate on them. The future at Howard is assured; indeed, the new Freedman's Hospital is an asset the like of which is in this country extremely rare. *It is greatly to be hoped that the government may display a liberal and progressive spirit in adapting the administration of this institution to the requirements of medical education.*

Meharry is the creation of one man, Dr. George W. Hubbard, who, sent to the south at the close of the war on an errand of mercy, has for a half-century devoted himself singly to the elevation of the negro. The slender resources at his command have been carefully husbanded; his pupils have in their turn remembered their obligations to him and to their school. The income of the institution has been utilized to build it up. The school laboratories are highly creditable to the energy and intelligence of Dr. Hubbard and his assistants. The urgent need is for improved clinical facilities — a hospital building and a well equipped dispensary. Efforts now making to acquire them, deserve liberal support.

The upbuilding of Howard and Meharry will profit the nation much more than the inadequate maintenance of a larger number of schools. They are, of course, unequal to the need and the opportunity; but nothing will be gained by way of satisfying the need or of rising to the opportunity through the survival of feeble, ill equipped institutions, quite regardless of the spirit which animates the promoters. The subventions of religious and philanthropic societies and of individuals can be made effective only if concentrated. They must become immensely greater before they can be safely dispensed."

SOURCE: Flexner A. *Medical education in the United States and Canada: A report to the Carnegie Foundation for the Advancement of Teaching.* Washington D.C.: Science and Health Publications, 1960, Chapter 14.

don't see color." They function with the belief that color or culture make no difference and that we are all the same. Culturally blind individuals are characterized by the belief that helping approaches traditionally used by the dominant culture are universally applicable; if the system worked as it should, all people—regardless of race or culture—would be served with equal effectiveness. This view reflects a well-intended liberal philosophy; however, the consequences of such a belief are to make settings so ethnocentric as to render them virtually useless to all but the most assimilated people of nondominant culture. The difficulty with this view from a treatment perspective is that it does not allow for modification of care to meet the needs of the patients. It also does not allow the collegial environment to be enriched by valuing another culture.

Cultural Pre-competence. As we move toward the positive end of the scale, we reach a position we will call cultural pre-competence. This term implies movement. The pre-competence agency realizes its weaknesses in approaches to individuals from various cultures and attempts to improve. Pre-competent individuals may be characterized by asking the question, "What can we do?" One danger at this level is a false sense of accomplishment or of failure that prevents an individual or setting from moving forward along the continuum. Another danger is tokenism.

Basic Cultural Competence. Culturally competent individuals and settings are characterized by acceptance and respect for difference, continuing self-assessment regarding culture, careful attention to the dynamics of difference, continuous expansion of cultural knowledge and resources, and a variety of adaptations to better meet the needs of all cultures.

Advanced Cultural Competence. The most positive end of the scale is advanced cultural competence, or proficiency. This point on the continuum is characterized by holding culture in high esteem. The culturally proficient institution or individuals seek to add to the knowledge base of culturally competent practice by conducting research, developing new therapeutic approaches based on culture, and pub-

lishing and disseminating the results of demonstration projects.

Q: Is it enough to engage in developing cultural competency? What about the reality of the dynamics that occur in cross-cultural interactions?

What occurs in cross-cultural interactions might be called the *dynamics of difference.* When an individual or institution of one majority culture interacts with individuals from another culture, both may misjudge the other's actions based on learned expectations. Both bring to the relationship unique histories with the other group and the influence of current political relationships between the two groups. Both will bring culturally prescribed patterns of communication, etiquette, and problem solving. Both may bring stereotypes with them or underlying feelings about serving, being served by, or establishing a collegial relationship with someone who is "different." Nonmajority culture individuals may exhibit behaviors which are uncomfortable to those of the majority culture. Tension and frustration may result. It is important to remember that this is creative energy engendered by the tension which is a natural part of cross-cultural relations.

We all must be constantly vigilant for the dynamics of misinterpretation and misjudgment. Without an understanding of cross-cultural dynamics, misinterpretation and misjudgment are likely to occur. It is important to note that this misunderstanding is a two-way process; thus, the label *dynamics of difference.* These dynamics give cross-cultural relations a unique character that strongly influences the chances for productive cross-cultural interventions. The health-belief model can be used as a schema for analyzing ways in which perceptions of illness and perceived benefits of treatment may differ between patient and physician.

Cultural Stereotypes. The following statements describe a variety of responses to pain that may be culturally determined, as perceived by a health care professional who may or may not be distorting reality through the lenses of cultural bias, and who is more comfortable with some responses than with others.*

- "Mr. Smith in Bay A is the ideal patient. He never has a single complaint of pain."
- "Mrs. Cohen in B is a real complainer. She is constantly asking for pain medication and putting on her light."
- "Mrs. O'Malley in C is an ideal patient. She never complains about pain. For that matter, she never complains."
- "Mr. Chen in D says nothing. I often wonder what he is feeling."
- "Mrs. Petrini in F dramatically cries every time I look at her and complains of pain at every opportunity."

Q: "But . . . we are not all alike" . . . what does this mean for the provider?

The above statements were written as stereotypic descriptions of behaviors observed concerning patients responses to the subjective feeling of pain. Social scientists, health care researchers, and other professionals maintain that the phenomenon is culture bound: how pain and discomfort—for that matter, most emotions—are presented varies among cultures. A person raised in one cultural background may be allowed the free and open expression of his feelings, whereas a person from another culture may have been taught that (for a multitude of reasons) he must never reveal his true feelings. However, intra ethnic variation should be considered.

Let us say that these statements were all made by the same nurse. Let us go one step further and say that each patient had the same procedure performed 30 minutes ago. It would not be unusual, within the limits of general expectations, to see the different patients from differing cultures and ethnic groups exhibit the behaviors described. The fact that culture plays a role in behavior during illness was aptly demonstrated and strongly documented by Mark Zborowski in his study on pain in 1952.[28] Briefly, his findings were that Jewish and Italian patients generally responded to pain in an emotional fashion, and they tended to exaggerate the response; "old Ameri-

can Yankees" tended to be more stoic; and the Irish tended to ignore pain. Presentations of this type of data can often lead to a major problem: *stereotyping*. Todd and Hoffman reported that patients of Hispanic origin were less likely to receive pain medication for the same injury in the ED. In his discussion stereotyping was postulated as a reason for the discrepancy.[29]

Finally, the provider should use this information about a patient's culture cautiously, much as he would any epidemiological generalization; first to match the individual patient with the general predictor, and then to perform the appropriate test (or tests) to see whether in fact the patient fits the pattern. Intraethnic variation must be recognized. Discussions with patients about their involvement and dependence on kin and friends within the ethnic group would serve to reveal their adherence to ethnic health orientations and probably behaviors as well.

Q: What are some strategies and guidelines for applying cultural competence and social science concepts at the bedside?

1. **Recognize intraethnic variation.** Although standards for health behavior may be shared among people of an ethnic category, each patient is an individual. Five factors have been identified that contribute to variation in health belief and behaviors of ethnic groups. These factors may serve as a "guide."[6] They have been shown to have independent effects on health behaviors.

a. Exposure to biomedical and popular standards of health care (level of formal education, generational removal from immigrant experience, limited migration to mother country).
b. Income.
c. Occupation (migrant, manual, sedentary).
d. Religion.
e. Area of origin of mother country.

2. **Elicit the patient's concept or model and stage of disease and illness.** The provider should take particular care to elicit the patient's concept of his problem in a way that is nonjudgmental and that communicates genuine interest in the response. This might be accomplished by the following kind of preliminary explanation: "I know that patients and

*From Spector RE. *Cultural diversity in health and illness*, 3rd ed. Norwalk, CT: Appleton-Century-Crofts, 1985.

doctors sometimes have different ideas about diseases and what causes them. So it's often important in treating a disease to get clear on how both the doctor and the patient think about it. That's why I'd like to know more about your ideas on [whatever disease or symptom is relevant to the situation]. That way I can know what your concerns are, and we can work together in treating your sickness." (Of course, clarification of patients' disease concepts may also be relevant to other clinical tasks, such as eliciting a history or explaining a diagnostic procedure, and the wording of the introductory comment would have to be modified accordingly.)

Following such an introductory statement, a patient's concepts of his or her disease might then be asking the following questions:

a. What do you think has caused your problem?
b. Why do you think it started when it did?
c. What do you think your sickness does to you? How does it work?
d. How bad do you think your illness is? Do you think it will last a long time, or will it get better soon in your opinion?
e. What kind of treatment would you like to have?
f. What are the most important results you hope to get from treatment?
g. What are the major problems your illness has caused you?
h. What do you fear most about your illness?

3. Consider issues which may influence a patient's explanatory model of illness. Although the five issues listed below may apply to *any* population, they are listed here for your special consideration of the unique ethnic or cultural interpretation in a given population for whom you may be providing care.

a. Relief of pain or other symptoms.
b. Anxiety provoking symptoms (respiratory for Puerto Ricans, weakness for Haitians/Mexicans).
c. Fear of treatment (blood loss among Chinese).
d. Interference with role responsibilities.
e. Interference with valued activities.

4. Consider common ethnic concepts of disease. Although specific conceptual differences occur among various groups, certain general ideas are somewhat consistent across groups. For providers who care for many ethnic groups, awareness of these broad concepts may be of value. These issues should

be given special consideration as you deliver your explanatory model and engage the patient in a treatment plan.

a. "Blood"—Quality and quantity (thick, thin, high, low).
b. "Hot/Cold"—Idea of bodily imbalance precipitated by a variety of situations or foods that alter the body's temperature.
c. Drafts—Often, but not necessarily, related to hot and cold beliefs. Idea of respiratory infection, muscle aches and spasms due to air currents when "pores are open," i.e., perspiration, after a shower.

5. Acknowledge and incorporate ethnic folk models of treatment to enhance medical practice.

6. Use of translators when any question of reliability or validity of information. AT&T 1-800 service can be of value. Ask translator to use patient's own words as much as possible. To use AT&T, obtain a client ID number and organization name and call 1-800-874-9426.

7. Consider that interaction norms may also be specific to certain ethnic or cultural groups. Again, giving this knowledge may be of unique value to the provider. Age and sex may often influence the patient's expectations and participation in the medical encounter.

Differences in culture will increase in our society. Physicians do not need to agree with the logic of beliefs or efficacy of the behavior, but they should acknowledge and respect the individuals with these beliefs. Shared decision making and better understanding will enhance our professional lives and improve quality of care.

Q: What are the implications for scholarly research?

We need to understand the importance and validity of cultural competence and other social science concepts for our practice. There is a small but growing body of epidemiologic research which demonstrates the effects of racial and ethnic discrimination, sexism, and social class on health and health care. These studies are challenging the methods, the concepts, the norms and the conclusions of traditional approaches to racial/ethnic disparities in health.

Table 14-1   *General Principles of an Intercultural Curriculum*

Demonstrates knowledge of basic intercultural concepts.

- Recognizes that American society is heterogenous and physicians and patients are often of different cultural backgrounds.
- Recognizes that culture is important in the identity of all patients as well as all physicians.
- Recognizes that the physician's own culture and the culture of medicine has an important impact on his/her relationship with patients.
- Recognizes that communication of cultural understanding and respect is essential for establishing rapport and confidence.
- Recognizes that culture-related concepts (for example, explanatory model of illness) and behaviors (such as religion, diet) affect patients' acceptance of and compliance with prescribed therapy.
- Recognizes that nonverbal and verbal communication may differ from culture to culture.
- Recognizes that each individual patient is a unique combination of cultural, family, social group, and idiosyncratic beliefs.
- Recognizes the importance of communicating with the patient in a language in which the patient is fluent.
- Recognizes and appreciates the role of the trained medical interpreter in the bilingual medical encounter, and the importance of using such personnel rather than family members whenever possible.
- Recognizes that culture-related stresses and tensions can induce illness.
- Recognizes possible culturally-related differences in clinical epidemiology of common illnesses.

Demonstrates intercultural knowledge by appreciating basic categories of cultural information; for particular cultural groups encountered frequently, develops a knowledge base in these areas.

- Demonstrates understanding and knowledge of the importance of:
  - Predominant cultural values
  - Traditional health practices and health beliefs

- Family structure: patriarchal versus matriarchal; nuclear versus extended; role of individual members
- Community structure, and the role of important community leaders
- Religious beliefs and their effect on health care beliefs and practices
- Customs and attitudes surrounding death
- Nature and significance of common verbal and nonverbal communication styles
- Common dietary habits, foods, and their nutritional content
- Awareness of "culture shock", particularly in relation to patients entering modern health centers
- Awareness of prevailing intercultural tensions and psychosocial issues

Demonstrates important intercultural attitudes.

- Recognizes importance of patient's cultural background and environment when constructing an approach to an illness.
- Acknowledges patient's role as an active participant in his or her own care and as an "expert consultant" in conveying cultural information.
- Works to overcome language and cultural barriers in providing care, and provides support and advocacy for patients.

Demonstrates basic intercultural skills.

- Communicates an interest in and respect for the patient's culture.
- Tactfully and respectfully elicits general cultural information (see Objective 2).
- Elicits patient's understanding of and beliefs about illness or health problems.
- Elicits and considers information regarding possible culture-related health problems.
- Interprets verbal and nonverbal behaviors in a culturally-relevant manner.
- Negotiates a culturally appropriate health care plan with patient and family as partners.
- Demonstrates the ability to work as a team with a medical interpreter in the bilingual medical encounter.

---

* This curriculum does not list specific cultural beliefs of particular ethnic or cultural groups. Rather, a set of general objectives to be mastered which includes both general principles and guidance for obtaining more specific information when appropriate.

SOURCE: Goldstein E, Bobo L, Womeodo R, Kaufmann L, Nathan M, Palmer D, Scott CJ, "Intercultural Medicine," in *A Curriculum for Internal Medicine Residency,* Norman M. Jensen and Judith A. Van Kirk (eds). American College of Physicians, Philadelphia, Pennsylvania [1995 in press].

Q: What can I do as a medical educator?

Principles of intercultural medicine should be integrated into the EM curriculum. Models exist and are available.[30,31] General principles that can be considered are noted in Table 14-1.

NOTES

1. Cross TL, Bazron B, Jacobs CG, Doller B. *Towards a Culturally Competent System of Care: A Monograph on Effective Services for Minority Children Who are Severely Emotionally Disturbed.* Washington D.C.: Child and Adolescent Service System Program (CASSP) Technical Assistance Center, Georgetown University, Child Development Center, 1989.

2. Fong C, Hua M, Jui J, et al. Factorial structure of the chinese scale of attitudes towards disabled persons: A cross cultural validation. *Int J Rehab Research* 1984; 7:317–19.

3. Estes G, Zitzow D. *Heritage consistency as a consideration in counseling Native Americans.* Presented at the National Indian Education Association, Dallas, Texas, November 1980.

4. Hanwood LT. Hypertension in minority populations: Access to care. *Am J Med* 1990; 88(b):175–205.

5. Fejos P. Man, magic and medicine. In I. Goldston (ed.). *Medicine and anthropology.* New York: International University Press, 1959.

6. Cruickshank JK, Beevers DG (eds.). *Ethnic Factors in Health and Disease.* Boston: Wright; 1989.

7. Senior PA, Bhopal R. "Ethnicity as a variable in epidemiological research. *BMJ.* 1994; 309:327–30.

8. Centers for Disease Control and Prevention. Use of race and ethnicity in public health surveillance. Summary of the DC/ATSDR workshop. Atlanta, Georgia, March 1–2, 1993, *MMWR* 1993; 42:1–16.

9. Edwards LD. A survey of correct practices in the U.S. regarding minorities and gender. In S Walker, C Lumley (eds.). *The relevance of ethnic factors in the clinical evaluation of medicine.* Boston: Kleuter Academic. 1994: 107–14.

10. Schermerhorn R. *Comparative ethnic relations: A framework for theory and research.* Chicago: University of Chicago Press, 1978.

11. Feinstein JS. The relationship between SES and health: A review of the literature. *Milbank Quarterly* 1993; 71:279–321.

12. Wright L. One drop of blood. *The New Yorker.* July 25, 1994, 46–55.

13. Krieger N, Rowley DL, Herman A, Avery B, Phillips MT. Racism, sexism, and social class: Implications for studies of health, disease, and well-being. *Am J Prev Med* 1993; 9(5):92–122.

14. Hutchinson J. AIDS and racism in America. *J National Med Assoc.* 1992; 84(2):119–24.

15. Adler NE, Boyce T (et al.). Socioeconomic inequalities in health. *JAMA* 1993; 269:3140–5.

16. Gebbie K. Community—you, me, or us: Prevention and health promotion. *Am J Prev Med* 1993; 9(5):321–3.

17. Yee DL. Healthcare access and advocacy for immigrants and other underserved elders. *J Health Care Poor Underserved* 1992; 2(4):448–64.

18. Kelley MA (et al.). Primary care arrangements and access to care among African-American women in three Chicago communities. *Wom Health* 1992; 18(4):91–106.

19. Petronis KR (et al.). Effect of race on access to recombinant human erythropoietin in long-term hemodialysis patients, *JAMA* 1994; 271(22):1760–3.

20. Russell K, Jewel N. Cultural impact of health care access: Challenges for improving the health of African Americans. *J Comm Health Nurs* 1992; 9(3):161–9.

21. Health Services Administration. Identification of problems in access to health services and health careers for Asian Americans. *Pub Health Rep* 1976; 1:637–41.

22. Huth EJ. Identifying ethnicity in medical papers. *Ann Intern Med* 1995; 122:619–21.

23. Cauldwell S, Popenoe R. Perceptions and misperceptions of skin color. *Ann Intern Med* 1995; 122;614–17.

24. Bergner L. Race, health, and health services. *Am J Pub Health* 1993; 83(7):939–41.

25. Pachter LM. Culture and clinical care: Folk illness beliefs and behaviors and their implications for health care delivery. *JAMA* 1994; 271:690–4.

26. Snow, LF. *Walking over medicine.* San Francisco: Westview Press, 1992.

27. Kleinman A (et al.). Culture, illness and care: Clinical lessons from anthropologic and cross cultural research. *Ann Intern Med* 1978; 88:251–58.

28. Zborowski M. Cultural components in responses to pain. *J Soc Iss* 1952; 8:16–30.

29. Todd KH, Hoffman J, et al. Ethnicity as a risk factor for inadequate emergency department analgesia. *JAMA* 1993; 269(12):1537–9.

30. Kristal L (et al.). Cross-cultural family medicine residency training. *J Fam Pract* 1983; 17(4):683–7.

31. Goldstein E, Bobo L, Womeodo R, Kaufman L, Nathan M, Palmer D, Scott CJ. Intercultural Medicine. In NM Jensen and JA Van Kirk (eds.). *A Curriculum for Internal Medicine Residency.* Philadelphia: American College of Physicians, 1995 (in press).

15

Asthma and the Unmet Needs of Minorities

RENATE AUSTIN

CONTENTS

- Prevalence
- Risk factors
- Discrepancies in incidence between minority and majority populations
- Causative agents
- Physician practice patterns
- Interventions
- Protocol

CHAPTER SUMMARY

Mortality rates for asthma are rising for the population as a whole, but the risk is greater for minorities and for those who are poor or have limited access to health services. In one study, mortality risk increased 33 percent among African-Americans between 1976 and 1991. Causative agents are thought to include lack of access to medications, deficits in asthma education outreach efforts, and physician inattention to compliance with protocols. Suggested interventions involve improvements in discharge planning and education, protocol development, and multidisciplinary and multispecialty collaboration.

INTRODUCTION

The distribution of health care is inequitable. Minorities of many different backgrounds appear to share a common burden of inequity, the lack of adequate health care because of discrimination, and lower socioeconomic status. Hispanic Americans may also have language and cultural barriers that impede their access to health care. In addition, minority groups experience an increased morbidity and mortality from a variety of illnesses.

Asthma, in particular, is often viewed as an indicator of unmet health needs among people of color. In 1990, 12.3% of the population was African American, 10% Hispanic, and 74% white.[1] Mortality rates were greatest among African Americans. White women have an average life expectancy of 78.9 years, compared with 73.4 for black women, and white men have an average life expectancy of 72.3 years, compared with 64.9 years for black men. Mortality rates for black men are comparable to those seen in developing countries, and men in Harlem have been shown to fare worse than men in Bangladesh.[2] In the late 1980s, the infant mortality rate for black Americans was 2.1 times higher than the infant mortality rate for white Americans, and the postbirth death rate was 2.0 times greater. In emergency medicine, we see the sequelae of these health care dilemmas, but we also have the opportunity to care for, teach, and make a difference in these patients' lives. As health professionals, it is our duty to investigate, to try to delineate the causes of these discrepancies, and, if possible, to find a solution that will alleviate this health care crisis.

Case #1

A 19-year-old black female presents to the emergency department with complaints of wheezing and shortness of breath. The patient had been feeling ill for several days and thought she was "catching a cold." The patient has a history of asthma but has not seen her primary care physician in over a year. She states that she usually receives her medical treatment from the local emergency department and was last seen in the emergency department for an asthma attack one month ago. Her last hospitalization for asthma was about 6 months ago. The patient admits to being intubated once in her life several years ago, but says she had been relatively asymptomatic with her asthma until 1 year ago. She denies any known allergies or precipitating factors which might lead to bronchospasm. The past medical history is significant only for asthma. She denies tobacco or illicit drug use but admits to social drinking. Her medications include a ventolin inhaler as needed, birth control pills, and motrin. The patient denies any known drug or seasonal allergies. She was afebrile, with a heart rate of 120 beats per minute and a respiratory rate of 30. She was in moderate respiratory distress and able to speak in short sentences. Physical exam revealed accessory muscle use with supraclavicular retractions. The lung exam showed inspiratory and expiratory wheezes bilaterally throughout all lung fields. The patient was treated with inhaled B-agonists without significant improvement. An IV line was started, and she was given prednisone. She was subsequently admitted to intensive care because of continued deterioration of her condition.

Q: What factors influence the prevalence of asthma?

It has been estimated that asthma effects 9.9 million people in the U.S. During the 1970s, there was a decrease in mortality from asthma by 7.8% per year,[3] but in the 1980s, mortality rose by 6.2% annually. Certain conditions increase asthma morbidity and mortality: (1) living in poverty (13.1%), compared to above-poverty levels (10.3%); receiving suboptimal care or having limited access to care; (2) being black (12.7%), instead of white (10.4%); (3) being young; (4)

being male (11.4%, compared to 9.7% for women); (5) living in the South (12.7%) and West (11.6%), instead of the Northeast (9.1%) or Midwest (8.6%); and (6) having a history of a previous life-threatening asthma episode or hospitalization for asthma within the last year.[4]

During the period between 1965 and 1983, the hospitalization rate for asthma increased 50% in adults and more than 200% in children. In addition, the hospitalization rates for nonwhites were 50% greater in adults and 150% higher in children.[5] A study in New York City looked at preventable hospitalizations—cases in which appropriate outpatient management could have possibly averted inpatient care—and found that households with annual income below $15,000 had admission rates up to 6.4 times higher than those in high-income areas.[6] Similar admission-rate patterns were found for other diseases such as diabetic ketoacidosis, hyperosmolar coma, bacterial pneumonia, and congestive heart failure. In New York City, Hispanics were also found to have a higher number of hospitalizations and increased mortality. From 1982 to 1986, the number of hospitalizations for Hispanics was 29,633 for asthma, compared with 9,887 for whites, and the asthma mortality for Hispanics was 1.3 per 100,000, which was 3 times the white rate.[7] The majority of asthma deaths occurred in persons aged 20 to 34, with 76.2% of the deaths occurring in blacks and Hispanics. A study in Chicago produced a similar mortality pattern, with the greatest risk occurring among 20-to-34-year-olds, and an increase in mortality of 337% among African Americans between 1976 and 1991.[8]

Q: Why is there such a discrepancy between the majority and minority population in regard to asthma morbidity, mortality, and hospitalization?

Poverty, racial discrimination, and environmental factors related to both of these conditions modulate any genetic predisposition to disease. Research design problems make it difficult to separate out the relative contributions of these interacting variables.

Q: What questions might have been asked about allergens that trigger bronchospasm?

Does someone at home smoke cigarettes? Is there an animal in the house? Other questions that must be asked concern accessibility to adequate health care. Many Americans, at least 12%, have no health care insurance at all, and a large percentage of them live at or near the poverty level. Minority patients may be at increased risk of morbidity and mortality from asthma because they do not have a primary care physician, or because work requirements and child care responsibilities or transportation problems interfere with the ability to seek timely care. Many of these patients acquire their health care from the emergency department. Unfortunately, the ED is not the optimum place for a patient to learn how to manage and control asthma because of the high volume of patients and the lack of continuity of care. It has been shown that when patients are educated about their disease, they tend to use the ED less frequently for mild exacerbations.

Another possible reason for increased disease among minorities may be differences in practice patterns for minority and white patients, as well as possible differences in the prescribing patterns for white and minority patients. In 1984, a telephone survey was done in New York City with primary care physicians.[9] This survey included questions about practice guidelines, ethnic backgrounds of patients, physician education, certification, clinical hours worked per week, medical journal subscriptions, and the percentage of patients using Medicaid and Medicare. It was found that physicians with 50% or more black or Hispanic patients were less likely to follow nationally established guidelines. Only 33% were board-certified, 27% were affiliated with a medical school, and 40% subscribed to the *New England Journal of Medicine*. On average, these physicians worked 39.8 hours per week and saw 104 patients during that time. Of the physicians whose practice consisted of 50% or more white patients, 57% were board-certified, 40% were affiliated with medical schools, and 64% subscribed to the *New England Journal of Medicine*. Their work week consisted of 46 hours of clinical practice, and they saw 86 patients during this time. This same group of physicians were also more

likely to recommend mammography screening, sigmoidoscopy, influenza immunization for the elderly, pap tests, and stool guaiac, compared with physicians who predominantly cared for black and Hispanic patients. This study did not include asthmatic patients and the management of their illness. One could postulate, however, that there would be more education about asthma among the physician group with predominantly white patients. The physicians who treated primarily minority populations may have believed that their patients could not afford preventive care or believed that patients with less education do not appreciate the importance of preventive medicine; or, the physicians who care for primarily black patients may have been less aware of current guidelines for medical practice. Whatever the explanation, this study provides some preliminary corroboration that health care provided to the minority population contributes heavily to the disparities in morbidity and mortality.

Another explanation for the increased severity of asthma among blacks is inadequacy of medication. A study investigated the use of medication for the management of childhood asthma in Michigan.[10] Black asthmatics were found to receive medical care more frequently, yet they obtained asthma medication less often when compared to other groups. When they did receive medication, it was frequently in the form of fixed-combination drugs, and steroids were prescribed less frequently. Systemic steroids were prescribed 13.4% of the time, an adrenergic inhaler 21.3%, sustained-release theophylline 55.6%, and a fixed-combination product 35.7%. The fixed-combination product consisted of a methylxanthine, a barbiturate, and an adrenergic sympathomimetic agent. Systemic steroids were given to 9.8% of urban black patients and to 18.8% of white urban patients. Adrenergic inhalers were prescribed for 18.1% of black urban patients, compared with 24% of white urban patients. Sustained-release theophylline was given to 54.5% of black urban patients and to 57.8% of white urban patients. Fixed-combination products were distributed to 28.2% of urban white patients and to 43.7% of urban black patients. In this study, urban and rural patients were separated in the statistical analysis, but it was difficult to compare data because of the small numbers of rural black residents.

The most striking difference in the study was between the medications received by black and white patients. Surprisingly, black patients continued to receive less effective medical therapy until Medicaid stopped reimbursing for products that were less efficacious.

Q: What can be done to reduce mortality and severity of illness among minority asthmatics?

A program was devised in New York City in the 1980s to see if intensive education and special treatment for the difficult asthmatic would reduce the number of hospitalizations for these patients. The emphasis in this program was on aggressive at-home management of asthma exacerbations and education about the disease. This program targeted patients who had previously had many hospitalizations for asthma. There was a threefold reduction in admissions, and there was a reduction in hospitalization length by twofold.[11]

This program was developed at Bellevue Hospital in New York, where there was a substantial number of asthmatics who required frequent admission. According to the protocol, the patient's first couple of physician visits consisted of interviews which lasted about an hour, in which the pathophysiology of asthma and its treatment were discussed. The following visits were scheduled for at least a half-hour. The information given was in the patient's primary language, and no written material was distributed to the patient. All of the patients in this program used B-agonists and inhaled steroids. In addition, they had oral steroids available for exacerbations. Each treatment plan was specifically designed for each patient's needs. There were a few patients on methylxanthines and a few patients on cromlyn sodium, but no one in this program showed any undesirable affects from the medications. The key to preventing severe asthmatic attacks was aggressive, early at-home management. Intensive education and individually designed treatment plans contributed to a reduction in the number of hospital visits, as well as a reduction in the number of asthma hospitalizations. Education about disease and prevention *can* make a difference.

In emergency medicine, we do not have the opportunity to sit down for an hour with one patient to explain the pathology of illness, nor do we have the accessibility to our patients to insure that they are properly educated in the management of their specific disease, but if we are aware of our limitations, it is possible to do a better job than we are currently doing. Our goal should be to advocate for preventive measures against disease entities that we encounter frequently. As emergency physicians, we are uniquely equipped to make substantial differences in our patients' lives. We are most often the physician of first encounter, and most often the only physician with whom the minority population gets acquainted.

We therefore have a challenge of the utmost importance. We must be primary care physicians as well as specialists. We must be the initiators of education about disease processes and their management. We must be patient advocates because we see that those who fall between the cracks of primary care eventually end up in our care. Asthma is a disease that most commonfolk do not respect as a life-threatening illness, but as emergency physicians, we know this is far from the truth. Many patients who we watch succumb to this illness are vibrant young people in the prime of their lives. If we are more diligent in our efforts to provide primary care as well as emergency services to these patients, we can contribute to decreasing the morbidity and mortality. If we are cognizant of the need for asthma education, we can easily provide this service while the patient is in the ED. We can also provide referrals and linkages to asthma clinics or primary care settings.

As part of our history and physical, we should inquire about patients' general health status and access to care, their history of education about asthma, and investigate the role of environmental elements. Pollution in the form of particulate matter has been shown to cause an increase in hospitalizations in children with bronchitis and asthma.[12] Total airborne particulate matter decreased by 20% between 1979 and 1988, but information on particulate matter that causes lower respiratory tract disease has not been available. Children whose mothers smoke have a higher incidence of reactive airway disease. A decrease in pulmonary function is associated with maternal smoking, and this causes increased risk of reactive airways in the first year of life. Mothers therefore need to be educated about the increased health risk to their children if they are smokers.

A study program was designed to improve the outcome of inner-city children with asthma.[13] The program focused on three main elements: (1) an individualized medication schedule; (2) patient and parent education about the disease to prevent wheezing and respond to it appropriately when it occurred; and (3) efforts to reduce patient noncompliance. The patients that were enrolled in this program were recruited from the ED to include all patients with and without a primary care physician. When information was elicited about medications, many preventable problems were identified. It was found that 47 of the patients had been given medications "as needed," 39 had been given medication on a continuous basis, and 2 patients were not prescribed any medication. Patients who received "as needed" medications received only theophylline, which does not work once wheezing has begun. Those patients who received continuous medication did not have any additional medications for acute exacerbations. When the parents were interviewed, it was found that 10% had no medication at home, and 63% said they could only get refills by going to the medical site. Almost all of the parents knew precipitating factors that caused their children to wheeze. However, half of them did not believe that asthma attacks could be prevented. Seventy-five percent of the households had a smoker in the house, and 71% of parents gave their children medication *after* wheezing began.

The parents were also questioned about their knowledge of asthma. After the nurse from the study group identified aspects of medical care that could be improved upon, changes were implemented. Parents were sent educational material about asthma, and primary care physicians were contacted regarding potential changes in patients' medication schedules. Parents were instructed in the correct use of medications, and the importance of primary care provider contact was stressed. Parents were also contacted every couple of months to check on medication needs and the patients' health status. After these interventions, 16% of problems with medication prescription had been improved, the rate of acute care visits fell 50%, and the rate of nonacute visits did not increase. This program confirms what has been seen in studies on adult asthmatics—that intensive education, individualized medication schedules, and close care fol-

low-up can decrease ED use in high-risk asthma patients.

Q: What interventions can the emergency physician make to help improve the health of our asthmatic patients?

In obtaining the history we should inquire about first diagnosis of asthma, history of intubations, history of ICU admissions, last admission to the hospital, last visit to the ED, history of steroid use, usual precipitating factors, present medication regime, smoking history, and whether or not patient has a primary care physician. We should also inquire about the ability to obtain medications once they are prescribed and the ability to complete follow-up care with a physician once an appointment has been made. Educational materials about the pathophysiology of asthma, its precipitants, warning signs, and treatment should be placed in the treatment area. If we find that the patient is unable to purchase the necessary medication, we should get social service assistance to provide it. The patient who has no primary care physician should be referred to a nearby primary health care facility. There should be contact with the physician within 72 hours. A nurse should try to follow up on all asthmatic patients who were seen within the prior week to ensure that they have not had a relapse and have proceeded with their plan of care. We should also establish a close relationship with the pulmonary department and have the ability to refer patients to them to obtain pulmonary function tests. We should attempt to identify patients at presentation in the ED who are at high risk and target these patients specifically for intensive education, medication management, and outpatient follow-up. In an attempt to identify patients at high risk, a questionnaire should be administered to all patients prior to discharge or admission, and specific discharge instructions and educational materials should accompany routine discharge information. Correct usage of medication should be demonstrated, and samples should be available for patients who need them. The peak expiratory flow rate should be measured pre- and posttreatment in all patients when possible, and results should be interpreted based on the average predicted norm for height and age. A file card should be kept in the department for patients who appear frequently in the ED with a summary of all pertinent information, including last ED visit, baseline PEFR, intubations, use of steroids and tapers, and any allergies that precipitate attacks. Patients who are at increased risk should be given peak flow meters, as this would give the patient a more accurate measurement of the status of their disease. Some patients have psychosocial issues which affect their ability to obtain health care, and these issues should be addressed. In addition, an association has been identified between depression and increased mortality from asthma.[13] If we observe mood alterations, we should refer our patients to a psychiatrist. If asthma is exacerbated by cocaine, heroin, or marijuana use, the patient should be referred for drug abuse treatment. We must make an attempt to address all the basic health needs of our high-risk asthmatic patients in order to change the current trend.

NOTES

1. Hall CB. A demographic profile of African Americans. In Braithwaite RL, Taylor SE (eds.). *Health Issues in the Black Community.* San Francisco: Jossey-Bass, 1992.
2. McCord C, Freeman HP. Excess mortality in Harlem. *NEJM* 1990; 322:173–7.
3. Weiss KB, Wegener DK. Changing patterns of asthma mortality. *JAMA* 1990; 264:1683–7.
4. Larsen GL. Asthma in children. *NEJM* 1992; 326:1540–5.
5. Evans R, Mullally DI, Wilson RW, Gergen PJ, Rosenberg HM, Grauman JS, Chevarley FM, Feinleib M. National trends in morbidity and mortality of asthma in the U.S. *Chest* 1987; 91:655–745.
6. Billings J, Zeital L, Lukomnik, Carey TS, Blank AE, Newman. Impact of socioeconomic status on hospital use in New York City. *Health Affairs* 1993; 12:162–73.
7. Carr, Zeital L, Weiss K. Variations in asthma hospitalizations and deaths in New York City. *AJPH* 1992; 82:59–65.
8. Targonski PV, Persky VW, Orris P, Addington W. Trends in asthma mortality among African Americans and whites in Chicago, 1968 through 1991. *AJPH* 1994; 84:1830–3.
9. Gemson DH, Elinson J, Messeri P. Differences in physician prevention practice patterns for white and minority patients. *J Comm Health* 1988; 13:53–64.
10. Bosco LA, Gerstmann BB, Tomita DK. Variations in the use of medication for the treatment of childhood asthma in the Michigan Medicaid population, 1980–1986. *Chest* 1993; 104:1727–32.
11. Mayo PH, Richmond J, Harris HW. The results of a program to reduce admissions for adult asthma. *Ann Int Med* 1990; 112: 864–71.
12. Gergen, Peter I, Weiss, Kevin B. Changing patterns of asthma hospitalization among children, 1979–1987. *JAMA* 1990; 264:1688–92.
13. Wisson LS, Warshon M, Box J, Baker D. Case management and quality assurance to improve care of inner city children with asthma. *Am J Dis Child* 1988; 142:748–52.

16

Hispanic Immigrants: Health Care Access and Outcome

CARLOS R. FLORES

CONTENTS

- Current status of the Hispanic population
- Health beliefs of Hispanics
- Informed consent
- Translation issues
- Cross-cultural similarities to other ethnic groups
- Access to health insurances
- Refugee status: victims of torture and war
- Recommendations for emergency medicine: need for cultural training, advocacy, manpower, and health policies

CHAPTER SUMMARY

American history has been shaped by different waves of immigrants. These immigrants have brought with them cultures rich in language, custom, beliefs, and traditions, which have been incorporated into this country's cultural mosaic. This cultural heritage has a significant impact, along with socioeconomic status, on the ability of immigrants to access health care and achieve satisfactory health outcomes. These communities pose a challenge to Western medicine. Health care providers need a better understanding of this cultural and socioeconomic heritage in order to communicate effectively with their patients. Recommendations include: advocacy on the part of health care providers, enhanced manpower, cross-cultural training, and broad health care policy changes. _____

INTRODUCTION

Immigration patterns continually change. As an immigrant community becomes a part of the political majority, other groups assume the role of newly arrived immigrants and minorities. Current advances in technology, travel, and communication have allowed some of these groups to keep close ties to their countries of origins, avoiding acculturation and continuing to live in this country in relative social, economic, and political isolation.

These communities are increasing in size. For example, between 1980 and 1990, the Hispanic population grew five to eight times faster than the non-Hispanic white population.[1,2] Currently, approximately 20 million Hispanics live in this country, and it is expected that by the year 2000, at the current growth rate, Hispanics will be the largest minority.[1,2] Immigrant community growth coupled with generally substandard economic status, housing, and education, and growing health care needs have created a formidable challenge for health care policy makers, physicians, and all health care professionals. In addition to these demographic factors, immigrants bring with them a cultural heritage that plays an important role in their perception of their health, their understanding and acceptance of Western medicine, and their health care needs.

Although Hispanics, Africans, Caribbean, and Middle Eastern peoples are usually considered single entities, there are major differences of social history and cultural identity among the many nationalities that compose each group. These differences among subgroups influence health behaviors, access to care, and, ultimately, health outcomes.[3] Immigrants from India are a good example of a complex, culturally diverse nation. There are approximately 16 recognized languages in India's constitution, with many others spoken throughout the country. Although most of the population is Hindu, India has a large Muslim population. Immigrants from India also differ in their level of education, from highly educated scientists to barely literate individuals, and in their level of income and acculturation.[4]

One solution has been to develop subcategories based on national origins to describe different subgroups. For example, Hispanics are divided into Puerto Ricans (Mainland and Islander), Mexican Americans, Cuban Americans, Central and South Americans.[5] Subcategories, in general, are problematic. They do not take into account acculturation and the fact that there are shared cultural ties among these groups that transcend their national origins and that have created shared political and economic agendas. The challenge lies in developing classification schemes that recognize distinctions in community practices but that also respect the need for these diverse communities to respond to broad problems with a collective voice.[3] For Western medicine to be successful, health care practitioners must understand these factors and the effect they have on health care beliefs and practices, health care access, and outcome.

DISEASE AND ILLNESS: CULTURALLY SPECIFIC MODELS FOR INTERPRETING SICKNESS

Sociologic research justifies the distinction between disease and illness. Disease is an abnormality in the structure and function of the human body. Illness, on the other hand, is what the individual suffers. It is the human experience of sickness, and it is culturally constructed. Modern (Western) physicians train in the diagnosis and therapy of diseases.[6] The doctor, not the patient, is the one who defines disease.[7]

It is not surprising that sickness is viewed differently by the physician and the patient. These disparate views of the same sickness can impact on health care delivery and outcome. Differences between the patient and the physician in interpretation and expectations about diagnosis and therapy, and about the nature of the physician-patient relationship, will, to an extent, be culturally specific.[4,6] It is therefore essential that clinical science investigate illness as well as disease, and clinical care should emphasize both perspectives.[6]

The cases described in this chapter will serve as an example of the complex picture of immigrant health, with emphasis on the effect of social, economic, and cultural factors on the ability of these communities to access our health care system. The concept of informed consent and special circumstances faced by immigrants will be discussed to emphasize additional factors which contribute to these communities' perception of and acceptance of medical care.

Case # 1

A 24-year-old Hispanic male was brought to the emergency department after his friends witnessed him having a seizure. He had been in good health, without known past medical illnesses or hospitalizations. He stated that he had been in this country for a few months and had worked at a variety of low-paying jobs. He was not taking any medicines and had no known allergies. During the initial evaluation, the patient had a generalized, tonic-clonic seizure followed by a brief post-ictal state. He became alert and oriented and was admitted to the hospital for further evaluation. Prior to the admission, during the registration process, it became apparent that the patient had used two different names. His friends had provided one name; he had provided another. He spoke limited English and the physician spoke limited Spanish. The clerical staff, serving as interpreters, asked his friends for clarification, but they could not provide additional information. The patient was assessed by a Hispanic physician who obtained a more detailed history and developed a rapport with the patient. During this conversation it became evident that the patient was an undocumented immigrant (did not have legal entry status) and did not have any medical insurance. The different names were provided because of his fear regarding his illegal immigration status.

Q: What is the current status of the Hispanic population in the United States? What effect does this have on their ability to access our health care system? What circumstances might emergency physicians keep in mind as they elicit histories from Hispanic patients or other immigrant groups?

The Hispanic population and its health care needs pose a complex health care challenge that requires consideration of the specific social, cultural, economic and institutional factors that contribute to the health status of each Hispanic subgroup.[2,8] Specifically levels of education, occupational achievement, and income must be understood as they directly affect health status.[9,10] As one of the largest groups of immigrants, Hispanics serve as an example from which observations can be made regarding health care of minorities and immigrants in this country.

Hispanic families are generally larger than those of non-Hispanic whites and are more likely to be headed by a woman.[1] But, there are variations between groups, with 43% of Puerto Rican families headed by a single woman and 19% of Central and South American families headed by a woman.[1] Hispanics, in general, have the lowest educational attainment.[1,2] Approximately 50% of all Hispanics graduate from high school, compared with 64% of African Americans and 78% of non-Hispanic whites.[1] This is significant, as it has been shown that levels of education are related to a variety of factors, such as health beliefs, health practice, distrust of doctors and health care personnel, and to gaps in health information and education.[5,9,11]

Hispanic families have a high rate of unemployment.[1,2] Approximately 10% of Puerto Ricans and Mexican American are unemployed, twice the rate of white Americans, versus 6% of Cuban Americans. Employed Hispanics have, in general, the lowest status occupations and are the lowest paid.[1] Many are employed in service and production industries or as laborers.[2,12,13] Approximately 9.5% of non-Hispanics live in poverty, whereas 25% of Mexican Americans live in poverty and 37% of Puerto Ricans live in poverty.[1]

Except for Cuban Americans, Hispanics are generally younger and are concentrated in groups that theoretically require fewer health services.[1,9] Their lower socioeconomic status, however, creates an above average need for services.[9] Mexican Americans and Puerto Ricans have a two to three times higher incidence of type-II diabetes, with Mexican Americans having a higher rate of retinopathy and end-stage renal failure.[5,9,14] Despite these facts, there continues to be inadequate screening in this population for early detection of diabetes and its complications.[9] Infant mortality rates are higher in Hispanics but show considerable variation between groups, with Puerto Ricans having a higher rate than Cuban Americans or Mexican Americans.[15] Hispanic women have a higher incidence of cancer of the cervix, perhaps as a result of inadequate access to preventive services.[5] Hispanics also suffer from excess incidence of cancer of the stomach, esophagus, and pancreas.[5] Finally, rates of alcoholism and drug abuse are higher among Hispanics, compared with those of non-Hispanic whites.[16]

Case Continuation

Before the patient was transported to his hospital bed, the emergency physician sat down with him to explain the possible causes of his seizures and prepare him for the diagnostic workup he would experience during his admission. The EP began by eliciting the patient's own health beliefs and attitudes toward Western medicine by asking how he understood what had happened to him. In addition, the practitioner mentioned that a lot of people take herbs for different illnesses and wondered what the patient had been doing for his health before he came to the ED. He also discussed the patient's fear related to his immigrant status, reassured him that he himself was glad to provide care, and provided the information that it was illegal to deny medical care to patients without papers.

Q: What are the cultural issues which may affect Hispanics' acceptance and interaction with Western medicine? What role do cultural factors play in this case?

Hispanics bring with them a myriad of cultural beliefs and traditions which affect their interpretation of sickness and their reaction to professional health practitioners in the United States.[17] In many instances, they reject what the established medical system can offer and instead seek health care within the informal system they brought with them from their country of origin.[18]

Puerto Ricans have brought with them what some have named the "Puerto Rican Syndrome," characterized by trembling, falling to the floor with seizure-like convulsions and semiconsciousness. This syndrome has no pathophysiologic basis and is felt to be a psychological expression of anger and/or libidinal conflicts. Spiritism, a doctrine based on the interrelationship between the material world and the spirits of the invisible world, plays a major role in the lives of some Puerto Ricans. The doctrine states that the spirits are able to make people sick or cure them.[18,19]

Some Mexican Americans continue the tradition of *curanderismo*. This type of folk medicine is based on a combination of Native American and medieval Spanish medicine and carries with it the belief that God can heal and that certain individuals have the gift to carry on God's healing.[7] For an individual to be healthy, a balance between the cold and the hot must be maintained. An imbalance will cause disease. Cold sicknesses require hot remedies, and hot illnesses require cold medications. The *curandero* prescribes a variety of herbal and traditional potions as well as prayers and other rituals to attempt to restore the balance.[17,18,20] The practice of *curanderismo* is not limited to any socioeconomic group. It seems to have participants at all levels, regardless of economic status, educational level, family size, or primary language.[21]

Intrinsic to *curanderismo* are a variety of folk conditions and mystical diseases. *Caida de la mollera*, or fallen fontanelle, for example, is thought to have several etiologies. It is believed that if a baby is removed too quickly from the mother's breast or the bottle, or if the baby is held incorrectly or dropped, the baby will suffer from *caida de la mollera*.[21] Children who present with crying spells, restlessness, vomiting, inability to suck, sunken eyes and decreased tearing, diarrhea, and sometimes fever are thought to have this diagnosis.[21] It is not unusual for parents to take these children to local healers for treatment and avoid professional care, with sometimes tragic outcomes as a result of untreated hypovolemic shock. Treatment for *caida de mollera* includes pushing the palate, holding the child upside down while striking the heels, or shaking the child.[21]

Empacho is a syndrome attributed to the inability of the digestive system to pass a chunk of food that causes severe abdominal pain. The treatment for *empacho* is based on body massages that seek to restore the balance of hot and cold in the body as well as a variety of herbal preparations. *Mal de ojo* has its origin in the evil eye concept. It is believed that if the patient is untreated, he will die, but sometimes the patient is not brought to the attention of a doctor for fear that the physician will miss the diagnosis and make the patient worse. *Susto*, an illness caused by exposure to a frightening experience, presents with languor, listlessness, insomnia, depression, and anorexia.[17,18,19,21] Treatment requires the *asustado* to speak openly about the events that led to the *susto*, followed by bed rest and a ritual that includes prayers, incantations, and *barridas* (sweeping of the body with an egg, a candle, or herbal teas).[21,22] *Santeria*, a blend of Christianity and West African religions, is practiced by some Cuban Americans.[18,19]

Relevant to this specific case is the notion that epilepsy is often considered to be a result of excess of cold and that it is best treated with plenty of hot chicken-pea soup.[20] In case #1, it was critically important for the physician to ascertain the patient's health beliefs and practices. The patient's acceptance of anticonvulsant medications in the form of distinct pills will depend on the ability of medical staff, including social workers, to make connections between the patient's prior health experience and the scientific concept on which treatment is based. This will have a major bearing on patient compliance and outcome. The physician needs to know the role folk medicine plays in the patient's attitude towards Western medicine. A precise, albeit concise, social-cultural history will guide the physician to tailor the therapeutic plan, anticipate discharge needs, and participate with the other members of the health care team in delivering the best care possible. This concept becomes even more consequential in the interaction between physicians and immigrant patients and their families.

Q: How can physicians and health professionals obtain a history and explain procedures and potential complications to a patient who does not speak English?

Health care professionals are frequently faced with the predicament of obtaining informed consent from a non-English-speaking patient. Written informed consent, to be valid, must satisfy two requirements. First, it must contain all the necessary information for the patient to make a reasonable, intelligent, and informed decision. Second, it must be understandable to the patient.[23] Studies have documented that consents, even in English, tend to be written at too high a reading level, and some are even at the level of a legal or academic journal. This, of course, makes them incomprehensible to the average English-speaking person and certainly does not meet the standard of informed consent.[23]

It is common for immigrants to be faced with complex decisions for themselves or for a relative that require a clear understanding of the nature of the disease, its manifestation, and the therapeutic regimen recommended. Cultural organization, the perception of illness, the expectations of the physician, and language barriers all make it very difficult for information to be conveyed clearly and appropriately.[17,4] The use of appropriate translators and interpreters then becomes essential. Obtaining a history in the patient's primary language is extremely valuable. Such a conversation permits information about cultural practices and beliefs to be extracted, yields a better understanding of the patient's symptoms and perception of the disease, and enables the physician to explain to the patient and family the nature of the illness and therapeutic plan.

Q: What about using family members or other hospital employees to translate?

Unfortunately, trained professional translators and interpreters are not always available.[17] Physicians then resort to using friends and family members as translators. This practice is full of practical and legal problems. It places patient confidentiality at risk and can be unsatisfactory to the patient, as it might disrupt cultural standards that dictate behavior between relatives and friends.[17] For example, immigrant cultures often have a strict family hierarchy that would make it very difficult to use children as interpreters. Placing the child in what might be interpreted as a position of control might be inappro-

priate.[17,24] The patient might be unable or unwilling to provide all the information required, and the child might, because of his age and cultural and language barriers, be unable to understand or explain to the patient the information he has been given.[17]

In many emergency department situations where formal translation services are unavailable, "nonprofessional staff" (clerks and janitors) are pressed into dual duty as translators. This practice creates several problems. First, there is a violation of patient confidentiality, since these individuals have had no formal instruction in medical ethics. Second, there may be problems in accuracy, since conveyance of medical information often requires understanding medical terminology. Third, translation creates an unfair burden on the hospital worker, who assumes a serious responsibility for which there is no compensation and reward and which takes him or her from normal duties.

Medical translation is a difficult art and best practiced by trained individuals. When this expertise is not available on a regular basis, it is necessary for the hospital to contract with telephone company translation services and to have printed instructions sheets and consent forms available in several languages.

It is clear that obtaining consent can be a complex procedure. Cultural differences between the patient and the practitioner make it difficult to explain necessary procedures and interventions. Religious beliefs might also play a role in obtaining informed consent. For Southeast Asian refugees, an invasive procedure can be especially frightening because of fear stemming from the belief that the soul is attached to the body and can leave, thereby causing illness or death.[25]

Cultural organization and value systems will mold an individual's response to death and to the inevitability of death, as is often encountered in patients with terminal diseases. These values, along with language barriers, interfere in the explanation of death by the physician, the understanding of death by the family, and the acceptance of culturally specific behavior by the physician.[17,24,25] Adequate translation services are particularly essential for communicating issues related to fears and deeply held values and beliefs that influence the appropriateness of the decision-making process.

Q: What are the implications of this case for patients from other ethnic backgrounds?

There are similarities between the effects of social, cultural, and economic factors on health care of Hispanics and of other immigrants. Immigrants from India, as noted, exhibit tremendous variability in their levels of education, employment, salary, and acculturation.[4] And, although Western medicine is the preferred type of medicine in India, East Indians also share a common health-related behavior derived from the traditional *Ayurvedic* principles. The interrelationship between the body and the universe is a fundamental principle of *Ayurveda*. A person is considered healthy when the body humors—wind, fire (bile), and water (phlegm)—are in harmony and ill when the humors are out of balance. This helps explain why the consumption of food, particularly the consumption of cold or hot food, is of great concern to this community. Additionally, the variability in language and the ease of expressing feelings and symptoms within the population makes it difficult to express precisely the patient's symptomatology.[4]

Iranian immigrants to this country also show variability in level of education and religion. Sensitivity is valued in Iranian society, but a sensitive person may become *naharat*, a term used to express undifferentiated, unpleasant, emotional, and physical feelings. The expression of *naharat*, which may arise from the process of immigration and uprooting from one's formal and customary society and the difficulties in learning the norms of a new society, coupled with financial stress and the separation of a family unit, may be expressed in verbal or nonverbal means and by somatization. Some Iranians, as do some Hispanics and East Indians, share a tradition of humoral medicine based on four elements—fire, air, water, and earth—and a balance between blood, red bile, phlegm, and black bile. There is also the concept of a balance of hot and cold foods that dictates health and illness.[26]

Afghan immigrants frequently suffer from depression. They seem to avoid psychotherapy, particularly if the issues surrounding their diseases reflect weakness, an issue they find hard to discuss. And, because of traditional male and female roles, women prefer to be examined by a female, particularly for gynecological or obstetrical matters.[27]

The case illustrates the effects that social, economic, and cultural factors have on the abilities of immigrants to gain access to our health care system. It is clear that many different factors will influence the patient's perception of good health, understanding of Western medicine and relationship with Western physicians. These same variables play a very important role in the physician's ability to understand the needs of the community and how best to serve that community within the structure of Western medicine and within the confines of a different culture.

Case # 2

A 31-year-old Central American black male presented to the emergency department for evaluation of fever, malaise, and a rash. The patient had a complicated history and was unable to describe his past medical history in detail. He suffered from an unknown vascular problem which left him paralyzed below the waist. He was on no medication, and he denied allergies to known medications. He was found to be febrile but with no source for the fever. On examination, the rash had vanished. He had a marked leukocytosis and anemia. The decision was made to admit the patient, but the ED was unable to find an accepting physician for 24 hours. It was only after administrative intervention that an accepting physician was found and the patient was admitted to the hospital.

Q: How easy is it for immigrants to obtain health insurance? What effect does this have on national and local policies regarding availability of health insurance?

In addition to cultural issues that affect their health care, many immigrants lack adequate health insurance to cover physician visits or hospitalization. Lack of health insurance coverage is a result of various factors. Immigrants suffer from a higher unemployment rate and, therefore, lack commonly found benefits such as health insurance.[1,2] Employment does not guarantee coverage, as many find employment in industries that do not provide coverage; and, if coverage is provided, it is usually basic in nature and not comprehensive.[2,5] Migrant workers because of the nature of the industry, and their fragile financial, political, and social status also lack health insurance.[12,13]

A study performed in Dade County, Florida, revealed that elderly immigrants, compared with their native-born counterparts, were less likely to have Medicare or private insurance. Being under 65 years of age and of a lower-income group were determinants in not being insured. The ability to be privately insured was influenced by race, income level, and level of education.[28]

Lack of insurance creates a significant barrier to primary care.[29] In a study of Hispanics in Orange County, California, insurance status was the strongest predictor of access to care. Uninsured Hispanics were least likely to have a regular source of care or to have visited a physician within the previous year. The study did not find any difference between illegal residents and citizens.[30] This lack of primary care forces individuals to gain access to our health care system via our emergency departments.[29,31] Patients who are older, unmarried, nonwhite, of lower socioeconomic class, or uninsured are more likely to be admitted through the emergency department.[31] Although data for all immigrants is not readily available, it is known that Hispanics, in general, gain access to the hospital via the emergency department.[8] These admissions are more expensive than similar elective admissions.[8,31]

Policies regarding national or state health insurance availability must take into consideration the present status of immigrant populations. Policies that restrict or limit health insurance on the basis of citizenship, length of immigration, or other factors might discriminate against immigrants. Providing health insurance to all immigrants will improve access, promote primary care, and, ultimately, improve the health status of these communities. Studies have shown that these individuals will participate in health insurance programs as long as the costs are manageable.[30]

These policies must include undocumented immigrants as well. From a public health point of view, any barriers to care for these individuals increase health risk for the entire population. Easy access prevents exacerbation of infectious and chronic conditions, reduces mortality, and, in the long run,

reduces the cost of care. In addition to humanitarian reasons for providing undocumented immigrants health care, it must be realized that these people are contributing to their communities through their labor (many pay social security and local, state, and federal taxes) and have earned the medical right to treatment when they are ill or in pain.

Case Continuation

Further discussion with the patient elicited information that he was a political refugee who had immigrated legally 3 years ago. He had been febrile for several weeks, and, when herbal remedies failed to cure him, his friends insisted he come to the hospital. In his own country, he had been tortured and spent 6 months in solitary confinement. He also reports that during his internment there, he was injected with malaria.

Q : What issues should be specifically addressed in the medical treatment of refugees?

Refugees are considered involuntary immigrants.[24] Their immigration was caused by a variety of social, political, and economic conditions in their country of origin.[17,18,24,32] This immigration is often sudden, and dangerous. Families are broken, and socioeconomic status can change quickly and precipitously.[27]

Many refugees are victims of trauma, including torture, which creates lasting scars on individuals. The survivors can have physical, psychological, or cognitive symptoms. Illnesses such as tuberculosis or malnutrition have been reported in this group. Severe bone fractures with poor treatment have caused long-lasting physical impairment. Sleep disturbances, irritability, depression, and suicide have all been reported.[27,32,33]

A study to evaluate the influence of culture on the receptiveness of victims of torture to various treatment modalities revealed significant differences between South American and Indochinese refugees. The authors noted that the differences were attributable to cultural factors. South American survivors were more receptive to psychodynamic therapeutic approaches than the Indochinese community, who were more appreciative of specific medication than their Hispanic counterparts.[32]

Research data suggest that treatment of these survivors should take into account the role of culture in the survivors' receptiveness to treatment. Additional research is required to better understand this field.[32,34]

CONCLUSION

The immigrant population has grown substantially throughout the last 20 years. Their current status, marked by lower levels of education, lower-income jobs, and lack of health insurance, results in a harsh political reality. These factors decrease their access to our health care system. While cultural factors do not necessarily impair access to health care, they do modify receptiveness to Western medicine.[30] Cultural factors also play a role in the ability of health care professionals to understand health care beliefs and practices among immigrant communities. Special circumstances, such as forced immigration and torture, should also be understood and treated in a culturally specific manner.

RECOMMENDATIONS

Emergency medicine's role includes

1. *Cultural training.* Medical schools and training programs should encourage cultural competence, and include education in the commonly practiced traditional and cultural beliefs in various countries and cultures. Access to our health care system, for some, is primarily via our emergency departments. Emergency physicians must strive to include cultural competence training into emergency medicine residency curriculums. This training, at a minimum, must be geographically specific but must also provide residents and students with a foundation upon which they can expand in the future, as their patients' problems and questions direct the course of their learning.

2. *Advocacy.* Health care professionals must serve as advocates for issues pertaining to immigrant health. Health care professionals are in an excellent position, with some additional education, to understand the needs of these communities and to articulate these needs, in careful detail, to the appropriate governmental and regulatory agencies.

Emergency medicine is in a pivotal position to enact change. As the only open door to our health care system for these vulnerable communities, emergency medicine becomes the central axle of a complex organization whose purpose is to provide for the welfare of us all. A strong, educated voice, pursuing research into the many factors that impede access, interacting with local, state, and national and federal organizations, and advocating for these communities, will find its rewards in the improvement of health care delivery to these communities.

3. *Manpower.* Medical school and training programs in the United States, through active recruitment of faculty and students, must strive to create a culturally diverse medical community. With this cultural diversity, medicine will be able to tackle the multitude of problems facing immigrant communities.

4. *Health insurance.* It is clear that one of the strongest deterrents to adequate health care is the lack of health insurance. A national policy that guarantees insurance to all (without exception) will provide perhaps the most important long-term solution to the issue of immigrant health.

NOTES

1. Amaro H. *In the midst of plenty: Reflections on the economic and health status of Hispanic families.* Presented at the American Psychological Association Convention, Washington, DC, August 14–18, 1992.
2. Furino A, Munoz E. Health status among Hispanics: Major themes and new priorities. *JAMA* 1991; 265:255–7.
3. Novello AC, Wise PH, Kleinman D. Hispanic Health: Time for Data, Time for Action. *JAMA* 1991; 265:253–5.
4. Ramakrishna J, Weiss M. Health illness and immigration: East Indians in the United States in cross-cultural medicine—A decade later. *West J Med* 1992; 157:265–70.
5. Council on Scientific Affairs. Hispanic Health in the United States. *JAMA* 1991; 265:248–52.
6. Kleinman A, Eisenberg L, Good B. Culture, illness and cure: Clinical lessons from anthropologic and cross-cultural research. *Ann of Intern Med* 1978; 88:251–8.
7. Hentges K, Shields C, Cantu C. Folk Medicine and medical practice. *Texas Medicine* 1986; 82:27–9.

8. Munoz E. Care for the Hispanic Poor: A growing segment of American society. *JAMA* 1988; 260:2711–12.

9. Ginzberg E. Access to health care for Hispanics. *JAMA* 1991; 265:238–41.

10. Pappas G, Queen S, Hadden W, Fisher G. The Increasing disparity in mortality between socioeconomic groups in the United States, 1960 and 1986. *NEJ* 1993; 329:103–9.

11. Andersen RM, Giachello AL, Aday LA. Access of Hispanics to health care and cuts in services: A state of the art overview. *Pub Health Rep* 1986; 101:238–52.

12. Mobed K, Gold EB, Schenker MB. Occupational health problems among migrant and seasonal farm workers in cross-cultural medicine—A decade later. *West J Med* 1992; 157:367–73.

13. Palerm JV. A season in the life of a migrant farm worker in California in cross-cultural medicine—A decade later. *West J Med* 1992; 157:362–6.

14. Stern MP, Haffner SM. Type-II diabetes and its complications in Mexican Americans. *Diab and Metabol Rev* 1990; 6:29–45.

15. Becerra JE, Hogue CJR, Atrash HK, Perez N. Infant mortality among Hispanics: A portrait of heterogeneity. *JAMA* 1991; 265:217–21.

16. De La Rosa M. Health care needs of Hispanic Americans and the responsiveness of the health care system. *Health and Social Work* 1989; May:104–13.

17. Haffner L. Translation is not enough: Interpreting in a medical setting in cross-cultural medicine—A decade later. *West J Med* 1992; 157:255–9.

18. Ruiz P. Cultural barriers to effective medical care among Hispanic American patients. *Annual Review of Medicine* 1985; 36:63–71.

19. Hurlbut KM. The immigrant patient. In *Emergency Care of the Compromised Host*. Herr RD, Cydulka RK (eds.). New York: Lippincott, 1994.

20. Ripley GD. Mexican-American folk remedies: their place in health care. *Texas Medicine* 1986; 82:41–4.

21. Marsh WW, Hentges K. Mexican folk remedies and conventional medical care. *AFP* 1988; 37:257–62.

22. Foreman JT. Susto and the health needs of the Cuban refugee population. *Topics Clin Nurs* 1985; 7:40–7.

23. Grunder TM. On the readability of surgical consent forms. *NEJM* 1989; 302:900–2.

24. Kisken PB, Kisken WA. Consent problems and the Southeast Asian refugee. *Wi Med J* 1990; November 639–46.

25. Klessig J. The effect of values and culture on life-support decisions in cross-cultural medicine—A decade later. *West J Med* 1992; 157:316–22.

26. Pliskin KL. Dysphoria and somatization in Iranian culture in cross-cultural medicine—A decade later. *West J Med* 1992; 157: 295–300.

27. Lipson JG, Omidian PA. Health Issues of Afghan refugees in California in cross-cultural medicine—A decade Later. *West J Med* 1992; 157:271–5.

28. Siddhasthan K. Health insurance of the immigrant elderly. *Inquiry* 1991; 28:403–12.

29. Burstin HR, Lipsitz SR, Brennan TA. Socioeconomic status and risk for substandard medical care. *JAMA* 1992; 268:2383–7.

30. Hubbell FA, Waitzkin H, Mishra SI, Dombrink J, Chavez LR. Access to medical care for documented and undocumented latinos in a southern California county. *West J Med* 1991; 154:414–17.

31. Stern RS, Weissman JS, Epstein AM. The emergency department as a pathway to admission for poor and high-cost patients. *JAMA* 1991; 266:2238–43.

32. Morris P, Silove D. Cultural influences in psychotherapy with refugee survivors of torture and trauma. *Hosp Comm Psychiatr* 1992; 43:820–4.

33. Chester B, Holtan N. Working with refugee survivors of torture, in cross-cultural medicine—A decade later. *West J Med* 1992; 157:301–4.

34. Gold SJ. Mental health and illness in Vietnamese refugees in cross-cultural medicine—A decade later. *West J Med* 1992; 157:290–94.

17

Gay and Lesbian Health Issues

NORMAN D. KALBFLEISCH
JOCELYN C. WHITE

CONTENTS

CHAPTER SUMMARY

The intent of this chapter is to establish greater understanding of the wide spectrum of sexuality and sexual behaviors. Strategies are reviewed that enhance the ability of the clinician to obtain an accurate sexual behavior history, where appropriate. Health care needs unique to patients who have same-gender sexual activities are discussed, as are the social and cultural contexts for gay and lesbian experience. The goal of this information is to help clinicians create a risk-free, accepting, and caring environment in the ED for gay, lesbian, and bisexual patients.

INTRODUCTION

Sexuality is a basic and essential biological phenomenon of the human condition, as primary as other survival drives, such as hunger or thirst. It is present as an integral component of people's thoughts, if not their actions, on a daily basis. Paradoxically, in our society, an individual's basic sexuality is seldom acknowledged or discussed without some degree of discomfort. Such discomfort is often heightened when more specific information, such as sexual orientation, is discussed.

Sexual orientation refers to a person's potential to respond with sexual excitement through attraction, fantasy, or behavior to people of the same sex (homosexual), opposite sex (heterosexual), or both sexes (bisexual). Any definition of sexuality based solely on behavior is bound to be deficient and misleading.[1] Sexual orientation can be viewed as having two components, behavior and identity, which may or may not be congruent in an individual. For instance, a man may have exclusively same-gender sexual behaviors but may not identity as gay. Conversely, a woman may consider herself to be a lesbian, but may not be sexually active or may be active with men. Thus, people may identify with one sexual orientation, yet their sexual behavior, either past or present, may not correspond to this orientation.

More people have homosexual feelings than engage in homosexual behaviors, and more engage in homosexual behaviors than develop lasting homosexual identification or relationships.[2] Studies show that 20 to 37% of men have had some same-gender intimate sexual contact, and 1.1 to 10% have an exclusively male sexual orientation. Studies also show that 16 to 20% of women report intimate same-gender sexual contact, and that 2 to 8% have an exclusively female orientation.[3]

Investigators believe that there is likely an underestimation of prevalence rates because participants must self-disclose behavior that in many states remains criminal. Demographic information such as marital status or the existence of children does not accurately predict sexual orientation. Bell and Weinberg reported that 20% of gay men, 33% of white lesbians, and 50% of black lesbians had been married.[4] Roughly 10% of gay men and 20% of lesbians are parents; most of their children were conceived in a heterosexual marriage that ended in divorce.

Sexual orientation appears to be determined by a complex interplay of both biological and environmental factors. Research on neuroanatomy, twins, and genetic mapping suggest a heritable physiologic basis for sexual orientation.[5] How each individual expresses that trait may be influenced by family attitudes, religious proscription, internalized conflicts, social attitudes, or merely fear of rejection.

In a broader context, sexual orientation and identity refers to the sense of emotional and psychological connection between an individual and a social or cultural group whose sexual orientation and values the person shares. Terms such as *gay* and *lesbian* describe individuals who identify in this context as homosexual. Lesbians and gay men are a diverse group of individuals from all racial, economic, geographic, religious, cultural, and age populations. Despite this diversity, gay men and lesbians have developed a culture of their own, replete with music, art, literature, history, spiritual beliefs, ethics, and politics. Many believe that the modern gay and lesbian era began in New York City in 1969, when clients of a bar called Stonewall, along with other community members, rioted in response to police harassment and brutality directed against the gay and lesbian community. The modern era marked by this event has seen an increase in the visibility and strength of the gay and lesbian community.

Many older men and women who developed their gay or lesbian identity before Stonewall may feel less connected to the larger gay and lesbian community. These older individuals may be more reluctant to reveal their identity even to peers because of experience with or fears of discrimination. Those individuals who developed their gay or lesbian identity in the years since the Stonewall riot often look to

the gay and lesbian community as an important source of support. For many individuals, it may provide an alternative family or kin group. Community resources also may be of use to health care providers looking for gay- and lesbian-sensitive referrals for social services, counseling, or peer support.

There are nearly 100 million patient encounters each year in emergency departments across the country. As emergency care providers, we acknowledge and appreciate the wide diversity of people who we evaluate and treat. Our departments are recognized as a safety net for those patients who, for many reasons, do not have access to ongoing primary care. We see a disproportionate number of racial, ethnic, and sexual minorities, legal and illegal immigrants, the disenfranchised and socially stigmatized, and the poor. We pride ourselves in serving anyone who seeks emergency medical care, prioritizing their care based on medical acuity, not ability to pay.

Regardless of practice size or location, emergency medicine clinicians evaluate and treat significant numbers of people who engage in same-gender sexual activity or who identify as gay or lesbian. Most of these people are not readily apparent. Those who identify as gay or lesbian are unlikely to feel comfortable in an emergency medical setting and so, when possible, may choose to remain invisible to clinicians. Those who are visible represent but a portion of the diversity of the population.

Case #1

Ken is a 32-year-old lawyer working at an agency in Washington, DC. Over the course of the last 5 months, he has noted a nonvolitional weight loss of 30 pounds. Although he was never significantly overweight, initially his close friends and colleagues thought be looked more fit. As the weight loss progressed, their unspoken concern was AIDS. Ken attributed the weight loss to excessive travel, workload, and worry about job loss with the changing administration. The fear of losing his job was disconcerting because he and his partner of 2 years had just purchased a home.

Ken had grown up in a small town in upstate New York and attended a local college. He was sexually active, primarily with women, but had a couple of sexual encounters with men. His sexual fantasies seemed primarily homosexual and were troubling to him. At this point in his life, he certainly did not identify as homosex-

ual, nor did he know gay men or women in a social context.

He was accepted into law school and married Kay. That marriage ended in divorce 3 years later, with joint custody of their two children. He had kept his fantasies and previous homosexual activity very private, not confiding in his former wife, his friends, or work colleagues. Early in the AIDS epidemic, he knew about the transmissibility of the virus. Most of the time he had practiced "safer sex," but there had been a few lapses, especially if he had been drinking.

Two and a half years ago, Ken met Larry, an artist and activist in gay rights. Soon thereafter, they moved in together. Both were monogamous after that point. Ken's parents and a sister seem comfortable with Ken being gay and living with Larry. The relationship between Larry and Ken's brother remains strained.

Although Ken and his partner Larry are able to talk about most every aspect of their joint lives, Ken's weight loss has been a subject Ken refuses to discuss. Secretly, Ken is very worried about AIDS. During the past several years, he had seen many of his friends become ill and die, despite aggressive medication regimens. At first, these losses had been very hard on him. More recently, he felt that he had grown accustomed to this cycle of loss. He became fatalistic about his own weight loss and assumed he was HIV-seropositive. New night sweats and groin adenopathy were also something he attributed to his presumptive AIDS. He presents in the emergency department (ED) with a syncopal episode after several days of abdominal pain, diarrhea, and anorexia.

Case #2

Matt is a 21-year-old male with an unremarkable past medical history who presents to an emergency department with a 10-day, nonproductive cough. He is accompanied by his friend Nancy. Because he has a prolonged cough, some of your history questions will be directed at assessment of risk factors for an immunocompromised state. You ask Nancy to leave the examination room. During your history, you determine that Matt has occasional, unprotected, high-risk, same-gender sexual activity and had a negative HIV test two weeks ago. Physical examination is unremarkable, oxygen saturation 99% on room air, CBC and chest radiographs are unremarkable. From a social context, he considers himself bisexual, lives at home, and does not discuss his sexuality

with his parents or his sexual partners. His medical insurance is through his parents. He is finishing college and has just been hired in his first full-time job.

Case #3

For the past 15 years, Kate and Helen have been partners. Six years ago, Kate developed breast cancer, which was relatively advanced by the time it was discovered. She had undergone radical mastectomy with six of eight lymph nodes in her right axilla positive for malignancy. Kate subsequently underwent radiation and chemotherapy, and her cancer is now in remission.

At the time of her initial surgery, Kate's parents found out about her "lesbian lifestyle." Considerable emotional turmoil and conflict ensued. Since that time, Kate's relationship with her parents has been strained. Her parents resent Helen's role. Kate has not completed an advance directive naming Helen as her attorney in fact in a durable power of attorney for health care, although it was her intention to have Helen be the decision maker for her.

In the past 2 weeks, Kate has been troubled by frequent headaches and intermittent blurred vision and clumsiness. Both women knew that this might mean the return of her breast cancer. Because of the estrangement that occurred with her family when she was ill previously, the couple decided not to keep Kate's family informed.

Helen was at work the day that Kate seized in a grocery store. Paramedics arrived, and she was subsequently intubated in the field and taken to the emergency department at an unfamiliar hospital. In the ED, next-of-kin were notified. Kate's mother and father arrived at the same time as Helen.

Although Kate has had a treating oncologist, she has been unable to find a primary care provider on her HMO panel who is sensitive and knowledgeable about the health needs of lesbians. She, therefore, has no primary care advocate who knows her wishes for end-of-life care.

Helen worries that Kate will die. She fears that she will not be treated as one of Kate's family members who is allowed in the room with Kate. She fears the doctors will not treat her and Kate with respect and kindness because they are lesbians. She fears that there will be open conflict with Kate's parents over care decisions. She also fears that when Kate dies, her own grief will be mixed with anger, frustration, and loneliness.

Q: These are disturbing personal stories, but what do they have to do with the way we practice medicine?

Establishing a doctor-patient relationship. Ken has delayed a medical evaluation for months and now presents with unstable vital signs. The emergency clinician's ability to obtain an accurate history and effectively treat Ken will be dependent to a large part on his or her ability to rapidly establish a patient-physician relationship. Providers who are uncomfortable working with lesbian and gay patients or who fail to recognize the sexual orientation of a patient will manage patients incompletely, and perhaps incorrectly. They will fail to obtain pertinent information or to recognize important elements of evaluation and treatment.

Developing a patient-physician relationship is harder in an emergency department than in other medical settings. Ken and Kate are both acutely ill. They have no prior experience with this emergency care provider or emergency department, and the physical layout of most EDs does not allow for confidential discussions. Had Ken established care with a primary care physician, many of his concerns could have been dealt with, allowing his evaluation to proceed. If Kate had found a sensitive provider, she and Helen would have had a familiar advocate in the ED. Those patients who do not obtain competent, sensitive primary care services, including screening, health risk counseling, and psychosocial counseling, are likely to have a lower health status than their heterosexual counterparts. They, like Ken and Kate, may be more likely to seek care in an emergency department for acute and advanced conditions.

Q: So, how do we establish a relationship with lesbian and gay patients?

Barriers to communication. Sensitive communication is the key to building rapport with lesbian and gay patients. Gathering information about a patient's sexual practices or sexual orientation is often the first stumbling block encountered by health care providers.[6,7] Many physicians do not obtain sexual histories on their patients.[8] Often, these physicians have the perception that patients would not accept such inquiry. They may believe that they were not trained

adequately in taking a sexual history, particularly from sexual minorities. Although many physicians believe that patients find questions about sexuality inappropriate, several studies have noted that up to 90% of patients believe that sexual history taking is appropriate.

Forty percent of physicians surveyed are sometimes or often uncomfortable in giving care to gay and lesbian patients.[10] Some believe homosexual behavior is morally wrong. Others may feel inexperienced in lesbian, gay, bisexual, and transgendered health issues or unsure what language to use to elicit information respectfully from patients. Often, important information is not shared.

Many lesbians and gay men are reluctant to share their sexual orientation with health care providers for fear of negative judgments and homophobic responses.[11–15] Sixty-one percent of lesbians report they are unable to come out to their physicians. Some patients fail to share this information even when asked directly. In one study, 44% of gay men did not tell their primary physician they were gay. Forty-four percent of the HIV-positive men did not reveal their status to their primary physician.[16]

Unpleasant experiences with health care providers have made lesbians and gay men more likely to avoid health care and routine screening. Patient concerns about negative experiences were recently corroborated in a survey of 711 gay and lesbian physicians. Sixty-seven per cent of the physicians reported knowing instances in which lesbian, gay, or bisexual patients received substandard care because of their sexual orientation. Sixty-four percent of the respondents believed that informing their own physicians of their sexual orientation increased their risk of substandard health care.[17]

Sensitive communication: sexual history. Men and women come in all shapes, sizes, ages, and colors. Their sexual practices, sexual orientation, and comfort with their own sexuality may vary over their lifetime. About the only assumption you can make as a provider is that the patient is or has been sexual; however, in rare circumstances, your assumption even on this point could be wrong.

When we take a sexual history, commonly used questions may set up barriers for patients and lead to inaccurate or incomplete information. "What form of birth control do you use?"; "Are you married?"; "Should I call your wife (or husband) and let her (or him) know you are in the ED?"; and "Is there a chance you could be pregnant?" are common examples. When lesbians or gay men hear these questions, they may not know how to respond because all the questions assume the patient is heterosexual. Because the options given do not necessarily pertain to a lesbian or gay patient, the patient must either provide false information, speak vaguely in the third person, or disclose his or her sexual orientation. Needing to give such an explanation can make the already challenging sexual history even more difficult for both parties. To avoid this awkwardness, patients may opt to play along with the assumption of heterosexuality.

Because sexual orientation cannot be reliably determined by just looking at someone, questions without heterosexual bias are important to use with all patients, not just those we "suspect" of being lesbian or gay. Gay men and lesbians themselves are no more accurate in their ability to "identify" gays or lesbians than their heterosexual colleagues.[18] "Over your lifetime, have your sexual partners been men, women, or both?" and "Are you sexually active? . . . Have your sexual partners been men, women, or both?" are examples of questions without heterosexual bias. In taking a sexual history, it is often helpful for providers to explain why they need information on specific sexual practices. Before culturing for STDs, providers may ask, "For many people, sexual intimacy may include mouth-genital, genital-genital, hand-genital, or genital-rectal contact. Should I culture your throat, rectum, and/or vagina (or penis)?"

If the sexual history is not germane to the patient's presentation in the ED, then the time it takes to obtain that history could be better spent elsewhere. In both Ken's and Matt's cases, however, an inquiry into sexual practices is important. For Ken, it may help to identify potential etiologies for his weight loss and diarrhea. For Matt, it will likely change the workup of his cough and his ED physician's recommendations for follow-up. For Kate, a sexual history at this time is irrelevant. A social history is the key to her visit.

Sexual history-taking from adolescents and young adults. Obtaining an accurate sexual history from young adults may be more difficult than for any other age group. Reasons include (1) discomfort in discussing sexuality with an adult medical professional; (2) frequent sexual experimentation, including high-risk and same-gender experiences; (3)

strong peer-pressure and perceived bias against homosexual behavior; (4) frequent use of intoxicants; and (5) young people's sense of invincibility.

Although 75% of older teenagers have been sexually active, many will deny sexual activity, even when pregnant or diagnosed with a sexually transmitted disease (STD).[19] Teenage boys who have same-gender sexual activity are more likely than other boys to report their initial sexual activity at a younger age (12.7 versus 15.7 years, respectively). Teenage girls who engage in same-gender activity also report their first sexual encounter at a slightly younger age than other teenage girls (15.4 vs.16.2 years, respectively).[20]

During the adolescent and young adult years, many people engage in sexual experimentation. Kinsey reported 37% of males and 20% of females had homosexual experiences resulting in orgasm during this period. Sexual activity or behavior during this time does not reliably predict future homosexual behavior or a gay or lesbian orientation as an adult.[21] During this period of sexual exploration, adolescents may engage in high-risk sexual behaviors, often under the influence of intoxicants.[22] Many adolescents and young adults have a sense of invincibility, yet 66% of cases meeting AIDs-defining criteria in 20 to 24-year-old men were as a result of sexual activity. Most if not all of these men became seropositive for HIV as teenagers. The 20-to-24-year-old and teenage age groups have among the highest rates of acquisition of the HIV virus.[23] Most studies on adolescent same-gender behavior have been of Caucasian boys who identify as gay. Less is known about lesbians, racial minorities, or the larger subset of adolescents or young adults who deny lesbian or gay orientation but who have same-gender sexual intimacy.[24]

Sensitive communication: the social-cultural history. Providers traditionally learn to ask about sexual orientation during the sexual history. Doing so, however, may increase provider and patient discomfort. This type of inquiry also limits opportunities to learn about sexual orientation only to those visits in which a sexual history is appropriate. In contrast, the social history is the more comfortable part of the interview in which to raise these issues. "Are you single, partnered, married, widowed, or divorced?" or "Are you in an intimate relationship with someone?" may provide useful information. "Who is in your immediate family?" or "If you become ill, is there someone important whom I should involve in your care?" are other useful questions without heterosexual bias.

By using questions without heterosexual bias in taking a social history, the provider can increase the comfortable opportunities for discussing sexual orientation issues. In asking about spouses, children, and support systems, providers and patients explore how patients are most likely to cope with illness. Providers can learn about the patient's family structure, any stressors the patient might have, and what personal and community resources the patient would be likely to draw upon.

Enhancing the relationship. Providers who show a nonjudgmental attitude and who use language without heterosexual bias are much more likely to develop trusting relationships with gay and lesbian patients. Providers can further improve the relationship in several simple ways: (1) offering to include a partner in the discussion; (2) ensuring that a gay or lesbian patient's partner is treated as would be any other spouse in the office or the hospital; (3) including partners in discussions of next-of-kin policies and advance directives; (4) using emergency, hospital, and office forms with words that do not assume heterosexual family structures; and (5) explicitly discussing medical record confidentiality with regard to sexual orientation documentation.

Medical record confidentiality. The emergency care provider should thoughtfully consider the implications of placing any documentation of specific sexual behaviors or sexual orientation in an emergency department record. When possible, these issues should be discussed with the patient. Medical records, although ostensibly covered by patient privacy and confidentiality rules, continue to be a legitimate concern of gay men and lesbians. Records, including ED documentation, have played pivotal roles in the denial of medical insurance, disability insurance, worker's compensation, tort claims, child custody or visitation rights, and in the ordering of dishonorable discharges from the military. As recently as the late 1980s, some health insurers denied insurance to men perceived as gay (because they were 30 years of age or greater and unmarried), regardless of their HIV status.[25]

In Ken's case, his ED provider should discuss with him what the provider would like to include in the medical record documentation and why. Probably, some medical record documentation that he has risk factors for HIV is warranted. Given permission, his social and cultural history should be documented in further detail, including whom he would like involved in his care.

In Matt's case, explicit documentation in his ED record of his sexual activity and HIV status is not necessary and may actually be deleterious. Since he is HIV-negative, his presentation is not due to an AIDs-defining illness. When he applies for health insurance with his new company, he may need to sign a medical release of information that will allow all his medical records to be reviewed. Medical insurance could be denied by explicit documentation of his sexual orientation or behavior in his ED chart. His job might be in jeopardy and he might be estranged from his family. Of course, regardless of what is placed in Matt's chart, Matt should be advised to obtain a primary care physician who can then counsel him about STD and HIV prevention.

Matt's primary care provider may choose to use a coded entry if Matt does not want his sexual activity specifically documented. Where this is an option, the code serves to remind providers of the patient's sexual history or sexual orientation but will prevent inadvertent breeches of confidentiality. Where a coded entry is not possible and sexual history or sexual orientation information is central to providing care, clinicians should inform the patient that this information is being placed in the chart and should discuss medical record confidentiality and release of information procedures.

Q: Are there any health issues unique to lesbians?

Lesbians are a diverse group in terms of sexual practices. They may be celibate or sexually active with women, men, or both. Most lesbians either are currently sexually active with women exclusively or are celibate.[26] In one study, 77% of lesbians had participated in heterosexual intercourse at least once in their lives.[27] The specific sexual practices of any individual patient determine her risks of a particular disease and are important in developing individual medical recommendations.

Unfortunately, there is limited population-based information about women who are sexually active with women. The few clinical studies available are methodologically flawed by sample bias or small sample size, and clinicians may not be able to generalize from these results. Specific information about cancer risks and screening in women sexually active with women is unavailable, but inferences can be drawn from larger epidemiologic studies.

Sexually transmitted diseases. STDs in women sexually active exclusively with women are less common than in either heterosexual women or in gay males. This may be due in part to the relative epidemiologic isolation of this population from men and the lack of penile-vaginal intercourse among lesbians. Anecdotally, younger lesbians, however, appear to be participating more frequently in heterosexual contact, sometimes with high-risk individuals, including gay men. Lesbian sexual practices include kissing, breast stimulation, manual and oral stimulation of the genitals and anus, friction of the clitoris against the partner's body, and penetration of the vagina and anus with fingers and devices. There are no gynecologic problems unique to lesbians, and none which occur more often in lesbians than in bisexual and heterosexual women.

Women sexually active exclusively with women appear to have a lower incidence of syphilis and gonorrhea than any other population except those who have never been sexually active at all.[27–29] Therefore, routine screening for these diseases in lesbians does not appear to be cost effective. Testing is appropriate, however, in the setting of other risk factors, particularly recent heterosexual contact. Other STDs common among heterosexual women are reported rarely in the lesbian population. Chlamydia, herpes, human papilloma virus (HPV), and pelvic inflammatory disease (PID) are uncommon in lesbians who have been sexually active exclusively with women, but are all theoretically transmissible.[27–29] Partners of infected women should be evaluated. Unlike the gay male population, enteric infections caused by Hepatitis A, amoeba shigella, and helminth's have a low prevalence in lesbians. Hepatitis B does not occur unless other risk factors are present.[28,30,31]

In contrast to STDs, bacterial vaginosis and vaginitis occur in lesbians, although bisexual women report vaginal candidiasis more often than lesbians, probably related to heterosexual contact.[13,27,29] Transmission between women seems possible. Trichomonas vaginalis has been found in women

sexually active exclusively with women.[27,29] Partners of lesbians with vaginal discharge should be evaluated and or treated.

HIV. To date, approximately 93% of lesbians with AIDS are intravenous drug users. Although woman-to-woman transmission of HIV has not been proven by DNA typing, transmission of the virus between women as a result of sexual contact only may have occurred in up to nine cases.[32,33] Exposure to menstrual or traumatic bleeding during sexual contact was probably the source of transmission in these cases. HIV has been cultured from cervical and vaginal secretions and cervical biopsies taken throughout the menstrual cycle; therefore, HIV theoretically may be transmitted by infected women who are not bleeding.[34]

Although transmission rates appear to be low, health care providers should counsel lesbians to avoid contact with cervical and vaginal secretions, menstrual blood, and blood from vaginal and rectal trauma in partners who have not tested negative for the virus. Methods believed to protect against transmission of HIV for oral-genital contact include latex squares, known as dental dams, and latex condoms or gloves cut open and laid flat. Plastic wrap is advocated as a moisture barrier. For vaginal penetration, latex gloves used on hands and condoms on sexual toys are appropriate.

Lesbians who undergo artificial insemination are also at risk for HIV infection.[35,36] Sperm banks routinely test donors for HIV infection at the time of donation and 6 months later before releasing the sample for use. This practice minimizes the possibility of transmission of HIV with frozen samples. When using fresh semen from donors, there is a high risk of HIV infection because of the delays in seroconversion. It is not recommended that women use fresh semen samples from donors because of this risk. When fresh samples must be used, it is advisable for the donor to undergo a 6-month testing cycle without the possibility of any HIV exposures during that time. Anyone who elects this route must understand that a negative test for HIV antibodies does not guarantee that an individual is free of transmissible virus.

Cancer. There are no population-based studies of cancer risk in lesbians. As a result, screening decisions should be based on individual risk factors using standard screening guidelines for women. However, depending on sexual and reproductive histories, the incidence of certain cancers in lesbians differs.

Cervical cancer may occur less commonly among lesbians than among bisexual or heterosexual women, as suggested by lower rates of abnormal Pap smears.[27,29,37] In women who have no history of abnormal Pap smear, dysplasia, or venereal warts and who have been sexually active exclusively with women, we recommend screening every 3 years, an interval similar to the American Cancer Society maintenance screening interval. Women with significant heterosexual contact or another known risk factor should be screened according to published guidelines.

Lesbians and single women over age 40 appear to smoke more, drink more, and have higher rates of obesity than the general population of women. They also appear to have fewer mammograms, clinical breast exams, and self-breast exams than the general population of women.[26,28,38–42] There is no specific information about breast, endometrial, ovarian, lung, colon, or head and neck cancer in lesbians. Physicians should emphasize the health risks of smoking and alcohol use in the lesbian population and strongly encourage smoking cessation.

Epidemiologic studies suggest an increased risk of breast cancer among nulliparous women, women who are older with their first birth, and women who have never breast-fed. Ovarian cancer has been reported to occur more frequently in women who have not used oral contraception and those who have not given birth. Endometrial cancer is also more common in nulliparous women. Because many lesbians fall into these categories, physicians should follow current guidelines on screening for these cancers.

Q: What role do homophobia and other psychosocial issues play in the care of lesbians and gay men?

In 1973, the American Psychiatric Association removed homosexuality from its list of mental disorders. Psychiatric and behavioral interventions used in the past to "cure" patients of homosexuality have proven neither effective nor necessary. Overall, mental illness is no more common in lesbians and gay men than in the general population. However, these individuals do face unique psychosocial issues and stressors that the heterosexual population does not.

The process of discovering one's sexual orientation and revealing it to others is known as "coming out" and may occur at any age. Stage theories for coming out have been well described and can be summarized as a four-step process: (1) awareness of homosexual feelings; (2) testing and exploration; (3) identity acceptance; and (4) identity integration and self-disclosure.[43]

The process of coming out involves a shift in core identity that can be associated with significant emotional distress, especially if family and peers respond negatively. Prevailing social attitudes also influence the experience of coming out. Societal and internalized homophobia often cause lesbians and gay men to perform a fatiguing "cost-benefit analysis" for each situation in which they consider self-disclosure. If the costs of self-disclosure are repeatedly high, the individual ultimately may become socially isolated or may deny the gay or lesbian identity.[43–45]

Most of the mood disturbance experienced by lesbians and gay men related to sexual orientation identity occurs in response to societal and individual homophobia. Controversy exists as to whether lesbians and gay men have a higher incidence of depression, anxiety, and substance abuse than the general population. Reports suggest that gay men have higher and heavier alcohol and drug use rates than the general population of men.[46] Recent studies suggest that lesbians have no higher rate of alcohol use than the general population of women.[47] There is little information on drug use among lesbians.

Alcohol and substance abuse put gay men and lesbians at risk for sexually transmitted diseases and HIV infection because intoxicated or drug-affected individuals may be less inclined to practice safer sex. Heavier alcohol and cigarette use also places these individuals at greater risk for lung cancer, head and neck cancer, and cardiovascular disease than the general population.

Domestic violence. Battery of lesbians and gay men by their partners exists. Although the prevalence of battery in gay and lesbian relationships is not known, it appears that the majority of incidents are related to alcohol or drug use.[48] Victims of domestic violence report that many shelters are not responsive to their specific needs as lesbians or gay men. Primary care and emergency care providers should screen all patients, including their gay and lesbian patients, for the possibility of domestic violence and be able to give patient referrals to lesbian- and gay-sensitive resources, including shelters and counselors.

Hate crimes.   Hate crimes, also known as *bias crimes*, are words or actions directed at an individual because of membership in a minority group. The U.S. Department of Justice reports that gay men and lesbians may be the most victimized group in the nation.[49] Studies report crimes ranging from verbal abuse and threats of violence to property damage, physical violence, and murder. The numbers of hate crimes reported by gay men and lesbians are increasing every year.[50] Perpetrators of hate crimes often include family members and community authorities. Many gay and lesbian adolescents leave home because of an abusive family member. Homeless gay, lesbian, and bisexual youth are of increasing social concern. When patients present with symptoms of depression, anxiety, or trauma, providers should consider violence, including hate crimes, as a possible correlate.

Adolescents.   Lesbian, gay and bisexual adolescents are particularly vulnerable to the emotional distress of coming out, and this distress can confound developmental tasks. Parental acceptance of the adolescent during the coming-out process may be the primary determinant of the development of healthy self esteem.[51] Health care providers need to screen for signs of sexual orientation confusion in their adolescent patients. These signs may include depression, anxiety, diminished school performance, alcohol and substance abuse, acting out, and suicidal ideation. Reports suggest that gay and lesbian adolescents may be two to three times more likely to attempt suicide than the general adolescent population, and that approximately one-third of all completed youth suicides occur in gay and lesbian teens.[52] Providers noting signs of depression or substance abuse need to consider sexual orientation confusion in the differential diagnosis.

Older adults.   Coming out can occur at any age, even among older individuals, and there are varying degrees of self-disclosure. Older individuals may be out to themselves and a partner or close friends, but to no one else beyond that support circle. Older lesbians and gay men are vulnerable to social isolation, and health care providers are often among the top three support resources for older individuals.[53,54]

In exploring the social support network for older patients, health care providers need to be alert to the possibility of lesbian or gay identity.

Parenting.   Surveys estimate that 6 to 14 million children have gay or lesbian parents. Gay men and lesbians may have children from previous heterosexual relationships or may have them through adoption, artificial insemination, heterosexual intercourse, or being foster parents. Among lesbians surveyed, artificial insemination is the preferred method of parenting. Adoption appears to be second, because of its difficulty. Parenting plays a role in the lives of many lesbians and gay men, and the decision to parent is usually a deliberate and carefully made one. Occasionally a lesbian couple and a gay couple will agree to parent together. Some members of society oppose parenthood for lesbians and gay men because of concerns about the psychological development and sexual orientation of the children. Studies have clearly shown that there are no differences in children raised by lesbians and gay men and those raised by heterosexual parents.[58-60] Open communication with children about parents' sexual orientation appears to be beneficial to family function, and children themselves appreciate it.[61]

A pregnant lesbian may find it difficult to get support for her pregnancy. The development of her identity as a mother may also be more complex. Health care providers can support a pregnant lesbian by showing nonjudgmental attitudes and encouraging acceptance of lesbian motherhood among members of the delivery team and child-bearing classes. Providers should encourage patients' partners, and donor fathers when appropriate, to participate in all phases of the fertility assessment, preconception and prenatal care, and delivery. Partners and donor fathers may also need emotional support after the delivery. Health insurance benefits for partners and their children are still difficult to obtain in most locations.

Q: Kate and Helen are partners. What does that mean in this "end-of life" situation?

During the process of working with Kate, the emergency clinician needs to respect Kate's partnership with Helen, even though it is not a legal marriage. A durable power of attorney for health care would have lent weight to having Helen act as Kate's surrogate decision maker. Helen's grieving process should be anticipated early on.

Partnering.   Like most heterosexuals, lesbians and gay men express the desire to find a partner and develop a relationship. And, like heterosexuals, lesbians and gay men can form and maintain long-lasting primary relationships. Gay men and lesbians may have commitment ceremonies, own homes together, share finances, and raise children.

Because of potential isolation from family, coworkers, and religious organizations, the relationship with a partner can be particularly important to a lesbian or gay man's psychological well-being. As a result, discord in the relationship or a health crisis may be even more stressful than it might be for the typical heterosexual couple.[62] In difficult times, an individual may have limited resources for solving the problem. Providers should be able to provide lesbian- and gay-sensitive therapy referrals when appropriate.

Durable power of attorney for heath care.   In recent years, discussions of the durable power of attorney for health care have become more common between patients and their providers. This document is particularly important for lesbians and gay men. Because they are unable to marry legally at this time, lesbians and gay men need to execute the document to appoint their partner as the surrogate health decision maker. Without such a document, the next of kin is the surrogate decision maker. Completing this document is the best way to avoid tragic decision-making conflicts between a partner and the estranged family members of seriously ill patients in a time of crisis. As with all patients, a discussion of the durable power of attorney for health care should be included in the preventive medicine checkup, and requests for existing advance directive documents should be made at the time of emergency visit. In the absence of such documentation, when at all possible, the individual whom the patient intends to be a surrogate decision maker, usually the partner, should be respected as such.

Grief.   Grieving the loss of a partner may be more difficult for a lesbian or gay man than for a heterosexual because of the potential that the lesbian or gay man has a smaller support system. Lesbians grieve the loss of partners and friends to breast cancer and other illnesses. Gay men and lesbians are particularly affected by the deaths of partners and many friends from AIDS. Some gay men and lesbians report losing 10 or more friends or family members in a single year. In cases such as these, grief or fatalism can become a life constant.

When a partner dies, the survivor, in effect, loses a spouse. Frequently, the family of the deceased partner excludes the survivor or will not allow him or her to take part as a spouse in the funeral. A close-knit network of surviving friends is often neglected when a grieving family takes over funeral plans. Primary care providers can assist surviving partners and friends in the grieving process in several ways. Providers can (1) assist the survivor to talk about the loss and express his or her feelings; (2) help the survivor to adapt roles and patterns of living; (3) encourage the survivor to develop new relationships and support structure; (4) identify and interpret normal grieving behaviors and time lines; and (5) provide ongoing support through the grief process. In some cases, the health care provider may be the only individual in whom the survivor can completely confide.[63]

CONCLUSION

Patients present to the ED with a wide spectrum of sexual behaviors. Individuals who engage in same-gender sexual activities have unique health needs. Accordingly, emergency providers need to identify these individuals by obtaining accurate sexual and social histories when appropriate.

Men and women who identity as gay, lesbian, or bisexual have social and cultural experiences that differ from those of heterosexuals. These experiences impact their interaction with health care providers. Emergency providers must be able to communicate sensitively with these patients by using language free of heterosexual bias. Emergency clinicians who can create a safe, accepting, and caring environment in the emergency department for people of all sexual orientations will be providing the highest-quality care for the community.

NOTES

1. Alper JS, Beckwith J. Genetic fatalism and social policy: The implications of behavior genetics research. *Yale J Biol Med* 1993; 66:511–24.

2. Lever J. Kanouse D, Rogers W, Carson S. Behavior patterns and sexual identity of bisexual males. *J Sex Res* 1992; 29:141–67.

3. Haas AP. Lesbian health issues: An overview. In A Dan (ed.). *Reframing women's health: Multidisciplinary research and practice.* Thousand Oaks, CA: Sage Publications, 1994.

4. Bell AP, Weinberg MS. *Homosexualities: A study of diversity among men and women.* New York: Simon & Schuster, 1978.

5. Bailey JM, Pillard RC. A genetic study of male sexual orientation. *Arch Gen Psychiatr* 1991; 48:1089–96.

6. White J, Levinson W. Primary care of lesbian patients. *J Gen Int Med* 1993; 8:41–7.

7. Office of Student Affairs. *A community of equals: A resource guide for the Temple medical community about gay, lesbian and bisexual people.* Philadelphia: Temple University School of Medicine, 1992.

8. Lewis CE. Are physicians addressing the issues? *J Gen Int Med* 1990; 5:78–81.

9. Ende J, Rockwell S, et al. The sexual history and general medical practice. *Arch Intern Med* 1984; 144:558–61.

10. Matthews WC, Booth MW, Turner JD. Physicians' attitudes toward homosexuality. *West J Med* 1986; 144:106.

11. Trippett SE, Bain J. Reasons American lesbians fail to seek traditional health care. *Health Care Wom Int* 1992; 13:145–53.

12. D. Brylace. *Michigan Lesbian Health Survey: A report to the Michigan Organization for Human Rights and the Department of Public Health,* 1990.

13. Johnson SR, Guenther SM, Laube DW, Keftel WC. Factors influencing lesbian gynecological care: A preliminary study. *Am J Obstet Gynecol* 1981; 140:20–8.

14. Stevens PE, Hall JM. Stigma, health beliefs and experience with health care in lesbian women. *Image* 1988; 20:69–73.

15. Warshafsley L. *Lesbian health needs assessment: Prepared for the Los Angeles Gay and Lesbian Community Services Center.* 1992.

16. Fitzpatrick R, Dowson J, Boulton M. Perceptions of general practice among homosexual males. *Br J Gen Pr* 1994; 44:80–82.

17. Schatz B, O'Hanlan K. *Anti-gay Discrimination in Medicine.* San Francisco: American Association of Physicians for Human Rights (AAPHR), 1994.

18. Berger G, Hank L, et al. Detection of sexual orientation by heterosexuals and homosexuals. *J Homosexuality* 1987; 13:83–99.

19. Seidman SN, Reider RO. A review of sexual behavior in the United States. *Am J Psychiatr* 1994; 151:330–341.

20. Diamond M. Homosexuality and bisexuality among different populations. *Arch Sex Beh* 1993; 22:291–310.

21. Committee on Adolescence, American Academy of Pediatrics. Homosexuality and adolescence. *Pediatr* 1992; 84:631–4.

22. Rotheram-Borus MJ, Rosario M, et al. Sexual and substance use acts of gay and bisexual male adolescents in New York City. *J Sex Res* 1994; 31:47–57.

23. CDC. *HIV/AIDS surveillance report.* Atlanta: Centers for Disease Control, 1993.

24. Remafedi G. Adolescent homosexuality: Psychosocial and medical implications. *Pediatr* 1987; 79:331–7.

25. Schatz B. The AIDS insurance crisis: Underwriting or overreaching? *Harv Law Rev* 1987; 100:1782–1805.

26. Ryan C, Bradford J. The national lesbian health care survey: An overview. In Shernoff, M, Scott, W (eds.). *The sourcebook on lesbian/gay health care,* 2nd ed. Washington DC: National Lesbian/Gay Health Foundation, 1988.

27. Johnson SR, Smith EM, Guenther SM. Comparison of gynecologic health care problems between lesbian and bisexual women. *J Repro Med* 1987; 32:805–11.

28. Robertson P, Schachter J. Failure to identify venereal disease in a lesbian population. *Sex Trans Dis* 1981; 8:75–6.

29. Degen K, Waitkevitz HJ. Lesbian health issues. *Br J Sex Med* 1982; May:40–7.

30. Walters MH, Rector WG. Sexual transmission of hepatitis in lesbians. *JAMA* 1986; 256:594.

31. Williams DC. Hepatitis and other sexually transmitted diseases in gay men and lesbians. *Sex Trans Dis* 1981; 8:330–2.

32. Chu SY, Buehler JW, Fleming PL, Berkleman L. Epidemiology of reported cases of AIDS in lesbians, United States. *Am J Pub Health* 1990; 80:1380–9.

33. Chu SY, Hammett TA, Buehler JW. Update: Epidemiology of reported cases of AIDS in women who have sex only with other women, United States, 1980–1991. *AIDS* 1992; 6:518–19.

34. Poole L. HIV Infection in Women. In Cohen, P, Sande, M, Volberding, P (eds.). *The AIDS knowledge base,* 4th

ed. Waltham, MA: The Medical Publishing Group 1990.

35. Arneta MRG, Maseola L, Eller A, et al. HIV transmission through donor artificial Insemination. *JAMA* 1995; 273(11):854–8.

36. Gulnan ME. Artificial insemination by donor. *JAMA* 1995; 273(1):890–1.

37. Sadeghi SD, Sadeghi A, Cosby M, Olincy A. Robboy SJ. Human papillomavirus infection: Frequency and association with cervical neoplasia in a young population. *Acta Cytol* 1989; 33(3);319–23.

38. National Health Interview Survey, 1985.

39. Skinner WE, Otis MD. Trilogy Project: Research in the lesbian and gay community, 14th National Lesbian and Gay Health Conference, Los Angeles, CA, July 1992.

40. National Health Study on Drug Abuse, 1992.

41. National Health Interview Survey, 1987.

42. National Health and Nutrition Examination Survey. 1976–80.

43. Sophie I. A critical examination of stage theories of lesbian identity development. *J Homosex* 1986; 12(2):39–51.

44. Stevens FE, Hall JM. Stigma, health beliefs and experiences with health care in lesbian women. *Image* 1988; 20(2):69–73.

45. Gonsiorek JC. Mental health issues of gay and lesbian adolescents. *J Adol Health Care* 1988; 9:114–22.

46. Stall R, Wiley J. A comparison of alcohol and drug use patterns of homosexual and heterosexual men: The San Francisco Men's Health Study. *Drug Alcohol Depend* 1988; 22;63–73.

47. Bloomfield K. A comparison of alcohol consumption between lesbians and heterosexual women in an urban population. *Drug Alcohol Depend* 1993; 33;267–69.

48. Schilit R, Lie G, Montague M. Substance use as a correlate of violence in intimate lesbian relationships. *J Homosex* 1990; 19(3):151–65.

49. National Gay and Lesbian Task Force. Anti-gay violence; causes, consequences, responses. Washington, DC:NG LTF, 1986.

50. Herek GH. Hate crimes against lesbians and gay men: Issues for research and policy. *Am Psychol* 1989; 44(6): 948–55.

51. Savin-Willians PC. Coming to parents and self-esteem among gay and lesbian youths. *J Homosex* 1989; 18(1–2):1–35.

52. Feinleib MR. *Report of the Secretary's Task Force on Youth Suicide.* Rockville, MD: U.S. Department of Health and Human Services, 1989.

53. Kehoe M. Lesbians over 65: A triple, invisible minority. *J Homosex* 1986; 12(3–4);139–52.

54. Quam JK, Whitford G. Adaptation and age-related expectations of older gay and lesbian adults. *Gerontol* 1992; 32(3);367–74.

55. Kirkpatrick M. Clinical implications of lesbian mother studies. *J Homosex* 1987; 14(1–2):201–11.

56. Zeidenstein L. Gynecological and childbearing needs of lesbians. *J Nurse Midwifery* 1990; 33(1):10–18.

57. Wismount L, Reame NE. The lesbian childbearing experience: Assessing development tasks. *Image* 1989; 21(3):137–41.

58. Green R. The best interests of the child with a lesbian mother. *Bull Am Acad Psychiatry Law,* 1982; 10(1):7–15.

59. McGuire M, Alexander NJ. Artificial insemination of single women. *Fertil Steril* 1985; 43:182–84.

60. Patterson CJ. Children of lesbian and gay parents. *Child Develop* 1992; 63;1025.

61. Brewaeys A, Olbrechts H, Devroey P, Van Steirteghem AC. Counseling and selection of homosexual couples in fertility treatment. *Hum Reprod* 1989; 4:850–3.

62. Kurdek LA, Schmitt JP. Perceived emotional support from family and friends in members of homosexual, married, and heterosexual cohabiting couples. *J Homosex* 1987; 14(3–4):57–68.

63. Fawzy FI, Fawzy NN, Pasnau RO. Bereavement in AIDS. *Psychiatric Med* 1991; 9(3):469–82.

18

Unmet Health Care Needs of Women

JUDITH A. LINDEN
JUDITH BERNSTEIN
GAIL D'ONOFRIO

CONTENTS

- Gender bias
- Detection bias
- Coronary artery disease (CAD)
- Evaluation and treatment in women
- Lung cancer in women
- Estrogen replacement therapy
- Alcoholism
- Mammography and Pap smear screening and referrals
- Female participation in research trials
- Domestic violence
- Role accumulation and health challenges

CHAPTER SUMMARY

Only recently has the impact of gender on medical decision making and treatment been emphasized in the scientific and general public literature. While women live an average of 7.5 years longer than their male counterparts, they more often experience chronic health problems, poor health, poverty, depression, and suicide attempts. Because they live longer, women more often suffer higher morbidity from chronic illnesses such as arthritis, osteoporosis, and bony fractures, dementia and Alzheimer's, depression, and collagen vascular diseases.[1,2] Women also suffer from underdiagnosis and suboptimal treatment of diseases that are believed to occur less frequently in women, such as ischemic heart disease and lung cancer. Research that includes female subjects and examines the differential effects of female gender and hormonal status is often sparse. This disparity exists in part due to exclusion, until recently, of women in childbearing years and older age groups from participation in research trials. Only recently have the unique manifestations of HIV and AIDS in women been appreciated and AIDS-defining illnesses in women been revised to include severe PID, refractory vaginal candidiasis, and invasive cervical cancer. Domestic violence remains a tragic but common presentation to the ED, which may be difficult to identify. While the presentation may be obvious if visible physical injury exists, more subtle manifestations include multiple vague somatic complaints.

Although the practice of emergency medicine places emphasis on the accurate and timely treatment of acute life- or limb-threatening illnesses, the recognition of abuse and chronic illnesses, and the need for counseling and referral for health maintenance are equally important to optimal care of the female patient.

Case #1

A 56-year-old female presents with epigastric pain that radiates to both shoulders, nausea, diaphoresis, and mild shortness of breath. On examination, her abdomen is mildly tender in the epigastrium and possibly the right

Figure 18-1 Heart Disease Mortality Rates for Females and Males: 1980s Crossover

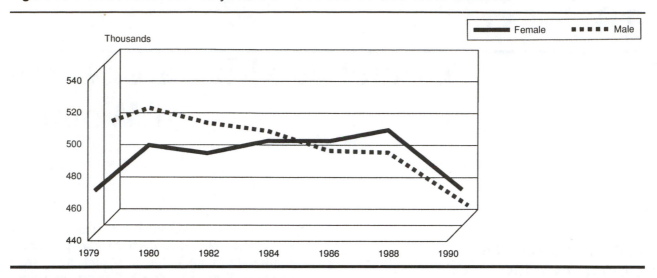

upper quadrant. Her cardiac exam reveals an S4 gallop but no murmurs. Her pulmonary exam is unremarkable, and the stool is hemoccult negative.

Q: Given the preceding information, what diagnoses should be considered?

Possible diagnoses include gastrointestinal disorders such as gall bladder and gastroesophageal reflux disease (GERD), peptic ulcer disease, and pancreatitis. Cardiac and pulmonary diseases, such as myocardial infarction, aortic dissection, and pulmonary embolism should be considered, given the patient's diaphoresis and shortness of breath.

Case Continuation

On further questioning, the patient states that she has had multiple, similar, but less severe episodes in the past few months, which are occasionally related to food. She does not smoke but has a history of hypercholesterolemia and borderline hyperglycemia. She is postmenopausal. The pain is somewhat worse when she is walking or carrying groceries. Given the high prevalence of gall bladder diseases in middle-aged women, her symptoms are attributed to gall bladder disease, or possibly dyspepsia. Maalox is administered, and liver enzymes, alkaline phosphatase, amylase, and right upper quadrant ultrasound are ordered.

While she is waiting for laboratory test results, her symptoms shift to the midsternal region. Since she is in so much distress and will probably be admitted, a decision is made by the RN to obtain an ECG, which reveals 2 to 3 mm of ST elevation in leads 2,3, and F, with reciprocal changes. At this point, she is asked about cardiac risk factors. Her father and sister had suffered myocardial infarctions in their fifties. She is also asked about the duration of her symptoms, which have lasted about 6 hours. She has been in the ED for 2 hours. She is given one baby aspirin and sublingual nitroglycerine. Thrombolytics and heparin are administered, and she is admitted to the CCU.

Q: At what point should an ECG have been obtained? What history might have contributed to an earlier diagnosis?

Some studies suggest that women presenting to the ED with atraumatic chest pain get ECG and thrombolytic therapy later than their male counterparts,[3,4] whereas other studies suggest women receive equitable care[5] or that the variation may represent overtreatment of men with low cardiac risk presentations.[6]

Although most physicians are trained to envision the typical high-risk cardiac patient as a 58-year-old man, women have now surpassed men in mortality from cardiac disease. Heart disease is the leading cause of mortality in women. (See Figure 18-1.) Female gender should not discourage the thorough historical evaluation and use of easily available tests such as ECG in the appropriate setting. Previous episodes, treatment, and exacerbating and remitting factors should be explored. An earlier diagnosis might have been made, if a more thorough history, including coronary risk factors and association of symptoms to exertion, had been elicited. An earlier diagnosis would have led to earlier consideration of thrombolytic therapy, an important factor in increasing myocardial salvage, preserving left ventricular function and decreasing morbidity.

Risk factors such as elevated cholesterol and triglycerides, low HDL, hypertension, and diabetes may have relatively more importance in the development of coronary artery disease (CAD) in women.[7,8] Data from the Framingham study suggest that whereas women tend to have higher HDL and lower triglycerides (TG) and total cholesterol levels than men, low HDL and elevated TG may be more powerful indicators of coronary risk in women than in men. For every 10 mg/dL decrease in HDL, women were noted to have a 40 to 50% increase in risk of coronary disease.[7] Menopausal status is important in evaluating coronary artery disease; after menopause, HDL levels decrease, while TG levels increase. Diabetes and asymptomatic hyperglycemia is associated with increased risk of coronary disease in women.[8]

Q: When the decision to administer thrombolytics is made, should the dosage and protocol be modified for gender, and will this patient be expected to respond similarly?

Fibrinolytic therapy significantly reduces mortality in women, as well as in men. Female patients have a slightly increased absolute risk of death from myocardial infarction but exhibit similar decreases in mortality from thrombolytic therapy.[9] There are a slightly significantly higher number of early deaths after thrombolytic therapy in women, compared with men, which may be secondary to the relatively older age of women presenting with MI or longer delay in receiving thrombolytics (7.0 hours for women versus 6.2 for men), according to a recent pooled data review of nine large thrombolytic trials.[9] The rate of bleeding complications may be somewhat

higher in women, particularly in older women. It is not clear whether this is because of more advanced age and higher prevalence of comorbid illnesses in the enrolled women or the lack of weight-based dosage calculations for thrombolytic therapy in women with smaller lean body mass. Current recommended thrombolytic doses do not differ based on gender or lean body mass.

Q: If the ECG had been normal and the etiology of her symptoms not attributed to CAD, what opportunities for primary prevention of CAD might be suggested by the ED physician?

In postmenopausal women, hormone replacement therapy favorably affects absolute lipid levels and lipid ratios.[10,11] Observational studies suggest a 35 to 50% decrease in risk of CAD in women receiving estrogen replacement therapy.[7,10–12] Estrogen therapy increases HDL levels but also increases triglycerides. Recent experimental evidence suggests that estrogen may have beneficial effects beyond improving lipid profile. Estrogen may increase relaxation in the muscularis layer of vascular walls and decrease prostacyclin production by vascular endothelium and thromboxane A2 production in platelets.[11] The addition of progestin reduces cardioprotection (since it decreases HDL and increases LDL levels), but it also decreases the risk of endometrial cancer (an effect of unopposed estrogen). A combined estrogen-progestin regimen has favorable effects on lipid profiles, but it does not increase the risk of endometrial cancer and is thus indicated for all women with uteri. There is currently no consistent evidence for any association of short-term, low-dose estrogen replacement therapy with an increased risk of breast cancer,[12] but there may be an increased risk for long-term use, especially if progestins are added.[13] Even if this evidence for elevated risk on long-term hormone replacement therapy (HRT) is confirmed, however, the risk to women of death from heart disease is still 10 times greater than the risk of breast cancer. Estrogen therapy prescribed for cardioprotection also decreases the risk of both cortical and trabecular fractures from osteoporosis but appears to have little effect on the risk of stroke.[12]

Women at risk for CAD appear to benefit from daily aspirin therapy. Aspirin therapy (1 to 6 aspirins per week) in women aged 34 to 65 years decreased the relative risk of myocardial infarction to 0.66 in a large uncontrolled prospective cohort study.[14] Prospective controlled trials in association with the Women's Health Initiative of the NIH are currently underway to determine the optimal dose of aspirin for primary prevention of heart disease and stroke in women. Smoking cessation, blood pressure control, weight loss, and diet modification are equally important factors in decreasing CAD in women. Moderate alcohol intake (1 to 3 drinks per week) may decrease the risk of death in women older than 50 years old and women with coronary risk factors.[15] Hypertension appears to be a more powerful risk factor for CAD in women than in men. Hypertensive women have four times the risk of heart disease, whereas hypertensive men have three times the risk of CAD.[16] There are few studies involving women, however, which explore the effect of blood pressure control on risk of cardiovascular disease. Recent studies that have demonstrated a positive effect of exercise on reduction in cardiac mortality, such as the large Harvard University Alumnus Study ($n = 17,321$), have, unfortunately, not included women.[17]

DISCUSSION

Sex describes anatomic, biologic, and physiologic attributes, while gender encompasses social and societal factors, which are, in part, shaped by environment and expectations. Gender bias may be described as differential diagnosis, evaluation, or treatment based on subjective assumptions and perceived gender differences, rather than on scientific or objective data. Gender bias in medical diagnosis and treatment has been identified in many areas of medicine. Four important areas in which gender bias has been identified include ischemic heart disease, renal transplant evaluation and receipt, lung cancer diagnosis,[18] and access to specialized alcohol treatment centers.

Renal Transplant Evaluation

Recent data suggests that male dialysis patients are more likely to be evaluated for and receive renal transplants. While controlling for comorbid illness and age, white women had only a 0.88 likelihood of being considered a renal transplant candidate, com-

pared with white men. Black men had a 0.77 likelihood, and black women had only a 0.66 likelihood of being identified as a transplant candidate.[19] In fact, male candidates were more likely to receive a renal transplant in every age category, although the disparities were most pronounced in the 40-to-60-year-old age group. These biases persisted even after accounting for the older age of female candidates. Further studies are necessary to determine if this disparity represents proper medical judgment or judgment decisions based on societal role and perceived social worth. Future modification in renal transplant evaluation might include a race- and gender-blind process.

Lung Cancer

Detection bias is used to describe the differential ordering of diagnostic tests, and, therefore, diagnosis rates, based on misconceptions about gender or other nonscientific patient characteristics. A prominent example of detection bias can be identified in the diagnosis of lung cancer. Male sex is generally considered an independent risk factor for lung cancer, although there is no scientific data validating this assumption. In fact, women comprise 39% of the lung cancer population.[20] The presumptive association of male gender with lung cancer may have been related historically to an increased prevalence of high-risk behavior in men (smoking and occupational exposure). The diagnosis of lung cancer is therefore more likely to be pursued in the male population, despite autopsy studies that suggest a large proportion of undiagnosed cases in women and nonsmokers.[21] Men who present with similar symptoms (cough, sputum), are two times more likely to have sputum pap smears ordered.[22] Once the prevalence of lung cancer in women is acknowledged, strategies for primary and secondary prevention in women can be vigorously pursued. Primary strategies include education and counseling young women about the dangers of smoking. Twenty-eight percent of women aged 25 to 34 currently smoke, and the highest increase in new smokers is among young women, who often use cigarettes for weight control.[23] Strategies for secondary prevention include liberal ordering of chest radiographs and sputum Pap smears in women with suspicious symptoms. The utility of screening chest radiographs in high-risk, asymptomatic populations remains controversial.[20,24]

Diagnosis and Treatment of Coronary Artery Disease

Coronary artery disease (CAD), although less common in younger women because of hormonal protection, can affect a significant proportion of older women, as well as younger women with a strong family history and risk factors. Unfortunately, women presenting with symptoms suggestive of CAD often receive less aggressive treatment than their male counterparts. As mentioned earlier, women often wait longer for ECGs and may receive less aggressive thrombolytic therapy. The issue of whether women receive less aggressive diagnostic studies and bypass surgery remains controversial. Some studies suggest decreased rates of cardiac catheterization for women, compared with their male counterparts after myocardial infarction,[25] whereas other studies suggest equitable treatment.[26] Some studies suggest decreased referral for coronary artery bypass grafting (CABG) in women,[27] whereas other studies suggest that men are referred too often for CABG and are more likely to be referred when the benefit is unclear.[28] These studies suggest that if the severity of coronary artery disease is controlled for, referral for CABG is equitable for men and women. The issue is further confounded by a reported increase in mortality in women who undergo CABG.[29] The increase in mortality may be due to anatomic considerations, increased disease severity at referral, older age, or increased number of comorbid illnesses.

These gender differences may represent undertreatment and referral of women, overtreatment of men, or appropriate care for both genders. Further research into gender differences is crucial to delineate among these possibilities. Lack of understanding of important physiologic differences, changes with age and hormonal status, and responses to treatment and medications highlight the difficulties in choosing appropriate treatment regimens for women. The need for more research which includes women, and explores these important gender differences is being addressed currently through the Women's Health Initiative of the NIH. A large amount of funding has been allocated to research projects that will study heart disease, stroke, cancer, osteoporosis, and the

Table 18-1 PMH: Female Gender-Sensitive Questions Regarding Alcohol Use

P = Do you carry alcohol in your **p**urse?

M = Does your drinking vary with your **m**enstrual cycle, or has it affected the regularity of your menstrual periods?

H = Has there been any physical violence in your **h**ome (spouse or child abuse), or has your drinking had an effect on your children?

* Adapted from Gore-Gearhart JG, Beebe DK, Milhorn HT, Meeks GR. Alcoholism in women. *Am Fam Physician* 1991; 44: 907–13.

effect of drugs, menopause, cigarettes, diet, and hormone replacement in women. Through this research, physicians will have a more sound scientific basis on which to make important treatment decisions in women.

Specialized Alcohol Treatment

Gender disparities also exist in the referral and treatment for alcoholism. Women may be less likely to seek treatment for alcohol abuse in specialized treatment centers, despite evidence for increased symptom severity.[30] Female alcoholics tend to conceal their drinking behavior by drinking at home.[31] Low self-esteem is common in women with alcohol problems, and older women alcoholics are at significant risk for suicide (see Chapter 19). Women tend to get more treatment in emergency care, primary care, and mental health centers, and are more likely to attribute their symptoms to depression or anxiety.[32] While the treatment of women in primary care and psychiatric settings may, in fact, represent more appropriate treatment, the reasons for underutilization of specialized alcohol treatment centers need to be explored further. Barriers to treatment include lack of financial funds and child care, as well as the stigma attached to female problem drinkers. Identification of alcohol problems in the ED may be an important first step in the diagnosis and treatment of alcoholism in women. Some suggested modifications of the "CAGE" questionnaire with respect to women are described in Table 18-1. These questions may increase the sensitivity of the CAGE questionnaire in the identification of female problem drinkers. The traditional Alcoholics Anonymous (AA) technique of confrontation and breaking down of defenses may be less effective in the treatment of female alcoholics.[33] Instead, a program focusing on the development of support networks and alternative activities and the provision of individualized counseling in a nonthreatening environment may be more effective.[34]

Case #2

A 57-year-old African American female presents with shortness of breath and lethargy, which has gradually increased over the past 2 months. The shortness of breath is increased on exertion but has recently progressed to dyspnea at rest. There is no chest pain, fever, sputum production, pedal edema. She had complained of low back pain intermittently for the past few months, which has been treated by her primary doctor with antiinflammatory medication and rest. She has noted polyuria (according to her family). The last 2 days she has been difficult to arouse, and she appears confused. On examination, she is lethargic but arousable. She is noted to have decreased breath sounds in the right base and dullness to percussion. Her neurologic examination is nonfocal.

Q: What diagnoses should be considered?

Infectious processes, including viral, bacterial, fungal, and Myocobacterium tuberculosis causing pulmonary or CNS infection need to be considered. Metabolic abnormalities, such as new onset diabetes with hyperglycemia and electrolyte abnormalities, are a possible etiology for her mental status changes and weakness. Toxic exposures to alcohol, drugs, or prescription medications should be explored fully. Malignancies (lung, metastatic breast, GI or GU metastases, lymphoma) as a cause of a pulmonary process and electrolyte abnormalities should be considered. Collagen vascular diseases (RA, SLE) can present with pulmonary and CNS findings.

Case Continuation

Laboratory tests reveal normal electrolytes, with a glucose of 140, a low normal potassium of 3.4, a normal BUN and creatinine, a calcium of 14.7, with an albumin of 3.8. The blood count and differential are normal except for a mild anemia. The chest radiograph reveals a large right pleural effusion, and a mass in the right upper lobe.

Q: What disease process can explain this presentation and findings? What further workup is warranted?

A malignancy with metastases or paraneoplastic manifestations could explain the findings of a lung lesion with an effusion and hypercalcemia. An infectious process cannot be ruled out at this point. Sarcoid remains a possible explanation for the lung findings and hypercalcemia. Spinal cord compression must be ruled out, given her back pain, and the possibility of metastatic cancer.

Q: What are the most likely malignancies in this 57-year-old woman? What further history, examination, and laboratory test should be obtained?

The two most common malignancies in a woman with this presentation are breast and lung cancer. While breast cancer is more common, lung cancer is more often lethal and is the leading cause of cancer-related deaths in female patients. A history of smoking or passive exposure to smoke or asbestos may be helpful, but, if absent, will not rule out lung cancer. A history of a recent mammogram, or lack of previous mammography, may be useful. Further examination including breast exam for masses, axillary adenopathy, and nipple discharge should be performed. A radiograph of the lumbar spine (and bone scan, if indicated) may be helpful in ruling out metastases as a cause of the back pain. CT scan myelogram or MRI is necessary if spinal cord compression is suspected.

Case Continuation

With saline diuresis, her calcium decreases to 12. She becomes more alert. A breast examination reveals a 2-x-2 cm hard mass in the upper outer quadrant of the left breast. A bone scan reveals metastatic disease in the left shoulder and lumbar spine. A thoracentesis and biopsy of the breast mass reveals infiltrating ductal carcinoma with metastases. The tumor is estrogen receptor negative. She is started on mithramycin to decrease her calcium, chemotherapy, and radiation to the back and shoulder.

She had no family history of breast cancer. She had a screening mammogram at age 40 but had not had one since. Her physician had not suggested a screening interval for mammography nor given her a direct referral.

Q: What is her prognosis, and how might an earlier diagnosis have changed her prognosis?

Her 5-year survival is approximately 10%. If the diagnosis had been made at an earlier stage, her survival may have been as high as 95% for small neoplasms.[35]

DISCUSSION

Early Detection of Treatable Forms of Cancer

Breast cancer is the most common cancer in women, but lung cancer carries the highest mortality. Among African American women, the incidence of breast cancer below the age of 50 is increasing at an epidemic rate. Mortality has more than doubled for African American women compared to white women, in part due to the late stage of diagnosis.[36] New research has also identified genetic differences in types of sporadic cellular change. African American women are more likely to have substitutions at the P53 regulating gene, whereas white women are more likely to have fragments. Substitution errors appear to give rise to more lethal cancers.[37]

Since early detection dramatically increases survival in patients with breast cancer, efforts to increase mammography utilization by the groups at highest risk are critically important. Direct referrals from the ED and distribution of literature describing the importance of mammography may increase understanding and utilization among women.

Cancer Screening

Clinical breast examination (CBE) and mammography contribute to earlier diagnosis and treatment of breast cancer and therefore increase survival rates.

Mammography is a relatively painless and available form of screening for breast cancer, yet many women are not screened according to current ACS guidelines. Confusion about appropriate intervals for screening exists even among professionals, partly because of the discrepancy between NCI guidelines, which recommend starting mammography at age 50, and guidelines from all other professional organizations, which recommend baseline mammography at 40.

Barriers to screening include patient based factors and provider referral behavior. Patient-based barriers to screening include knowledge deficits, fear (of incurable and deadly illness), cultural barriers, and lack of financial resources. A recent study suggests that the two most common reasons that women gave for not having a mammogram were that they had no problem (thus didn't see the need), and their physician had not recommended it to them.[38] Many women are not aware of the necessity of mammography even when asymptomatic (found in up to 40 percent of women surveyed).[39] This indicates a misunderstanding of the preventative nature of a screening test. Many women who have had one mammogram are not aware of recommended regular screening intervals. For women covered under Medicare, the allowable benefit of one screen every 2 years is less than optimal; this is the group at highest risk, and yearly screening is preferable.[40,41]

Fear represents a barrier to many women. Fear of the risks of radiation and the diagnosis of cancer (which might necessitate mutilation of the body) may further impede screening efforts. A woman may view screening tests as harbingers of illness and death, not as a means of early treatment and cure. Cultural differences may exist: One study which evaluated attitudes of African American women to cancer screening found that many doubted that there was a cure for cancer.[42]

Patient-based financial factors, including poverty and lack of insurance or financial resources for screening tests, represent a large barrier to compliance with screening recommendations. Uninsured and Medicare patients present with significantly more advanced disease and a risk of death that is 49% greater for uninsured women and 40% greater for Medicare-insured women, compared with insured cohorts.[43] Current co-payments required by Medicare for mammograms decrease compliance with screening recommendations (approximately $20 per mammogram after the $100 deductible is met).[44] This issue is salient, because women are overrepresented in uninsured and underinsured populations, secondary to part-time and temporary employment, often described as "a women's career pattern."[45] Recent efforts to increase screening of underserved women include funding through programs like the CDC National Breast and Cervical Cancer Screening Program.

Provider-based factors include referral patterns that are not in compliance with ACS guidelines for mammography and inadequate patient education. Many patients fail to follow screening recommendations because their physician has not emphasized the importance of screening examinations.[46] Significant age and racial biases exist, with fewer mammograms ordered on older women and women of color.[47] Several studies have demonstrated that most women would be willing to undergo screening examinations, if recommended by their physician.[48] Male physicians and older physicians appear to be less likely to comply with screening recommendations.[49] The odds ratio of an eligible woman with a female physician having a mammogram and PAP smear was 1.41 and 1.99 respectively, compared with those with a male physician.[50] This difference was less pronounced among OB/GYN practitioners and more pronounced in family practitioners.[51]

While the primary role of the ED physician is to treat acute illness, the routine inclusion of some pertinent questions regarding screening examinations (or lack thereof) in the history, and a brief explanation as to the importance of routine screening might increase interest and compliance with screening recommendations. The necessity of routine Pap smears and mammograms can be emphasized while palpating the abdomen or performing a pelvic examination.

The feasibility of screening for cervical cancer in the ED has recently been suggested,[52] but implementation on a large scale remains difficult given time constraints and difficulty with follow-up; suggestions are offered for solving these problems in Chapter 33. Women at highest risk for cervical cancer are often medically underserved and use the ED for primary care. Hispanic women, for example, often have low rates of insurance coverage and therefore have reduced access to private physicians.[53] As a result, they have a mortality rate from cervical cancer that is twice that of white women. Pap smear screening in

the ED is an opportunity that we cannot afford to miss.

Case #3

A 32-year-old female presents to the ED with the chief complaint of not "feeling well." On questioning, she admits to extreme fatigue but denies fever, chills, anorexia, weight loss, or other constitutional symptoms. Further review of symptoms reveals no pertinent positive findings. Physical examination is essentially unremarkable. Laboratory tests, including a CBC and electrolytes, are within normal limits. Thyroid function tests have been ordered.

Q: What issues should be considered in a woman who presents to the ED with multiple, vague, somatic complaints?

Domestic violence and sexual assault should be considered, when obvious organic pathology is ruled out. Substance abuse and depression can also present in a similar manner.

Case Continuation

When the physical examination and laboratory results fail to reveal an etiology for the woman's complaints, a red flag is raised and the physician considers the possibility of domestic abuse. She returns to discuss issues with the patient in further detail. The physician discusses her concerns of possible domestic violence with the psychiatric social worker, who also evaluates the patient.

The prevalence of acute domestic violence in females presenting to the ED is reported to be 6 to 30%,[54] with a lifetime prevalence rate of 53%.[55] Over 4 million women are assaulted every year by their male partners. The recognition of domestic violence and sexual assault in the ED can be difficult, since the presentation is often in the form of vague symptoms such as fatigue, poorly localized pain, or a variety of somatic complaints. The EP is afforded the unique opportunity to identify domestic violence and sexual assault, since many abused women receive their care in the ED during crisis situations. A high level of vigilance and increased attention to privacy and proper questioning during the examination is necessary. While consideration of domestic violence and sexual assault in women presenting to the ED is crucial, these issues are discussed in further detail in Chapter 10.

Case Continuation

The patient denies current domestic assault, and after the social worker discusses the issue with the patient, she agrees that she is probably not being actively battered. The physician then returns to talk with the patient again, since she still does not have a clear sense of why this patient is presenting to the ED. When the woman is asked in detail what might be causing her fatigue, she states that she can think of no obvious reason. On further questioning, the patient admits that she works full-time as a nursing assistant, is the primary caregiver for her four children, aged 2 through 12, and takes care of the house (including cooking and cleaning). She also looks in daily on her elderly parents, shops for them, and takes them to doctors. She admits that she has very little time to herself and little time to rest or exercise.

The modern woman faces many challenges as she attempts to maintain multiple roles in her career and motherhood/household/familial responsibilities. Multiple roles can be viewed in a positive way as role accumulation or enrichment, but overload results in role strain, burnout, and significant depression.[56] Physical and mental exhaustion is often the result of maintaining multiple roles. Six percent of women "moonlight" by holding more than one full-time job, compared with 2% two decades ago. This is approximately equal to the percentage of men who currently moonlight.[57] Women tend to have more household responsibilities and are often expected to maintain the household *and* family.[56] The result can be physical manifestations of inadequacy and exhaustion. On the positive side, women are more likely than men to seek help for signs and symptoms of burnout; they are more likely to present sooner for help, often in the form of physical symptoms.

Waitzkin, in *The Politics of Medical Encounters,*[58] discusses methods physicians can use to encourage discussion of these problems and alternative solutions:

> Patients experience these contextual issues as personal troubles that they express, directly or in passing, in conversations with their doctors. The structure of medical discourse tends to marginalize such troubles through subtle messages that reinforce adherence to mainstream expectations. . . . Spe-

cifically, doctors should let patients tell their stories, with fewer interruptions, cut-offs or returns to the technical. Especially at the beginnings of encounters, patients should have the chance to present their narratives in an open-ended way.

The patient in the preceding case scenario was seeking permission to rest—and did so, in assuming the sick role. The patient was given permission to discuss the stresses (physical and emotional) in the context of her ED visit for physical illness and was given a short respite from work and referral to counseling. She felt much better, and thanked the physician for her time.

CONCLUSION

Scientifically and sociologically based gender differences exist and may have important implications for optimal treatment of the female patient in the emergency department. Comprehension of scientifically based gender differences is necessary for the proper treatment of patients of both genders. Gender biases also exist and may represent significant barriers to optimal treatment. Recognition of the pitfalls of gender and detection bias is crucial. This is especially pertinent with reference to evaluation of chest pain and treatment of cardiac disease in the ED.

Encouragement of female participation in large clinical research trials is crucial to the development of an adequate database from which to make important clinical decisions. This can only be developed if an active effort is made to include women in research trials. Beyond simply identifying and treating acute illnesses that commonly affect women, the emergency visit can be used as an opportunity to educate a large population of women on Pap and mammogram screening recommendations and importance, which can be incorporated into routine history and physical examination, as is commonly done for smoking status. It is particularly important, when evaluating the health of women, to approach their problems from a broad perspective. Symptoms of illness cannot be separated, as we have learned from the experience of sexual assault, domestic violence, coronary disease, and HIV disease, from the social context. Improvement in women's status in society is also essential for good health. Jobs, insurance coverage, education, freedom from gender and racial or ethnic discrimination, social support, and physical and emotional safety are basic necessities for health. Much has been accomplished in this last decade, yet much remains to be done.

NOTES

1. Hebert LE, Scherr PA, Beckett LA, et al. Age specific incidence of Alzheimer's disease in a community population. *JAMA* 1995; 273(17):1354–9.
2. Verbrugge LM. Gender and health: An update on hypotheses and evidence. *J Health and Soc Behav* 1985; 26:156–82.
3. Maynard C, Althouse R, Cerqueira M, et al. Underutilization of thrombolytic therapy in eligible women with acute myocardial infarction. *Amer J Cardiol* 1991; 68:529–30.
4. Jackson RE, Peacock WF. Gender bias in thrombolytic therapy (abstract). *Ann Emerg Med* 1993; 22(5):463.
5. Silbergleit R, McNamara RM. Effect of gender on the emergency department evaluation of patients with chest pain. *Acad Emerg Med* 1995; 2:115–19.
6. Green LA, Ruffin MT. A closer examination of sex bias in the treatment of ischemic cardiac disease. *J Family Practice* 1994; 139(4):331–6.
7. Kuhn FE, Rackley CE. Coronary artery disease in women—Risk factors, evaluation, treatment and prevention. *Arch Intern Med* 1993; 153:2626–36.
8. Pan WH, Cedres LB, Liu K, et al. Relationship of clinical diabetes and hyperglycemia to risk of coronary heart disease mortality in men and women. *Amer J Epidemiol* 1986; 123(3):504–16.
9. FTT Collaborative Group. Indications for fibrinolytic therapy in suspected acute myocardial infarction: Collaborative overview of early mortality and major morbidity results from all randomized trials of more than 1000 patients. *Lancet* 1994; 343:311–22.
10. Nabulsi AA, Folsom AF, White A, et al. Association of hormone replacement therapy with various risk factors in post menopausal women. *NEJM* 1993; 328(15):1069–75.
11. Grady D, Rubin SM, Petitti DB, et al. Hormone therapy to prevent disease and prolong life in post-menopausal women. *Ann Intern Med* 1992; 117(12):1016–37.
12. Stampfer MJ, Colditz GA, Willette WC, et al. Postmenopausal estrogen replacement therapy and cardiovascular disease. *NEJM* 1991; 325(11):756–62.
13. Colditz GA, Hankinson SE, Hunter DJ, Willett WC, et al. The use of estrogens and progestins and the risk of breast cancer in postmenopausal women. *NEJM* 1995; 332:1589–93.
14. Manson JE, Stampfer MJ, Colditz GA, et al. A prospective study of aspirin use and primary prevention of cardiovascular disease in women. *JAMA* 1991; 266(4):521–7.
15. Fuchs CS, Stampfer MJ, Colditz GA, et al. Alcohol consumption and mortality among women. *NEJM* 1995; 332(19):1245–50.
16. Kitler ME. Differences in men and women in coronary artery disease, systemic hypertension and their treatment. *Am J Cardiol* 1992; 70:1077–80.
17. Lee IM, Hsieh CC, Paffenberger RS, Jr. Exercise intensity and longevity in men: The Harvard University Alumni health study. *JAMA* 1995; 273:1179–84.
18. Council on Ethical and Judicial Affairs, AMA. Gender disparities in clinical decision making. *JAMA* 1991; 266(4):559–62.
19. Soucie JM, Neylan JF, McClellan W. Race and sex differences in identification of candidates for renal transplantation. *Amer J Kidney Dis* 1992; 19(5):414–19.
20. Strauss GM, Gleason RE, Sugarbaker DJ. Screening for lung cancer re-examined. A reinterpretation of the Mayo Lung Project randomized trial on lung cancer screening. *Chest* 1993; 103(4):337s–341s.
21. McFarlane MJ, Feinstein AR, Wells CK. Clinical features of lung cancers discovered as postmortem "surprise." *Chest* 1986; 90(4):520–3.
22. Wells CK, Feinstein AR. Detection bias in the diagnostic pursuit of lung cancer. *Amer J Epidemiol* 1988; 128(5):1016–26.
23. Collins KS, Rowland D, Salganicoff A, et al. Assessing and improving women's health. In Costello, C, Stone, AJ (eds.). *The American Woman 1994–5—Where Do We Stand?* New York: WW Norton, 1994.
24. Smith EB. Primary cancer of the lung in women. *J Nat Med Assoc* 1989; 81(9):945–7.
25. Ayanian JZ, Epstein AM. Differences in the use of procedures between women and men hospitalized for coronary artery disease. *N Engl J Med* 1991; 325:221–5.
26. Krumholz HM, Douglas PS, Lauer MS, et al. Selection of patients for coronary angiography and coronary revascularization early after myocardial infarction: Is there evidence for gender bias? *Annal Intern Med* 1992; 116:785–90.
27. Bickel NA, Pieper KS, Lee KL, et al. Referral patterns in coronary artery disease treatment: Gender bias or good clinical judgment? *Ann Intern Med* 1992; 116:791–7.
28. Chiriboga DE, Yarzebski J, Goldberg RJ, et al. A community wide perspective of gender differences and temporal trend in the use of diagnostic and re-vascularization procedures for acute myocardial infarction. *Am J Cardiol* 1993; 71:268–73.

29. Khan SS, Nessim A, Gray R, et al. Increased mortality of women in coronary artery bypass surgery: Evidence for referral bias. *Ann Intern Med* 1990; 112:561–7.

30. Roman PM. *Women and alcohol use: A review of the research literature.* Rockville, MD: NIAAA, 1988.

31. Gore-Gearhart J, Beebe DK, Milhorn HT, et al. Alcoholism in women. *AFP* 1991; 44(3):907–13.

32. Weisner C, Schmidt L. Gender disparities in treatment for alcohol problems. *JAMA* 1992; 268(14):172–6.

33. Kasl CD. *Yes you can! A guide to empowerment groups based on the 16 steps.* Lolo MT: Many Roads One Journey, 1995.

34. Fredriksen KI: North of the market: Older women's alcohol outreach program. *Gerontologist* 1992; 32(2):270–2.

35. Tabar L, Fagerberg G, Duffy SW. Update on the Swedish two-county trial of mammographic screening for breast cancer. *Radiol Clin North Amer* 1992; 30:187–210.

36. Eley JW, Hill HA, Chen VW, et al. Racial differences in survival from breast cancer. Results of the National Cancer Institute black/white cancer survival study. *JAMA* 1994; 272:947–54.

37. Ross RK. Endogenous hormones and breast cancer risk. *Epidem Rev* 1993; 15:48–65.

38. NCI Breast Cancer Screening Consortium: Screening mammography: A missed opportunity? *JAMA* 1990; 264(1):54–8.

39. Smith RA, Haynes S. Barriers to screening for breast cancer. *Cancer Suppl* 1992; 69(7):1968–78.

40. Burg MA, Lane DS. Mammography referrals for elderly women: Is Medicare reimbursement likely to make a difference? *Health Serv Res* 1992; 27:505–16.

41. Morrison AS. The efficacy of screening for breast cancer in older women. *J Gerontol* 1992; 47:80–4.

42. Gregg J, Curry RH. Explanatory models of cancer among African American women at two Atlanta neighborhood health centers: The implications for a cancer screening program. *Soc Sci Med* 1994; 39(4):519–26.

43. Ayanian JZ, Kohler BA, Toshi A, et al. The relation between health insurance and clinical outcomes among women with breast cancer. *N Engl J Med* 1993; 329:326–31.

44. Bluestein J: Medicare coverage, supplemental insurance, and the use of mammography by older women. *N Engl J Med* 1995; 332(17):1138–43.

45. Golden C. Understanding the gender gap. New York: Oxford University Press, 1990.

46. Commission on Women's Health. *The Commonwealth Fund survey of women's health.* New York: Commonwealth Fund, 1993.

47. Peters RK, Bear MB, Thomas D. Barriers to screening for cancer of the cervix. *Prevent Med* 1989; 18:133–46.

48. Rakowski W, Rimmer B, Bryant S. Interpreting behavior and intention regarding mammography by respondents in the 1990 National Health Interview Survey of health promotion and disease prevention. *Pub Health Rep* 1993; 108:605–24.

49. Franks P and Clancy CM. Physician gender bias in clinical decision making: Screening for cancer in primary care. *Med Care* 1993; 31(3):213–18.

50. Fox SA, Siu AL, Stein JA. The importance of physician communication on breast cancer screening in older women. *Arch Intern Med* 1994; 154:2058–68.

51. Lurie N, Slater J, McGovern P, et al. Preventative care for women—Does the sex of the physician matter? *N Engl J Med* 1993; 329(7):478–82.

52. Hogness CG, Engelstad LP, Linck LM, et al. Cervical cancer screening in an urban emergency department. *Ann of Emerg Med* 1992; 21(8):933–9.

53. Perez-Stabile ES, Marin BV. Behavioral risk factors: A comparison of Latinos and non-Latino whites in San Francisco. *Am J Pub Health* 1994; 84:971–6.

54. MMWR: Emergency Department response to domestic violence—California, 1992. *JAMA* 1993; 270(10): 1174–5.

55. Abbott J, Johnson R, Koziol-McLain J, et al. Domestic violence in an emergency department population: Incidence and prevalence. *Acad Emerg Med* 1994; 1:34.

56. Moen P. *Women's two roles: A contemporary dilemma.* New York: Auburn House, 1992.

57. Cowley G, Hares M, Rogers A. The breaking point. *Newsweek* 1995; 56–61.

58. Waitzkin H. *The politics of medical encounters: How patients and doctors deal with social problems.* New Haven: Yale University Press, 1991.

19

Caring for the Older Patient

ELAINE W. ROUSSEAU
ARTHUR B. SANDERS

CONTENTS

- Demographics
- Differences in presentation
- Evaluation of diagnostic tests
- Deviation from baseline status: assessment tools
- Discharge planning

CHAPTER SUMMARY

America's population has been growing older throughout the twentieth century. Both the number and proportion of older people have been steadily increasing. This change is the result of a decline in fertility, a decline in mortality rates among those aged 65 and older, and the improved management of infectious diseases which has led to decreased infant and childhood mortality.[1]

This chapter presents an overview of demographic changes and their effect on health care delivery. Older persons are a special population often needing more comprehensive assessment in the emergency department than younger adults. A model identifying principles for the emergency care of older patients is presented that differs from traditional approaches to emergency medicine. This geriatric model was developed to take account of the complex presentation of illness in older people: differences in symptom patterns and normal laboratory values for some diagnostic tests; effects of polypharmacy and co-morbid diseases; psychosocial, functional and cognitive impairments; the adequacy of the patient's social support system; and the need to assess important conditions in the older person's life.

INTRODUCTION

The older population in the U.S. has been steadily increasing from 4% of the total population in 1900 to 13% in 1990. This trend will continue well into the twenty-first century. It is projected that one in five Americans will be 65 and over by 2030. Moreover, the older population is itself getting older. In 1993, the young-old group, those aged 65 to 74, was eight times larger than in 1900, while the oldest old, those 85 and over, was 27 times larger.[2] The oldest old are three times more likely to lose their independence and seven times more likely to enter a nursing home than the young old.[3] This decline in mobility and health with advancing age greatly increases the need for health care.

This demographic shift has had and will continue to have a major impact on health care utilization in the United States. Cross-sectional data reveal that more than four of five people aged 65 and over have at least one chronic condition, and multiple chronic conditions are commonplace.[4] The prevalence of chronic conditions results in greater health services utilization. On average, those 65 and over visited a physician eight times per year, compared with five visits by the general population.[5]

Emergency department utilization is also affected by the increasing numbers of older persons.

Data from 1990 reveal that 15% of ED visits were by those aged 65 years and older. Forty-six percent of these patients received comprehensive ED evaluation,[6] compared with 13% of nonelderly patients. Older patients were more apt to be admitted to the hospital (32% versus 6%), admitted to intensive care beds (7% versus 1%), and arrive by ambulance transport (30% versus 9%) than were nonelderly patients aged less than 65 years.[7] In another study, it was reported that older persons more frequently presented with co-morbid diseases (94% versus 63%) than did adult controls aged 21 to 64 years. The time from ED arrival until disposition was longer for older adults (3 hours and 5 minutes), compared with 1 hour and 29 minutes for younger adult controls. The frequency of ordering x-rays (77% versus 52%) and laboratory tests (78% versus 53%) was greater for those aged 65 and over than for adult controls.[7]

How does this increased use of the ED affect practicing emergency medicine physicians? In a survey of 1,000 members of the American College of Emergency Physicians, it was reported that for each of seven clinical presentations, 45% or more of the physicians had more difficulty in the management of older compared with younger patients. Inadequate research efforts and educational opportunities both in CME and residency were reported for geriatric emergency care. This lack of training may partially explain why physicians reported being less comfortable in the clinical evaluation and management of geriatric patients.[8]

Directors of emergency medicine residencies were also surveyed, with results similar to those of the practicing physicians. The directors reported that teaching of geriatric emergency medicine was inadequate and that national research efforts were insufficient. Residency directors also reported that older patients were more difficult to manage on four of seven medical complaints.[9]

What happens to the older persons themselves when they visit the ED? High levels of fear and anxiety were experienced by older persons. Anxiety was not allayed until they were informed of the seriousness of their condition and plans for both treatment and disposition were discussed. Frequently, the elderly were too cold while waiting in the exam room and reported having difficulties hearing and understanding nurses and physicians.[10] Older patients also have more difficulty with self-care than do younger adult controls after discharge

from the ED.[11] Staff need to be more sensitive to the concerns of older persons seen in the ED and must consider potential difficulties with self care in developing and communicating discharge plans.

Case # 1

Ms. Jones is an 85-year-old female who presents to the emergency department with a 2-day history of "not feeling well." She says that she is ordinarily active and energetic, but for the past 2 days is "just not feeling herself." On further questioning, she says she may be a little weak and dizzy but otherwise cannot further clarify her complaint.

Q: How do you evaluate this complaint?

The Geriatric Emergency Medicine Task Force of the Society for Academic Emergency Medicine has assessed the ED care for older patients and concluded that the traditional geriatric emergency medicine biomedical model does not work well for many older patients.[12] Older patients are a special population and often need a more comprehensive assessment. Table 19-1 lists a set of principles for the emergency care of older patients that was developed by the Task Force.[13]

The first principle (complex presentation) is illustrated by Ms. Jones's case. Older persons may complain of vague or imprecise symptoms such as "weakness" or "not feeling right." These complaints often frustrate busy emergency health care professionals. The fact that common diseases present atypically in older patients makes these vague complaints such as "not feeling right" important because they may indicate serious diseases. For example, most older patients with acute myocardial infarction do not present with chest pain. Acute appendicitis in older persons may manifest as vague abdominal pain rather than right lower quadrant pain with anorexia, nausea, and vomiting.

In Ms. Jones's case, principle IX (knowledge of the older person's baseline functional status) is essential for evaluating the complaint. This can best be assessed through the use of standardized tools. A number of tools are routinely used for assessing functional status in older patients. These include the Activities of Daily Living (ADL) Scale and Instrumental Activities of Daily Living (IADL) Scale (Figures 19-1

Table 19-1 Principles of Geriatric Emergency Medicine

I   The older person's ED presentation is frequently complex.

II   Common diseases present atypically in older persons.

III The confounding effects of co-morbid diseases must be taken into account.

IV   Elderly patients are frequently taking multiple medications (polypharmacy).

V   Many older persons have impairment of their cognitive function.

VI   Some diagnostic tests may have normal values that are different in older persons.

VII Older persons have decreased functional reserve.

VIII Older persons may not have adequate social support systems and may need to rely on caretakers.

IX   A knowledge of the older person's baseline functional status is essential for evaluating new complaints.

X   Health problems in older patients must be evaluated for associated psychosocial adjustments.

XI   The emergency department encounter is an opportunity to assess important conditions in older persons' lives.

SOURCE: Reprinted with permission from Sanders Arthur B. (ed.). *Emergency care of the elder person.* St. Louis, MO: Beverly Cracom Publications.

---

and 19-2). The ADL scale evaluates basic functions of daily living, including bathing, dressing, toileting, transfer, continence, and feeding—all necessary for independent living. Problems with any of these tasks are correlated with significant morbidity and mortality.[14] The presentation of a patient with a new ADL impairment is a medical emergency that needs prompt workup for etiology. For example, we may determine that Ms. Jones had previously needed assistance with bathing and dressing because of severe arthritis but was independent with regard to toileting, transferring, and feeding. If at presentation in the ED, Ms. Jones now has additional problems with toileting, the etiology of this impairment must be investigated. Higher levels of function are assessed with the IADL scale(Instrumental Activities of Daily Life), which includes assessment of ability to use the telephone, shop, do housework, and handle finances.[15] Although these factors are more subtle, a change in the IADL abilities can also be the only symptom of a serious disease.

Case Continuation

Using the ADL/IADL scales helped the ED team to classify Ms. Jones complaint. In her usual state of health, Ms. Jones is independent with regard to bathing, dressing, toileting, transferring, and feeding. She uses the telephone herself and prepares her own meals. She does not drive, however, and her daughter does the grocery shopping and checks on her daily. She also has outside help with the housework, laundry, and handyman activities. Ms. Jones takes her own medicine without help and manages her financial affairs herself. Over the past 2 days, several factors have changed. Ms. Jones has been unable to prepare her own meals. She doesn't feel that she can think straight enough to make any financial decisions. She is able to take her medicines and use the telephone, but has noted two episodes in which she "lost her urine" before she could get to the bathroom. This has not happened to her for "a long time." In summary, one notes a decrease in functional activities over the past 2 days.

Q: How does one evaluate a decline in functional activities in the older patient in the emergency department setting?

Once we have defined the patient's problem as one of functional decline a more comprehensive history is important. Was the decline acute or chronic? When was the last time the patient could do the specific activity such as laundry, shopping, dressing, feeding, and so on? The more acute the time course, the more likely it is that the patient is suffering from an acute disease state which could be reversible.

Environmental and social factors in the patient's history must also be assessed. Has something changed in the living environment? Has the housekeeper who usually does some of these chores changed? A review of the patient's co-morbid diseases is essential to understanding functional decline (Principle III). Is the decline a worsening of a chronic disease, such as congestive heart failure or chronic obstructive pulmonary disease? Further, older patients are frequently taking multiple medications (principle IV). Have the medications changed? Are there new over-the-counter medications? Is it possi-

Figure 19-1 Activities of Daily Living (ADL) Scale—Evaluation Form

Name _____   Day of Evaluation _____

For each area of functioning listed below, check description that applies. (The word "assistance" means supervision, direction or personal assistance.)

Bathing—Sponge bath, tub bath or shower.
- ☐ Receives no assistance (gets in and out of tub by self if tub is usual means of bathing).
- ☐ Receives assistance in bathing only one part of the body (such as back or a leg).
- ☐ Receives assistance in bathing more than one part of the body (or nor bathed).

Dressing–Gets clothes from closets and drawers, including underclothes, outer garments and using fasteners (including braces, if worn).
- ☐ Gets clothes and gets completely dressed without assistance.
- ☐ Gets clothes and gets dressed without assistance, except for assistance in tying shoes.
- ☐ Receives assistance in getting clothes or in getting dressed, or stays partly or completely undressed.

Toileting—Going to the "toilet room" for bowel and urine elimination; cleaning self after elimination and arranging clothes.
- ☐ Goes to "toilet room," cleans self, and arranges clothes without assistance. (May use object for support such as cane, walker or wheelchair and may manage night bedpan or commode, emptying same in morning.)
- ☐ Receives assistance in going to "toilet room" or in cleansing self or in arranging clothes after elimination or in use of night bedpan or commode.
- ☐ Doesn't go to room termed "toilet" for the elimination process.

Transfer
- ☐ Moves in and out of bed as well as in and out of chair without assistance. (May be using object for support, such as cane or walker.)
- ☐ Moves in and out of bed or chair with assistance.
- ☐ Doesn't get out of bed.

Continence
- ☐ Controls urination and bowel movement completely by self.
- ☐ Has occasional "accidents."
- ☐ Supervision helps keep urine or bowel control; catheter is used or person is incontinent.

Feeding
- ☐ Feeds self without assistance.
- ☐ Feeds self except for getting assistance in cutting meat or buttering bread.
- ☐ Receives assistance in feeding or is fed partly or completely by using tubes or intravenous fluids.

SOURCE: Reprinted with permission from Katz S. Assessing self-maintenance: Activities of daily living, mobility and instrumental activities of daily living. *J. Am Geriatr Soc* 1983; 31:721–7.

ble that the symptoms represent a medication effect or toxicity?[16]

Cognitive impairment may also play a role in functional decline. Cognitive impairment is more common in older patients (principle V). It is possible that the inability to do some tasks such as use the telephone, manage financial matters, shop, or prepare meals may be manifestations of cognitive impairments. Thus, it is essential to evaluate the patient for cognitive impairment, including delirium (acute

Figure 19-2 Instrumental Activities of Daily (IADL) Scale
Self-Rated Version Extracted from the Multilevel Assessment Instrument (MAI)

1. Can you use the telephone:
   without help; 3
   with some help; or 2
   are you completely unable to use the telephone? 1

2. Can you get to places out of walking distance:
   without help; 3
   with some help; or 2
   are you completely unable to travel unless special arrangements are made? 1

3. Can you go shopping for groceries:
   without help; 3
   with some help; or 2
   are you completely unable to do any shopping? 1

4. Can you prepare your own meals:
   without help; 3
   with some help; or 2
   are you completely unable to prepare any meals? 1

5. Can you do your own housework:
   without help; 3
   with some help; or 2
   are you completely unable to do any housework? 1

6. Can you do your own handyman work:
   without help; 3
   with some help; or 2
   are you completely unable to any handyman work? 1

7. Can you do your own laundry:
   without help; 3
   with some help; or 2
   are you completely unable to do any laundry at all? 1

8a. Do you take medicines or use any medications?
   Yes   If yes, answer Question 8b. 1
   No   If no, answer Question 8c. 2

8b. Do you take your own medicine:
   without help in the right doses at the right time; 3
   with some help if someone prepares it for you and/or reminds you to take it; or 2
   are you/would you be completely unable to take your own medicine? 1

8c. If you had to take medicine, can you do it:
   without help in the right doses at the right time; 3
   with some help if someone prepares it for you and/or reminds you to take it; or 2
   are you/would you be completely unable to take your own medicine? 1

9. Can you manage your own money:
   without help; 3
   with some help; or 2
   are you completely unable to handle money? 1

SOURCE: Adapted with permission from Lawton MP, Brody EM. Assessment of older people: Self-maintaining and instrumental activities. *Gerontologist* 1969; 9:179–86. Copyright © The Gerontological Society of America.

confusional state) as well as early dementia. A recommended screen for evaluating cognitive impairment in the ED setting is the use of orientation to person, place, and time, followed by three-item recall at 1 minute. If the patient fails the test of orientation or recall, a formal mental status test should follow.[17] The use of the Folstein Mini-Mental State Examination (Figure 19-3) is useful in ED settings to help distinguish organic from nonorganic impairment.[18] The Confusion Assessment Method (CAM) Scale (Figure 19-4) may be used to assess ED patients for delerium.[19]

Case Continuation

Ms. Jones has a normal three-item recall and orientation. There have been no changes in her home environment or social support system. She cares for herself and is generally independent. Her daughter lives about 1 mile away. The symptoms evolved over a 2-day period. Ms. Jones takes an ACE inhibitor for blood pressure control and one aspirin a day. She takes no other medicines and, other than hypertension, has no co-morbid diseases.

Q: What is the differential diagnosis when an older patient presents to the ED with functional decline?

The differential diagnosis of functional decline in elderly patients should follow from the history and physical exam. A complete physical exam with attention to focal neurological signs as well as mental status exam would be important. Deficits in the exam may point to a specific problem. Issues to consider are the following:[16]

- Is this an exacerbation of a known chronic disease such as congestive heart failure, chronic obstructive pulmonary disease, and so on?
- Does this represent an atypical presentation of myocardial ischemia?
- Does this represent sepsis from an occult infection?
- Is this an acute neurologic process such as stroke or subdural hematoma?
- Is this an acute abdominal process such as mesenteric infarction?
- Is this related to medications that the patient has taken?

- Does this represent a psychological illness such as depression?
- Are there environmental or social factors involved in the functional decline?

In the emergency department, work up would generally include electrocardiogram, blood tests to evaluate electrolytes, an evaluation of renal and liver functions, a complete blood count, and a urine analysis to rule out occult infection. Consideration must be given to a CT scan of the head if there is any chance of a subdural hematoma. Patients who have cognitive changes, neurologic signs, or frequent falls while taking anticoagulants are particularly susceptible to subdural hematomas.

If the patient is to be discharged home with functional decline, arrangements must be made for a safe environment. Principle VIII emphasizes the need for adequate social support systems by many older persons. Thus, one must do formal discharge planning for older patients with changes in their functional status to assure their health and safety when released from the emergency department.[13] Even a simple injury like a Colles' fracture in the dominant arm of an older patient may severely reduce the ability to perform activities of daily living. The fracture may be appropriately treated with reduction and casting, but how does this disability affect the older person's ability to function? Can she prepare meals, eat, take medications, and so on with a cast on her arm? If the person as a whole in his home environment is not addressed, a simple reversible injury such as a Colles' fracture can begin a spiral of functional decline resulting in poor nutrition, immobilization, secondary infections, and decompensation because of inability to take medications or comply with follow-up appointments.

Social service involvement is often an important part of discharge planning. An assessment by a home health nurse can usually be arranged from the ED with planning for essential support services such as meals and transportation to doctors' appointments. If these issues cannot be satisfactorily arranged, admission to the hospital may be necessary for the health and safety of the patient.

Case Continuation

Ms. Jones' physical exam is unremarkable. Her orientation and three-item recall are normal. The history, how-

Figure 19-3 Mini-Mental State Examination (MMSE)

Add points for each correct response.		**Score**	Points
Orientation			
1. What is the:	Year?		1
	Season?		1
	Date?		1
	Day?		1
	Month?		1
2. Where are we?	State?		1
	County?		1
	Town or city?		1
	Hospital?		1
	Floor?		1
Registration 3. Name three objects, taking 1 second to say each. Then ask the patient to repeat all three after you have said them. Give one point for each correct answer. Repeat the answers until patient learns all three.			3
Attention and Calculation 4. Serial sevens. Give one point for each correct answer. Stop after five answers. Alternate: Spell WORLD backwards.			5
Recall 5. Ask for names of three objects learned in Question 3. Give one point for each correct answer.			3
Language 6. Point to a pencil and a watch. Have the patient name them as you point.			2
7. Have the patient repeat "No ifs, ands or buts."			1
8. Have the patient follow a three-stage command: "Take a paper in your right hand. fold the paper in half. Put the paper on the floor."			3
9. Have the patient read and obey the following: "CLOSE YOUR EYES." (Write it in large letters.)			1
10. Have the patient write a sentence of his or her choice. (The sentence should contain a subject and an object and should make sense. Ignore spelling errors when scoring.)			1
11. Have the patient copy the design. (Give one point if all sides and angles are preserved and if the intersecting sides form a quadrangle.)			1
	Total		30

Source: Reprinted with permission from *J Psychiatr Res* Volume 12, Folstein MF, Folstein SE, McHugh PR. Mini-mental state: A practical method for grading the cognitive state of patients for the clinician. 1975, Elsevier Science Ltd., Pergamon Imprint, Oxford, England.

Figure 19-4 Confusion Assessment Method (CAM) Scale

		BOX 1

I. **Acute Onset and Fluctuating Course**

    a. Is there evidence of an acute change in mental status from the patient's baseline?

-OR-

    b. Did the (abnormal) behavior fluctuate during the day, that is tend to come and go or increase and decrease in severity?

                         No - 1   Yes - 2

II. **Inattention**

Did the patient have difficulty focusing attention, for example, being easily distractible or having difficulty keeping track of what was being said?

                         No - 1   Yes - 2

		BOX 2

III. **Disorganized Thinking**

Was the patient's thinking disorganized or incoherent, such as rambling or irrelevant conversation, unclear or illogical flow of ideas, or unpredictable switching from subject to subject?

                         No - 1   Yes - 2

IV. **Altered Level of Unconsciousness**

Overall, how would you rate the patient's level of consciousness?

- Alert (normal)   - 1

- Vigilant (hyperalert)   - 2
- Lethargic (drowsy, easily aroused)   - 3
- Stupor (difficult to arouse)   - 4
- Coma (unarousable)   - 5

Do any checks appear in this box?   No - 1   Yes - 2

If all items in Box 1 are checked and at least one item in Box 2 is checked, the diagnosis of delirium is suggested. → Exclude patient from study. If patient does not meet criteria for delirium, continue with enrollment interview.

Source: Adapted with permission from Inouye SK, van Dyck CH, Alessi CA, et al. Clarifying confusion: The confusion assessment method—A new method for detection of delirium. *Ann Intern Med* 1990; 113:941–8.

ever, does point to a possible area of concern with the two episodes of urinary incontinence. Blood and urine tests are done, and the CBC shows a hematocrit 32%, with 14,700 WBCs and 10% bands. Electrolytes, glucose, BUN, creatinine and liver function tests are all within normal limits. Urine analysis shows 30 WBC/hpf and 4+ bacteria.

Q: What lab tests are altered with age?

Principle VI of geriatric emergency medicine emphasizes that some diagnostic tests have normal values in older patients while others may be different. For example, in Ms. Jones's case, it is important to know that the hemoglobin and hematocrit do *not* change with age.[20] Thus, Ms. Jones's blood work shows an anemia which needs to be explained. In addition, the white blood count does *not* change. Thus, her elevated white blood cell count with the appearance of band forms is significant. It is important to know that other laboratory values *do* change with age. For example, glucose tolerance decreases and the sedimentation rates may show mild elevations.[20] Ms. Jones shows evidence of pyuria and bacteriuria. Asymptomatic pyuria and bacteriuria do not necessarily need to be treated. In this case, however, the bacteremia and pyuria may not be asymptomatic. Her elevated white count and left shift with band forms are consistent with an acute infectious process. One can postulate that Ms. Jones's urinary tract infection with systemic symptoms may be the cause of her functional decline.

Older persons are more susceptible to infections. Once they get infections, they are more susceptible to complications caused by a decreased functional reserve (principle VII). Because of a declining immune system as well as co-morbid diseases, older persons have a higher morbidity and mortality than younger adults with similar infections. Infections can present in older persons atypically.[21] In fact, it is not uncommon for patients with sepsis to present with vague symptoms such as fatigue, weight loss, confusion, or just "not feeling well." Up to one-third of older patients presenting with serious infections, including bacteremia, pneumonia, and urinary tract infections, are not febrile.[21]

Urinary tract infections are common in older persons, and the most frequent source of bacteremia.

Anatomic and functional changes with age predispose both men and women to urinary tract infections. Older persons, especially those with chronic infections, can have complicated etiologies with organisms that include pseudomonas, proteus, klebsiella, and enterobacter.[21]

Case Continuation

Ms. Jones is thought to have a urinary tract infection that is causing her functional decline. She is also noted to have an anemia that needs further workup. The question of inpatient or outpatient treatment is discussed with Ms. Jones and her daughter. Because of Ms. Jones's functional decline, leukocytosis, and left shift, she shows signs of systemic toxicity and possible sepsis. Blood cultures are drawn to assess the patient for bacteremia. It is decided that the patient would benefit most from in-hospital treatment with intravenous antibiotics. After 48 hours in the hospital, Ms. Jones returns home on oral antibiotics. Her activity of daily living returns to her baseline status.

CONCLUSION

This case is familiar to many people who have worked in emergency departments. It illustrates many of the principles of geriatric emergency medicine. Emergency health care professionals must understand that older patients are a special population and need to have a more comprehensive evaluation than younger patients with the same complaint. While this can often be frustrating for emergency health care workers, once these principles are understood, diagnostic workup and treatment should follow. Older patients should have mental status evaluations and functional assessments as part of their ED evaluation. Use of standardized tools such as the Activity of Daily Living (ADL) Scale or the Instrumental Activity of Daily Living (IADL) Scale will facilitate both information transfer and comparison of functional activity over time. These tools are especially useful in evaluating patients who reside in the nursing home. The older person frequently presents atypically with common diseases such as pneumonia or urinary tract infection, myocardial infarction, appendicitis, or subdural hematoma. One must always be aware of the confounding effects of co-morbid diseases and medication interaction as the cause of the patient's symptoms. Some diagnostic tests may have their normal values altered with age, whereas others do not change with age.

Older persons are particularly susceptible to disease and injury because they have decreased functional reserve. When they are injured or have an infection, they are susceptible to complications such as multiorgan failure. It is, therefore, critically important that emergency health care professionals make the diagnosis early so that treatment is initiated promptly. Finally, older persons may need evaluation of their social support systems and activities at home. The use of community resources, social services agencies, as well as home health nurses, can facilitate discharge planning and home treatment of older patients.

NOTES

1. Moritz D, Ostfeld A. The epidemiology and demography of aging. In Hazzard WR, Andres R, Bierman E, Blass JP (eds.). *Principles of geriatric medicine and gerontology.* New York: McGraw-Hill, 1990:146–56.
2. *Profile of older Americans.* American Association of Retired Persons and the U.S. Administration on Aging, 1994.
3. Soldo B, Manton K. Dynamics of health changes in oldest old: New perspectives and evidence. *Milbank Memorial Fund Quarterly* 1985; 63:20.
4. *Aging America: Trends and projections.* U.S. Senate Special Committee on Aging, American Association of Retired Persons, Federal Council on the Aging, U.S. Administration on Aging, 1991.
5. National Center for Health Statistics. *National hospital discharge survey: Annual summary, 1987.* Vital and Health Statistics Series 1989; 13:99.
6. Strange GR, Chen EH, Sanders AB. Use of emergency departments by elderly patients: Projections from a multicenter data base. *Ann Emerg Med* 1992; 21: 819–24.
7. Singal BM, Hedges JR, Rousseau EW, et al. Geriatric patient emergency visits part I: Comparison of visits by geriatric and younger patients. *Ann Emerg Med* 1992;21:802–7.
8. McNamara RM, Rousseau EW, Sanders AB. Geriatric emergency medicine: A survey of practicing emergency physicians. *Ann Emerg Med* 1992; 21:796–801.
9. Jones JS, Rousseau EW, Schropp MA, Sanders AB. Geriatric training in emergency medicine residency programs. *Ann Emerg Med* 1992; 21:825–9.
10. Baraff LJ, Bernstein E, Bradley K, et al. Perceptions of emergency care by the elderly: Results of multicenter focus group interviews. *Ann Emerg Med* 1992; 21: 814–18.
11. Hedges JR, Singal BM, Rousseau EW, et al. Geriatric patient emergency visits part II: Perceptions of visits by geriatric and younger patients. *Ann Emerg Med* 1992; 21:808–13.
12. Sanders AB. Care of the elderly in emergency departments: Conclusions and recommendations. *Ann Emerg Med* 1992; 22:830–4.
13. Sanders AB (ed.). *Emergency care of the elder person.* St. Louis: Beverly Cracom, 1995.
14. Katz S. Assessing self maintenance: Activities of daily living, mobility and instrumental activities of daily living. *J Am Geriatr Soc* 1983; 31:721–7.
15. Lawton MP, Brody EM. Assessment of older people: Self-maintaining and instrumental activities of daily living. *Gerontologist* 1969; 9:179–86.
16. Lachs MS. Recognizing and managing functional decline in the older emergency department patient. In Sanders AB (ed.). *Emergency care of the elder person.* St. Louis: Beverly Cracom, 1995.
17. Bernstein E. The emergency department assessment of the older person. In Sanders AB (ed.). *Emergency care of the elder person.* St. Louis: Beverly Cracom, 1995.
18. Folstein MF, Folstein SE, McHugh PR. Mini-mental state: A practical method for grading the cognitive state of patients for the clinician. *J Psychiatr Res* 1975; 12:189–98.
19. Inouye SK, van Dyck CH, Alessi CA, et al. Clarifying confusion: The confusion assessment method—A new method for detection of delirium. *Ann Intern Med* 1990; 113:941–8.
20. Kane RL, Ouslander JG, Abrass IB. *Essentials of clinical geriatrics.* New York: McGraw-Hill, 1994.
21. Evans R. Infections in the elderly. In Sanders AB (ed.). *Emergency care of the elder person.* St. Louis: Beverly Cracom, 1995.

20

Prisoners' Health

JAY M. BARUCH
LEWIS R. GOLDFRANK

CONTENTS

- Deficiencies in prison health care
- Health rights
- Right to refuse
- Barriers to a therapeutic patient-physician relationship
- Scope of the problem; prison health issues
- Impact on the community
- Guns in the hospital; prisoners and violence in health care settings

CHAPTER SUMMARY

The prison population in the United States is growing at an alarming rate, with over 1 million men and women currently incarcerated in state and federal correctional facilities. Prisoners have very high rates of HIV, TB, hepatitis, addictions, chronic diseases, mental illness, victimization and suicide. These conditions challenge the resources of prison facilities and the communities to which they return. Prisoners have a constitutional and ethical right to health care, and these rights include informed consent, confidentiality and the right to refuse care. The emergency department (ED) is often the usual site of care in the community for prisoners, but getting patient trust and cooperation in these circumstances is difficult.

The emergency physician who tries to provide quality care is often confronted with serious deficiencies in the prison health care system and must take into account the medical capability of each particular jail's receiving facility in order to develop an appropriate discharge plan. There is both a necessity and an opportunity for public health intervention.

Case #1

A 24-year-old man, recently arrested, presented to the Bellevue Emergency Department with the chief complaint, "I'm a diabetic and I need my insulin." His blood glucose was 300mg/dL, but urinalysis failed to show the presence of ketones. The patient was not clinically dehydrated, and electrolytes revealed a normal anion gap. The patient was given insulin and two liters of normal saline intravenously and observed for several hours. The repeat blood glucose was 160mg/dL and he was sent back to the holding cell to await arraignment. In the holding area there was no access to insulin. Two days later, the patient returned, still in police custody, with an altered mental status. He was tachypneic, dehydrated, and acidemic, with a blood sugar of 545mg/dL. He was admitted to the intensive care unit for treatment of diabetic ketoacidosis.

Q: What are the requirements of a prebooking exam?

The American Medical Association has established strict standards regarding the prebooking exam. Essentially, the physician should diagnose, treat, and arrange follow-up for any trauma or illness that may place the prisoner at harm, or any contagious disease that poses a risk to other prisoners as well. The exam also establishes baseline data on each prisoner.

Q: What might the physician have anticipated about the likelihood of the patient receiving insulin?

In New York City, arrested persons are eventually taken to a central holding area, central booking, to be processed and to await arraignment before a judge. In central booking, there are two nurses who do a very basic medical assessment and triage patients with complex medical problems to the Bellevue Emergency Department. These nurses are not permitted to dispense medications, not even insulin or acetaminophen. Nor do they check finger stick blood sugars for diabetics or evaluate patients with asthma. Prisoners who have been evaluated and sent back to central booking with prescriptions generally receive no therapy until they have been arraigned and either transferred to a jail where there are appropriate medical personnel or released back into the community and are free to fill the prescriptions themselves.

Although the ED has an important role in the acute management of prisoners, it cannot remedy the larger deficiencies of the prison health care system. At Bellevue, Keller et al. reported that 38 of the 54 admissions for diabetic ketoacidosis among prisoners occurred because prisoners with a history of insulin-dependent diabetes had not received insulin during the period immediately following arrest. The mean number of days from arrest until hospitalization was 2.5. Seven of the recently arrested prisoners had been initially treated at local hospitals and returned to the prison holding areas where they did not receive insulin and later returned in diabetic ketoacidosis.[1]

Q: How might this problem be handled differently by the emergency physician?

Efforts have been made to reduce the possible consequences resulting from the therapeutic vacuum that exists while arrested individuals await arraignment in central booking or in other holding cells. Ideally, persons are to be arraigned within 48 hours after being arrested. If individuals are unable to be present at the courthouse because of serious illness or injury, arraignment can take place at the hospital. The physician's options, especially when treating diabetic prisoners, are more complicated. The emergency physician can either admit each diabetic, which is unreasonable, especially if access to insulin is the sole justification, or observe the patient in the ED and then give a dose of NPH insulin before discharge, hoping it will hold the patient for the duration of the prearraignment period. In any case, it is imperative that physicians be aware of the specific capabilities of the detention or holding facility to which the prisoner will be transferred when planning discharge. If the protocols and capacities of the referring facility are unknown to ED providers, a phone call to discuss the feasability of the discharge plan with jail personnel is imperative. It is also helpful to arrange tours of the prison infirmaries that send patients regularly to the ED, and set up regular meeting with prison health providers to establish protocols and solve problems.

Case #2

A 24-year-old man, a Department of Corrections prisoner, presented with back pain, chest pain, abdominal pain, leg pain, and shortness of breath. He had used intravenous heroin "a long time ago," but didn't know if he was HIV positive. He cursed at the physician while being examined. The exam was normal except for total body tenderness. The lab work, chest radiograph, and electrocardiogram were all normal. During a repeat examination the patient tried to punch the physician when she palpated his abdomen. He said he wanted to vomit. An hour later, he yelled at the nurses requesting food. Finally, he admitted his real complaint: there was a hunger strike at prison and he hadn't eaten in 2 days, and he wanted to eat without being discovered by other prisoners. The prisoner was offered food but was made aware of the other prisoners around him and the presence of numerous corrections officers in the ED. The prisoner refused the food and asked to be discharged back to jail.

Q: What are some of the barriers to developing a positive physician-patient relationship?

When the patient is a prisoner, the physician-patient relationship is often undermined by doubt, a faltering trust that emanates from both parties. The prisoner's perception of the physician is clouded by a certain distrust. The physician is perceived as another representative of the prison system, an ally of the correctional staff. The community physician's place in the prison-health continuum may not be understood. Regardless of any personal beliefs or prejudices, physicians are obligated morally not to judge prisoners, to approach them with empathy and consideration, and to serve as healing agents to the best of their abilities. The obvious logistical limitations associated with caring for a patient who is a ward of the state should be the only apparent differences in type of care.

There may be different belief systems and socioeconomic, racial, religious, or gender biases that further distance the prisoner and physician. Doubt about where a physician's loyalty lies establishes a barrier to communication. Thus prisoners may not be forthcoming with medical histories; for example, the patient with a fever and cough who has concealed his positive HIV status to avoid stigmatization in prison; the assaulted or sexually abused prisoner who denies everything out of respect or fear for the code in prison; the diaphoretic and agitated patient who denies use of crack cocaine that he had acquired illicitly in prison and smoked hours before.

The perceptions of health care workers towards prisoners are often tainted by negative moral judgements that can also interfere with physician-patient communication and accurate diagnosis. What we tolerate as permissible is often rooted in a certain societal value structure; especially when patients are involved in high risk activities which inevitably result in illness or injury. Do we subconsciously create a hierarchy of culpability for disease? Does incarceration enhance this image of culpability for illness? Is the intravenous drug injector who is imprisoned for activities related to his substance abuse any more responsible for his HIV-positivity than a person who is HIV-positive as a result of unsafe sex? Or more culpable for his illness than a two-pack-a-day cigarette smoker with emphysema? The danger to a thera-peutic relationship is that patients may feel humiliated (in the vernacular, "less than") as a result of provider communications that project shame and blame toward prisoners for their illness.

Q: What are some of the issues related to confidentiality in caring for patients in custody?

The absence of confidentiality also impedes communication. Prisoners are often evaluated side-by-side, or in the presence of the corrections officers who guard them. This lack of privacy discourages the disclosure of sensitive and perhaps valuable information, even if the prisoner is willing to trust the examining physician. This is particularly the case when prisoners are assaulted by correctional officers.

Q: How should the physician evaluate possible malingering behavior or nonmedical motivation for an ED visit, as evidenced by the patient in this case study?

The emergency physician needs to suppress any biases towards prisoners, because the situation may not be as it first seems; the perceived malingering or manipulative prisoner may be manifesting behavior resulting from underlying mental illness, or reacting to abusive treatment by guards. The physician also needs to be sensitive to the contribution from the prison environment itself. Hours of inactivity encourage prisoners to focus attention on minor symptoms, and the fear of dying behind bars is universal.[2] For prisoners there are many possible secondary benefits for seeking health care in off-site facilities, besides the evaluation and treatment of illness or pain. These other motivations include getting out of work, seeking medication, meeting other prisoners, escaping boredom for a few hours, and escaping prison.[3]

Q: What health rights does the prisoner have?

Do prisoners have a "right" to health care? Rights are claims that individuals make on others or society. They are inviolable and others cannot interfere with them. The justification for these claims is based on legal principles, moral principles, and less formal but very real rules and laws derived from unique value constructs, like "rules of the street." Does the need or desire for health care transform itself into a right to health care? Are prisoners entitled to health care out of a sense of justice? Out of guilt? Because although imprisoned, they retain their status as human beings? What is society's obligation to people who show no respect for established moral and legal laws? Can the convicted murderer or rapist argue for unbridled access to health care based on the same principles he has abrogated, disrespected, and dismissed? Practitioners will answer these questions in accordance with their own religious, moral and ethical beliefs.

Regardless of any moral argument, there is a legal precedent demanding the humane rendering of health care to all prisoners. The U.S. Supreme Court has decreed that "deliberate indifference to the serious medical needs of prisoners constitutes the unnecessary and wanton infliction of pain . . . proscribed by the Eighth Amendment."[4] The Eighth Amendment prohibits cruel and unusual punishment.

Prisoners may have lost their right to liberty, but not to health care and the freedom to make essential decisions about their health. Since prisoners have this "right" they may sue for deprivation of their civil rights under the Civil Rights Act. Prisoners are dependent upon prison officials for the most basic health care. There are many variables involved in access to health care. Guards may refuse to inform staff of the inmate's request; the medical system may refuse to respond, or respond inadequately to the request. Since the prisoner has no alternative access pathways, a delay in evaluating a serious illness is equivalent to a denial of care. Prisoners can state a claim for violation of their rights if care is denied, delayed, or grossly negligent.[5]

Q: Can prisoners refuse care, and what can the emergency physician do if the patient refuses necessary treatment?

As autonomous decision makers regarding their own health, prisoners have a firm right to informed consent. Information about procedures or treatment, the benefits and risks, as well as possible alternatives and their respective benefits and risks should be presented to them in appropriate lay language. The

prisoner has the right to refuse treatment. The same standards apply to all patients, whether or not they are incarcerated. If the patient is considered to have sufficient capacity to make the decision, respect for autonomy dictates that patient's preference be honored.

Often a compassionate, open discussion is all that is necessary to achieve agreement with the diagnostic or treatment plan. If the individual still refuses, the discussion and final decision should be carefully recorded in the medical record. The prison system may encompass a locked prison ward as part of the hospital, and some patients who refuse treatment may be admitted upstairs to the prison ward in the hospital so they may be observed, and not sent back to a facility where emergency treatment may be difficult to obtain should the patient's medical condition deteriorate.

The physician must be prudent and sensitive to the prisoners' needs when there is refusal of care. Is it truly a rejection of all care, or a refusal of the specific kind of care offered? In an editorial on the rights of prisoners with AIDS, Dubler stated most succinctly, "If a patient with AIDS is shackled to a hospital bed, is the refusal of care a choice of death or a disinclination to suffer the pain and humiliation which accompany the care offered?"[6] Dubler also stated that because of the peculiar nature of prisons, with various intimidations and pressures from both prison staff and peers, it is often difficult to delineate true voluntary from involuntary behavior in the prison setting; in addition, there is often great difficulty distinguishing refusal of care from denial of care. These issues complicate the assessment of prisoners' medical problems; and communication may be even further compromised because the doctor-patient relationship is negatively altered by the correctional setting.

EPIDEMIOLOGY AND SCOPE OF THE PROBLEM

The prison population in the United States is growing at an alarming rate. A recent survey conducted by the Bureau of Justice Statistics reported that as of June 30, 1994, there were 1,012,851 men and women incarcerated in state and Federal prisons.[7] This surge in the prison population has greatly surpassed the rate of growth of the general population. In June

1994, there were a record 373 people in prison for every 100,000 residents in the United States, compared to 1980, when there were 139 people incarcerated for every 100,000 residents. This rise reflects a trend of escalating violence in society, an increase in drug offenses and violent crimes, and mandatory sentencing for drug offenders. These statistics do not include those people incarcerated in local jails, like Rikers Island in New York, which had a population census of approximately 16,000 people in October, 1994.[8]

The Bellevue Hospital ED evaluates approximately 4,380 prisoners per year from local jails, including Rikers Island (personal correspondence, Deputy Warden of Bellevue Hospital Prison Ward). Many of the issues discussed in this chapter derive from personal experiences with treating incarcerated patients. Although certain problems may be particular to the New York City corrections system, they are reflective of broader, pervasive themes that are applicable to all incarcerated persons and the prison health system as a whole. For the purpose of this discussion, jails are defined as city- or county-operated facilities to detain persons awaiting trial or to hold convicted persons serving sentences of less than 1 year. Prisons house convicted felons serving sentences greater than 1 year in duration.[9] Unless specifically stated, *prisons* will refer to both prisons and jails.

The soaring number of people in prisons presents challenges to the health care system. Largely as a result of mandatory drug sentencing, the proportion of drug offenders in the Federal Bureau of Prisons is expected to increase from 47% in 1991 to 71% in 1995.[10] In 1989, 1 in 3 female and 1 in 5 male prisoners in local jails were held on drug charges, three-fourths of whom were African American or Hispanic.[11]

HEALTH ISSUES IN THE PRISON MICROCOSM

The poor and undereducated are generally over represented among the inmate population. Inmates from more underprivileged socioeconomic backgrounds commonly have a long history of inadequate health care, a consequence of growing up in neighborhoods in which clinics are often overcrowded, inefficient, and insufficiently funded and

there are other financial, social, and cultural barriers to health care. In addition, the drug lifestyle responsible for many incarcerations involves risks: from the drugs themselves and from diseases associated with shared needles—for example, hepatitis and HIV; from chronic ailments including malnourishment, joblessness and homelessness; and from the unique moral law and high-stakes economics of an environment in which violence is common.

The prison environment itself jeopardizes the health of inmates. Overcrowding in jails and prisons is a worsening problem, mostly as a result of mandatory sentencing for drug offenders. By the end of 1990, prisons in the United States are expected to be 18 to 29% above capacity, and the federal prison system is estimated to be 51% over capacity.[12] Prison overcrowding not only contributes to a higher risk of communicable diseases, like tuberculosis, hepatitis, and HIV, it also results in the confinement together of a large number of people with an already high incidence of drug abuse, antisocial behavior, and mental illness. In addition, the boredom and tension that characterize the prison environment contribute to further violence.

Health services vary from 2.8 to 18.9% of the state correctional department budgets.[13] With more people being incarcerated, these allocations must increase. Health care budgets, however, are not increasing proportionately to the growing demands of a population predisposed to health problems.[14]

The incidence of AIDS was far greater in state and federal correctional facilities (202 per 100,000 inmates) in 1989 than in the general population of the United States at that time (14.6 per 100,000 people).[15] In addition, data from the National Commission on AIDS revealed that 28% of all adult and adolescent AIDS' cases reported from 1981 through 1989 involved intravenous drug abuse. The Commission stated that under the present policy of mandatory drug sentencing, 70% of all prisoners will be drug abusers, and the HIV disease problem will intensify in the prisons.

Tuberculosis has returned to the forefront as a public health priority, especially in prisons where there is a high incidence of drug use and HIV in an overcrowded environment. The incidence of a positive tuberculin skin test in persons with HIV is 500 times that of the general population, and among those persons who have a positive tuberculin test and who have HIV, 8% develop active tuberculosis each year.[16] In New York prisons, the cases of tuberculosis among inmates increased from 15.4 to 105.5/100,000 persons from 1976 through 1986, with 56% of these cases occurring in inmates infected with HIV.[17] Of great concern is the growing incidence of multidrug-resistant tuberculosis in the community and especially in prison systems. Since 1990, multidrug-resistant tuberculosis in the New York prison system has resulted in 14 deaths, including 13 inmates and 1 correction officer. As a result of these outbreaks, New York has established mandatory tuberculosis screening for all inmates and staff.[18]

The medical problems of prisoners represent only one of the challenges to the health care system; another formidable challenge is the increased prevalence of mental illness in this select population. A study in 1991 reported that 5.5% of all federal inmates have an Axis I disorder, and this excluded those patients whose problem involved alcohol and drugs.[19] In addition, a significant number of inmates remain untreated because of inadequate resources. An estimated 10,000 inmates, or approximately 15% of New York State's 66,283 inmates, have mental disorders. The percentage of mental health professionals in prisons has increased 15% since 1987, yet the inmate population has increased by almost two-thirds in that time.[20]

In 1990, the Bureau of Justice Statistics reported that 30% of inmate deaths in larger jails were a result of suicide. In a 1986 study, the suicide rate in detention facilities was approximately nine times greater than in the general population.[21] This same study showed that 51% of suicides occur within the first 24 hours of incarceration and 29% within the first 3 hours.

IMPACT OF PRISON HEALTH ISSUES ON THE COMMUNITY

Because of the short duration of jail sentences, there are nearly 10 million inmates released back to the community each year. The health problems of released prisoners must be viewed from a public health perspective, especially when there is a high prevalence of medical and mental illness. The American College of Physicians issued a policy statement in 1993 identifying the public health opportunity associated with incarceration. "Because of the high yearly turnover (approximately 800% and 50% in jails and

prisons, respectively), the criminal justice system can play an important role both during incarceration and in the immediate post-release period. . . . Taking advantage of the period of confinement would serve both the individual and society by controlling communicable diseases in large urban communities."[22]

Although the law dictates that prisoners have a "right" to health care, there is controversy as to where those rights should be exercised. Ideally, most health services should be handled at the correctional institution. The major advantages to an on-site medical service are the establishment of a medical record that ensures continuity of care, especially for patients with chronic diseases like hypertension, diabetes, and HIV, the recruitment of practitioners with interest and expertise in correctional health, the availability of medications, and the more timely response to emergencies and assessment of complaints. Establishing an on-site facility with a formal sick-call, with the necessary diagnostic equipment, staff personnel, and access to consultants could be very difficult, however, especially for smaller facilities.

Treatment of prisoners in the community ED presents many potential problems. Security is a major issue. Precautions to prevent the possibility of escape include adequate supervision by guards and the establishment of specific procedural protocols for handcuffing prisoners. Handcuffs must often be removed and reapplied to facilitate a physical exam, phlebotomy, or the performance of an ancillary test such as ultrasound or CAT Scan. The safety of the staff or other patients in the ED may thus be compromised. There is also reticence in the community about waiting and being treated alongside prisoners. The establishment of hospital holding areas or the priority triage of prisoners are possible solutions. Emergency departments are confronted with the difficult task of balancing the demands of a diverse community in such a way that they provide optimal medical care without losing sensitivity to the social and psychological needs of each individual.

PRISONERS AND VIOLENCE IN THE COMMUNITY HEALTH CARE SETTING

Unfortunately, behavior patterns that may be essential for survival in prisons but maladaptive in the health care setting are often acted out in the ED. Recently, in New York, there have been instances in which guns have been fired by prisoners in the emergency department or outpatient clinic areas; the episodes all involved weapons stolen from guarding law enforcement officers. In May 1994, a nurse's aide in the Bellevue Emergency Department rushed to help a prisoner who appeared to be having a seizure. The prisoner wrested a weapon from a guarding police officer and discharged it, and the bullet struck the nurse's aide in the wrist. Several weeks later in the clinic area of Kings County Hospital in Brooklyn, a prisoner seized a gun from a corrections officer, shot a second officer in the chest and abdomen, and tried to escape with shackled ankles through a populated waiting area, brandishing his gun, before he himself was fatally shot in the chest. A few years ago, a prisoner in the Bellevue Emergency Department grabbed a policewoman's gun when she leaned over the stretcher to adjust the handcuff and shot himself in the head.

On many nights in the Bellevue Emergency Department, there are so many prisoners at one time that there are more officers from the Department of Corrections than there are health care staff. In the typical frenetic atmosphere of an inner-city ED, staff must weave in between a forest of officers, loaded weapons at their sides, in the rush to provide efficient care to all. Inherent in such perpetual movement is the dangerous potential for distraction. For some prisoners who may often "have nothing to lose," a loaded weapon in the holster of an officer is more than a mere flirtation; it is an overt enticement for potentially tragic consequences.

There are solutions to this problem, but budget restraints, punitive attitudes toward prisoners, and bureaucratic ennui make a weapon-free emergency department a very complex goal. Officers are required to unload their weapons when escorting patients in the psychiatric emergency departments of New York City; this policy might also work well in the medical ED, especially with the significant percentage of mental illness in the prison population.

An environment must be created to make officers more accepting of the need to unload their weapons. Potential solutions include (1) installing metal detectors, (2) using high-tech guns with a computer chip that only allows the owner to fire the weapon (3) reducing access to the ED to control flow of patients and visitors, and (4) devising alternative venues to care for those prisoners with less severe problems so as to minimize overcrowding.

CONCLUSION

The complex interweaving of medical and social factors in the diagnosis, treatment, and follow-up of incarcerated patients presents a significant challenge to ED practitioners. What the physician may perceive as a simple complaint may be only the surface representation of multifaceted systemic and patient problems. And, sometimes even the simplest of problems, as viewed through the lens of medical logic, is not amenable to treatment in the jail context. Prisoners cannot be held accountable for the diagnostic conundrum confronting the physician, who may become easily frustrated and dismiss confusing complaints as attempts at secondary gain. It is not easy to approach the patient with openness of mind, and knowledge and experience do not necessarily make treating prisoners any easier. Nor does a legal obligation necessarily translate into a willingness of personnel in community emergency departments to provide this care. Negative personal biases may affect a practitioner's ability to conform to accepted moral principles. Some prisoners may be very difficult: rude, demanding, even violent. In an already stressful environment, such behavior may place incredible burdens on the patience of ED staff, whose tolerance may be thinned by their own personal moral conflicts and opinions concerning their roles in caring for the demanding needs of the community.

The penal system is often so labyrinthine that evaluating and treating the prisoner in the emergency department is the easiest part. Of more pressing concern is what happens before and after: Are prisoners who complain of pain or illness receiving medical attention? And, after they leave the emergency department, will the recommendations and treatment strategies be followed? Direct contact on a regular basis between ED staff and jail infirmary personnel may facilitate follow-up and improve outcomes.

Convicted prisoners have been punished with loss of liberty, not with denial of medical care. Prisoners have a constitutional right to health care; their health care needs must be addressed since they do not have the freedom to seek care elsewhere.

As mentioned previously, prisoners frequently come from socioeconomically deprived backgrounds, and exhibit a high prevalence of drug abuse, communicable disease, and mental illness. A great number will eventually be returned to those same communities, where their health needs may not be adequately met. When prisoners present to the ED, emergency physicians have a window of opportunity to provide infectious disease detection and treatment and to recommend alcohol and other drug counseling and mental health services. The large prison population is a part of the social community.

As members of that broader community, physicians can advocate for reforms. In particular, attempts at health care reform, now primarily occuring at the state level, must not ignore the more than 1 million prisoners. In the broad perspective, society as a whole will benefit from adequate health care for prisoners and will only suffer if the issues and problems are not adequately addressed.

NOTES

1. Keller AS, Link RN, Bickell NA. Diabetic ketoacidosis in prisoners without access to insulin. *JAMA* 1993; 269:619–21.
2. Thorburn KM. Croakers's dilemma: should prison physicians serve prisons or prisoners. *West J Med* 1981; 134:457–61.
3. Anno BJ. *Prison health care: Guidelines for the management of an adequate delivery system.* National Institute of Corrections, U.S. Department of Justice, March 1991.
4. *Estelle* v. *Gamble*, 429 US 97 (1976).
5. Winner EJ. An introduction to the constitutional law of prison medical care. *J Prison Health* 1981; 1:67–84.
6. Dubler NN. Editorial: Patient rights in an emerging AIDS crisis. *J Prison Jail Health* 1988; 7:3–7.
7. Holmes SE. Ranks of inmates reach one million in a 2-decade rise. *The New York Times*, October 28, 1994, p. A1.
8. Horowitz C. Is Rikers about to explode? *The New York Times*, October 10, 1994, pp. 29–37.
9. American College of Physicians. The crisis in correctional health care: the impact of the national drug control strategy on correctional health services. *Ann Intern Med* 1992; 117:71–7.
10. National Commission on Acquired Immune Deficiency Syndrome. *Report: HIV disease in Correctional Facilities.* Washington, DC: The Commission, March 1991.
11. Bureau of Justice Statistics. *Prisoners in 1990.* Washington, DC: U.S. Department of Justice, 1991.
12. Bureau of Justice Statistics. *Drugs and Jail Inmates, 1989.* Washington, DC: U.S. Department of Justice, 1991.
13. Anno BJ. The cost of correctional health care: results of a national survey. *J Prison Jail Health* 1991; 2:105–34.
14. American College of Physicians. The crisis in correctional health care: The impact of the national drug control strategy on correctional health services. *Ann Intern Med* 1992; 117:71–7.
15. Acquired immunodeficiency syndrome in correctional facilities: A report of the National Institute of Justice and the American Correctional Association. *MMWR* 1986; 35:195–9.
16. Barnes PF, Bloch AB, Davidson PT, Snider DE Jr. Tuberculosis in patients with human immunodeficiency virus infection. *N Engl J Med* 1991; 324:1644–50.
17. Braun MM, Truman BI, Maguire B, DiFernando GT Jr, Wormser G, Broaddus R, et al. Increasing incidence of tuberculosis in a prison inmate population. Association with HIV infection. *JAMA* 1989; 261:393–97.
18. Mandatory Testing for TB in Prisons Begins with Guards. *The New York Times*, November 19, 1991, sect. B (col. 3).
19. General Accounting Office. *Mentally Ill Inmates: BOP Plans to Improve Screening and Care in Federal Prisons and Jails.* Washington, DC: General Accounting Office, 1991, GAO/GGD-92-13.
20. Foderara LW. For Mentally Ill Inmates, Punishment is Treatment. *The New York Times*, October 6, 1994, p. A1.
21. Hayes LM, Rowan JR. *National Study of Jail Suicides: Seven Years Later.* Alexandria, VA: National Center on Institutions and Alternatives, 1988.
22. Glaser JB, Greifinger, RB. Correctional health care: A public health opportunity. *Ann Intern Med* 1993; 118: 139–45.

21

Food- and Water-Borne Illnesses

JEFFREY BRUBACHER
LEWIS R. GOLDFRANK

CONTENTS

- Range of the problem
- Illustrative cases
- Magnitude of the problem
- Water purification
- Quality control of drinking water
- Food processing and standards
- Emergency department role

CHAPTER SUMMARY:

Biological and chemical contamination of food and water pollution can cause outbreaks of illness ranging from individual symptoms to epidemic proportions. Contamination of food and water may involve an improperly stored meal and affect a single family, or it may involve a community water supply or widely distributed food product and threaten hundreds or even thousands of people. Illness from contaminated food or water ranges from self-limited symptoms caused by simple bacterial toxins all the way to life-threatening infections with invasive organisms. Food may be contaminated with organic toxins, including *botulinum toxin, aflatoxin,* and *ciguatoxin. Scombrotoxin* (histamine), the causative agent of scombroid, may be formed in the meat of improperly refrigerated fish. Food may contain traces of pesti-

cides or growth hormone used to increase yield, and chemical agents used as food additives (e.g., nitrates, monosodium glutamate, tartrazine, and sulfites) may cause disease. Poisonous plants and mushrooms may also be misidentified and eaten by amateur botanists.

Pollution exposes us to a huge variety of contaminants, many of which are difficult to measure and have unknown effects on our health. Heavy metals, chloroform, and polychlorinated biphenyls are common industrial pollutants that can affect our water and food. Because of specialized treatment requirements, the water used in our hospitals may be contaminated even when the community water supply is safe.

This chapter provides an overview of the epidemiology of food- and water-borne illnesses and the regulation processes in place to limit them. The emergency department response to this problem is discussed. For more detail about the clinical features and medical management of the vast range of illnesses that may be spread by contaminated food or water, the reader is referred to standard texts.[1,2]

Case #1

Two teenaged sisters presented to a pediatric emergency department in Montréal, Quebec, with GI symptoms, weakness, and cranial nerve palsies. They were visiting Canada from Hong Kong with their parents and had developed symptoms while travelling to Quebec from Vancouver, British Columbia. A presumptive diagnosis of botulism was made based on these classic symptoms, and they were admitted to the pediatric ICU where they later developed respiratory insufficiency requiring in-

tubation. Type B botulinum toxin was isolated from the serum of one of the girls.

Q: Are other persons are at risk? What steps should be taken to assess them?

The family had been eating in restaurants during their visit. The patient's parents had eaten the same meals as the two sisters. The parents were assessed at an adult emergency department and the mother was found to have symptoms of botulism. The Vancouver Health Department was notified and active surveillance in Vancouver soon revealed an additional 22 persons with symptoms consistent with botulism.

Q: How can the source of this outbreak be identified?

Interviews by the Department of Health with each of the 22 patients revealed that they had all eaten food at the same family-style restaurant in downtown Vancouver. Following this, persons who had eaten at that restaurant during the same time period without developing illness were sought to act as controls. Interviews with cases and controls showed an association between developing botulism and eating either the beef dip sandwich or a steak sandwich. In fact, all 22 cases had eaten one of these two sandwiches. However, 4 of the controls had also eaten one of these sandwiches. Further questioning revealed that all of the cases but none of the controls had eaten garlic-buttered bread with their sandwich.

Restaurant employees stated that unopened bottles of the chopped garlic used to make the garlic-buttered bread were stored unrefrigerated before being opened for use, despite the manufacturer's instructions to keep the bottles refrigerated even before opening. They also reported that one particular bottle had recently been discarded because of a bad odor. The contents of this bottle appeared to have been used in preparation of the meals eaten by the symptomatic cases.

The remaining bottles of chopped garlic in the restaurant were all tested and found not to contain any botulinum toxin nor *C. botulinum*. However, when other bottles of the same production lot were inoculated with *C. botulinum*, botulinum toxin was produced within 2 weeks when stored at 25°C. The

mean pH of the product was relatively alkaline (5.4) and contained no chemical or acid additives.

Q: Are other persons eating the same chopped garlic product also at risk?

Because the implicated bottled garlic was not stored according to the manufacturer's instructions, it was felt that the product itself did not pose a risk if stored properly. No further cases were reported due to exposure to this product after the suspect bottle was discarded. Nevertheless, it is possible that failure to follow the proper storage instructions could result in a similar disease outbreak in the future.

After the publicity generated by this outbreak, additional cases were recognized among people who had eaten at the restaurant before the implicated bottle was discarded. In all, there were 36 cases of botulism in three countries: Canada, the Netherlands, and the U.S. Some patients had been ill for over a month before the first cases were recognized. These patients had been given various diagnoses including Myaesthenia Gravis, psychiatric illness, viral syndrome, and Guillain-Barré syndrome.[3–5]

Case #2

During a single day, over 40 children attending an elementary school visited the school nurse complaining of headache, vomiting, and blue lips and hands. All of these visits occurred during or shortly after lunch period. Forty-nine children were seen by physicians, and, of these, a total of 29 were proven to have an elevated methemoglobin level (> 2%). Methemoglobin levels were either normal or unavailable in the remaining 20. Fourteen children had methemoglobin levels above 20% and were hospitalized. All children recovered without sequelae.

Q: How should this outbreak be investigated?

The Department of Health was notified and began investigations. Additional cases were sought by contacting local hospitals. The 29 children with documented methemoglobinemia served as cases and an additional 52 children selected sequentially from the school roster who had not become ill served as controls. All but one of the cases were in the first three grades in school, whereas the controls were distributed evenly among grades one through five. It was found that all 29 cases but only 33% of controls had eaten soup from the school cafeteria prepared that day. No other food item on the menu that day was implicated.

The following day, the school was visited by the local health department. They learned that two large pots of soup had been prepared sequentially by diluting canned soup with water from both the hot- and cold-water taps in the kitchen sink. The children in grades one through three were seated and served from one of the two pots while the older children stood in line and were served from the second pot of soup.

Q: No cases of methemoglobinemia caused by canned soup from this manufacturer had been reported. How might the soup have become contaminated? Should other soup cans from the same production lot be recalled?

Water for the kitchen's hot-water tap could be heated by passing through coils in the school's boiler. It was discovered that the boiler had been turned on for the first time that season on the morning in question. Inside the boiler tank, the coils were immersed in water treated with a special anticorrosive boiler treatment solution. The treated water in the boiler tank did not come in contact with water inside the coils. However, the tap for introducing the boiler treatment solution was in close proximity to the tap for accessing the potable water in the heating coils. Neither was labeled.

It was conjectured that, instead of being placed into the boiler tank, the treatment solution may have been inadvertently added to the boiler's hot-water coil tap, which was in contact with the school's potable water lines. Four sets of samples were taken for analysis: (1) treated water in the boiler tank; (2) the boiler treatment solution; (3) water from the kitchen's hot and cold taps; and (4) the leftover soup. These samples were analysed in the Health Department laboratories.

Q: What substances should be looked for by the laboratory?

The boiler treatment solution contained nitrite and sodium metaborate as its major components. The leftover soup contained high concentrations of nitrite (459 ppm) and of sodium metaborate. Undiluted soup from the same lot had only 2 ppm of nitrite. Water from the hot water tap had detectable levels of nitrite, whereas cold water samples did not, demonstrating that the treatment solution was actually added to the hot water system. Water from the boiler tank had only 11 ppm of nitrite, whereas water from a properly conditioned boiler tank would be expected to have 300 to 500 ppm. This discrepancy showed that if, in fact, the solution had been added, it was *not* added in the approved place—the boiler tank.

Based on this evidence, it appears that boiler treatment solution had been mistakenly added to the hot-water coil tap within the boiler instead of into the boiler tank. This boiler treatment solution remained in the hot-water coils until the boiler was restarted and hot water was used for soup preparation. The first samples of water from the hot-water tap on that day would have had the highest degree of contamination with the nitrite rich boiler treatment solution, explaining why the first pot of soup resulted in methemoglobin production in those who were served from it.[6,7]

Questions for Further Consideration

- Could these cases have been adequately managed without involving the health department?
- As a physician managing one of the patients in these cases, would you have recognized the potential magnitude of each outbreak?
- Both of these cases involved food prepared from a widely distributed commercial product (bottled garlic and canned soup). Should the products have been recalled pending definite confirmation that they were safe?
- If recall was appropriate, at what point in time should such recall have occurred?

Table 21-1 Water-Borne Disease Outbreaks in the U.S., 1985–1992

Responsible Agent	Cases No.	Cases (%)
Parasitic		
Giardia lamblia	2,730	(4.0%)
Cryptosporidium	16,551	(24.1%)
Total parasitic	19,281	(28.1%)
AGI (see footnote)	19,142	(27.8%)
Bacterial	3,732	(5.4%)
Chemical		
Nitrates	4	(<0.1%)
Chlorine	31	(<0.1%)
Flourine	314	(0.5%)
Other	49	(0.1%)
Total Chemical	398	(0.1%)
Viral	6,409	(9.3%)
Other	93	(0.1%)
Total	68,734	(100%)

Outbreaks of disease caused by water intended for drinking that were reported to the CDC from 1985 to 1992.[27–29;11] There may be a significant number of unreported outbreaks, so the actual number of water-borne disease outbreaks is probably much greater than reflected here. This does not include disease caused by recreational water use such as swimming. Note that for many outbreaks, the etiology was not determined; these are represented as "AGI" . . . acute gastrointestinal illness of unknown etiology.

MAGNITUDE OF THE PROBLEM

Waterborne Illnesses

For the 7-year period from 1986 through 1992, over 100 disease outbreaks caused by water intended for drinking (affecting over 47,000 people) were reported to the CDC. Protozoal parasites were responsible for the majority of outbreaks. The largest U.S. outbreak of water-borne disease, caused by *Cryptosporidium* contamination of the Milwaukee water supply,[8] caused a diarrheal illness in over 400,000 persons. Common bacterial pathogens include *Shigella* species, *Campylobacter*, and *E. coli* 0157:H7. Viruses are occasionally implicated. Many disease outbreaks have no proven pathogen. Chemical contamination of drinking water is relatively rare. Nitrate contamination of private wells is probably the most common clinically apparent cause of chemical water contamination. Another type of chemical contamination is exemplified by the occurence in Hooper Bay, Alaska, in 1992 of overflouridation of the town's drinking water. Nausea, vomitting, diarrhea, and tingling of the face and extremities were observed in an estimated 296 patients, and there was one death.[9] The *MMWR* reports from 1986 through to 1992 are summarized in Table 21-1.

Foodborne Illnesses

During the 5-year period from 1983 through 1987, the CDC received reports of a total of 2,397 food-borne disease outbreaks affecting 54,540 people and causing 137 deaths. The majority of cases and most of the deaths were caused by bacterial pathogens. *Salmonella* species caused more cases of food-borne illness and more deaths than any other bacterial pathogen. *Shigella* species, *Staphylococcus aureus*, and *Clostridium perfringens* each caused a significant number of cases. Viruses (predominately Hepatitis A and Norwalk virus) accounted for 5% of cases and one death. Chemical contamination resulted in 2% of cases and three deaths. Common chemical agents causing foodborne disease included ciguatoxin, scombrotoxin, heavy metals, and various toxins found in poisonous mushrooms. Parasitic pathogens were identified in less than 1% of cases. The CDC's five year survey is summarized in Table 21-2.[10] The CDC believes that the majority of food-borne disease outbreaks go unreported and that sporadic food-borne disease (which is not included in their report) is far more common than food-borne disease outbreaks.

Famous Outbreaks of Food-Borne Illness

The relative rarity of chemical contamination of food products in recent CDC reports belies the potential

Table 21-2 Food-Borne Illness, by Etiology, in the U.S., 1983–1987

Responsible Agent	Cases		Deaths	
	No.	(%)	No.	(%)
Bacteria				
Salmonella sp.	31,262	(57.3%)	39	(28.5%)
Shigella sp.	9,971	(18.3%)	2	(1.5%)
S. aureus	3,181	(5.8%)	0	
C. perfringens	2,425	(4.4%)	2	(1.5%)
C. botulinum	140	(0.3%)	10	(7.3%)
Total bacterium	50,304	(92.2%)	132	(96.4%)
Chemical				
Ciguatoxin	332	(0.6%)	0	
Scombrotoxin	353	(0.6%)	0	
Total chemical	1,244	(2.3%)	3	(2.2%)
Parasitic				
T. spiralis	188	(0.3%)	1	(0.7%)
G. lamblia	15	(<0.1%)	0	
Total Parasitic	203	(0.4%)	1	(0.7%)
Viral	2,789	(5.1%)	1	(0.7%)
Total	54,540	(100%)	137	(100%)

Food-borne illnesses reported to the CDC for which an etiology was discovered; combined totals from 1983 to 1987 inclusive.[10] Note that these data reflect only those outbreaks that were both reported and for which an etiology was found, and, as such, the data underestimate the actual number of disease outbreaks.

for huge epidemics of food-borne illness caused by accidental or intentional chemical contamination. Mass production and global distribution of food products make it possible for contaminated food to affect thousands of persons before the source is identified and corrected.

In the 1930s, an estimated 50,000 persons living in the U.S. developed muscle pain and weakness after consuming a popular beverage known as Jamaica ginger extract, or "Jake." It was discovered that one of the manufacturers had changed the formula, replacing castor oil with the cheaper triorthocresyl phosphate, and this proved to be the causative agent.[11,12] Since the 1930s, triorthocresyl phosphate has caused sporadic epidemics, including a 1959 outbreak in Morocco that was caused by contaminated

olive oil and that involved an estimated 10,000 people.[13]

In 1955, 12,131 infants in Japan developed an illness consisting of anorexia, anemia, rash, diarrhea, vomiting, bloating, and fever. There were 130 fatalities. The cause of the illness was traced to accidental arsenic contamination of powdered milk intended for bottle feeding.[14] In 1971, methylmercury-treated grain that was intended for planting was instead baked into bread and consumed in Iraq. Over 6,500 people were admitted to hospitals with paresthesias, headaches, ataxia, dysarthria, and blindness. There were 459 deaths.[15]

Fish caught in waters contaminated with mercury are other potential sources of methylmercury poisoning. A famous outbreak of methylmercury poisoning from contaminated fish affected thousands of people living near Minamata bay in Japan in the 1940s.

The toxic oil syndrome that affected almost 20,000 people in Spain in 1981 consisted of fever, cough, and pulmonary infiltrates, followed by gastrointestinal symptoms and eosinophilia. Many people recovered after several weeks, but approximately one-fourth went on to develop severe neuromuscular symptoms, including myalgias, weakness, muscle atrophy, paresthesias, and dysesthesias. The illness was linked to rapeseed oil contaminated with an aniline derivative. Inexpensive rapeseed oil intended for industrial use had been "de-denatured" with 2% aniline and sold as "olive oil" for human consumption.[16]

An eosinophilia-myalgia syndrome consisting of debilating myalgias and eosinophilia as well as arthralgia, rash, peripheral edema, and cough affected over 1,500 people in the U.S. in 1989. This syndrome was caused by a dimer of L-tryptophan which contaminated certain tryptophan preparations.[17-19]

Municipal Water Supply

The major sources of potable water for municipal usage are surface water and groundwater. Rainwater is generally insufficient for community requirements. The cost of desalination makes saltwater sources prohibitively expensive, and reuse of waste water, especially for nonpotable uses, becomes increasingly attractive.

Surface waters found in lakes and rivers have been the traditional water sources for large cities. Unfortunately, large watersheds are frequently contaminated with microorganisms and chemical waste from upstream industrial and agricultural activity. Purification methods are ineffective in removing synthetic chemicals from industrial pollution. Smaller, upland watersheds are less polluted and provide higher-quality water. Groundwater is formed as rainwater and runoff percolate through the ground. Groundwater is relatively free of microbial contamination but more heavily mineralized than surface water. Pollution of groundwater is becoming a problem, and once a groundwater aquifer is contaminated, it will remain polluted for many years.

Water purification serves to remove or destroy microbial contamination, improve taste and clarity, and remove chemical contamination. Removal of suspended particles and colloidal material is achieved by coagulation, flocculation, and sedimentation. After addition of coagulants such as aluminum sulfate or ferric sulfate, the water is gently stirred in flocculation tanks, where particles clump together into flocs, which settle out in the sedimentation tanks. The next step is filtration of the water to remove small flocs and microorganisms. Typically, a bed of sand or other fine particles about 1 meter deep is used for this purpose. Following filtration, most water sources require disinfection to remove remaining bacterial and parasitic contamination. Chlorination is the most widely used disinfection method. Aeration of the water adds oxygen and removes dissolved carbon dioxide and hydrogen sulfide, which results in improved taste and color.

Quality Control of Drinking Water

Under the Safe Water Drinking Act of 1986, the United States Environmental Protection Agency (USEPA) is authorized to set standards for drinking water contaminants. There are two categories of drinking water regulations; the National Primary Drinking Water Regulations, which regulate levels of toxic contaminants, and the National Secondary Maximum Contaminant Levels, which are concerned with aesthetic qualities such as color, odor, and taste. The National Primary Drinking Water Regulations consist of two tiers of regulations: Maximum Contaminant Levels (MCLs), which are enforceable standards, and Maximum Contaminant Level Goals (MCLGs), which are nonenforceable goals. MCLs are compromises between health risk and technical and economic reality, whereas MCLGs represent a theoretical near-zero risk level. MCLs have been established for metals, pesticides, radioactive contaminants, and organic compounds.[20]

Maintaining our drinking water free of pathogenic microbes is exceedingly important for preventing illness. The total coliform count is used as a marker of water quality; absence of coliforms correlates well with absence of pathogenic bacteria, and presence of coliforms indicates inadequate water decontamination. Fewer than 5% of the water samples may be positive for coliforms. Any positive sample must be tested for fecal coliforms and *E. coli* and be repeated within 24 hours. Fecal coliforms or *E. coli* must be reported to the state agency.

Results from coliform counts require approximately 24 hours. This means that a breach of water purity could go undetected for an unacceptably long period of time. Surrogate "real time" measures of bacteriological safety have been developed. These include water turbidity and chlorine concentrations.[2,21]

Purified water is distributed by a series of pumps and water mains. This system must be adequate to provide service during peak demand and must have enough interconnections to maintain service with minimal interuption should repair of one section be required. Contamination with surface water or cross-connections with nonpotable water lines may result in contamination.

Even when the municipal water supply is adequately treated, chemical or microbial contamination can occur in the hospital water system. Water used in hospitals is often demonstrated to be contaminated only when hardware becomes colonized with microorganisms. This was the cause of an outbreak of *Pseudomonas aeruginosa* sepsis in a burn unit[22] and of several outbreaks of *Legionella pneumophilia*, or Legionnaires' disease.[23] Ethylene glycol contamination of the water used in hemodialysis units has occurred as a result of cross-connection with the air conditioning system.[24] In another hemodialysis unit, malfunctioning of a deionization device caused fluoride contamination of dialysis fluid, resulting in three deaths.[25] Minimizing the impact of such outbreaks requires early recognition and correction of the problem. Interim solutions range from using an alternate water source or closing certain units to evacuating the hospital. Permanent solutions require cooperation between clinicians and laboratory and maintenance personnel to facilitate early detection and correction of the problem. Hospital disaster plans should incorporate strategies for such eventualities.

Food Processing and Standards

Unsafe food products can result from microbial contamination, unsafe food additives, or contamination with environmental pollutants. Organic toxins such as botulinum toxin, aflatoxins, and scombrotoxin may result from improper food storage or preparation. Pesticides, antibiotics, and growth hormones may persist. The greatest impact on public health is from microbial contamination caused by unsanitary or improper food handling or storage.

Commercial food products are widely distributed, giving them the potential for causing international disease outbreaks. Raw materials may come from multiple suppliers and be mixed together in bulk before distribution and processing. Contamination of food from one source may result in an entire lot being contaminated. This was suspected to play a role in a 1993 outbreak of bloody diarrhea caused by hamburger patties contaminated with *E. coli* 0157:H7. This outbreak affected more than 500 persons in the western United States and caused 4 deaths. Over 90 restaurants were implicated and 250,000 hamburgers were recalled.[26]

Food safety in the United States is regulated by the Food and Drug Administration (FDA) and the U.S. Department of Agriculture (USDA). The FDA regulates food additives, including coloration agents, pesticide residues, and potential harmful packaging materials. Food additives are allowed without testing if they were in use in 1958 when the *Food Additives Amendment* of the FDCA was passed. These additives are classified as *Generally Regarded as Safe*. Newer additives must undergo extensive testing before being approved. The USDA monitors all agricultural products with visual inspection of live animals, carcasses, and individual organs. This inspection detects unsanitary conditions, and the USDA will prohibit the sale for food of animals that appear diseased or carcasses or organs that appear deformed or unsanitary. Inspection for microbial contamination is not part of this process. Eggs and poultry undergo similar inspection procedures.

In addition to inspecting the raw products, food processing plants are monitored to ensure sanitary plant conditions, minimization of food handling, and achievement of proper temperatures for cooking and for refrigeration. Certain foods, such as milk, are regulated more closely than others due to differing public health risks.

The efficiency of the regulation is reflected in the fact that the majority of food-borne disease outbreaks reported to the CDC are not caused by unsafe food sources but rather from improper handling or storage by restaurant, school or institution.[10]

EMERGENCY DEPARTMENT ROLE

The emergency department goals for managing patients with suspected food- or water-borne illnesses are multifaceted. Medical care of the patient is the first priority. Specific management of the wide variety of possible diagnoses is discussed in standard medicine and toxicology texts.

Recognition that a patient's symptomatology may be caused by exposure to pathogens or chemical contaminants in drinking water or in a food product is the single most important diagnostic hurdle. With this recognition comes the responsibility to search for other persons who have already been exposed, to notify those at risk, and to eliminate the source of the problem. The department of health will play a key role. Data collection is necessary to increase the practitioner's understanding of the problem, as an aid in decision making, and as a means of gauging the effectiveness of efforts at prevention. Patient and public education has the goal of reducing the incidence of food- and water-borne illnesses.

Recognizing Food- and Water-Borne Illnesses

Illness caused by food and water contaminants may occasionally be easily diagnosed based on a classic presentation. Unfortunately, in most cases the exposure history is not appreciated by the patient or not volunteered and the symptoms are nonspecific. Asking about recent meals and other family members with similar symptoms may give the information needed to make a diagnosis. Diagnosing an outbreak of illness caused by a community-wide exposure (e.g., contaminated drinking water) requires a search for other persons with similar symptoms and a high index of suspicion. Informal consultation with other emergency department staff may reveal that they are also seeing many patients with similar complaints. This process may be formalized by maintaining a departmental database that will allow early recognition of such trends. The health department may already be investigating similar reports from other centers or may have received notification of potential problems at the water treatment plant and be on the lookout for disease outbreaks.

Mini epidemics of "stomach flu" are common and do not necessarily imply a food or water source.

The cost of investigating every such outbreak is not warranted. In certain circumstances, however, investigations such as stool cultures may be justified. Food handlers, health care workers, day care workers, and residents of institutions all constitute groups in which stool cultures for definitive diagnosis of diarrheal illnesses is required for public health concerns. On occasion the microbiology laboratory should be asked to look for organisms requiring special isolation techniques. Examples include *Cryptosporidium* in cases of failure of the water filter system or *E. coli* 0157:H7 in cases of invasive diarrhea suspected to be spread by contaminated ground beef.

Exposure Interview

Once the presence of a food-borne disease outbreak is suspected, the exposure interview serves to determine which of multiple food items is responsible. To do this properly all potentially exposed persons both with and without symptoms are interviewed to determine which food items they ate and which they did not eat. The attributable risk for a given food item is the difference between the attack rate in those who ate that item and the attack rate in those who did not eat that item. The food with the highest attributable risk is probably the culprit. Often this can be confirmed by laboratory testing. For this process to be accurate, all potentially exposed persons both with and without illness must be interviewed.

The fact that most people with illness ate a specific food item may mean that the item in question was the culprit or may simply reflect the fact that the item was popular. If the exposure interview is limited to persons with disease symptoms this distinction will not be made. The necessity of interviewing unaffected persons as well as time and manpower considerations limit the ability to conduct useful emergency department exposure interviews. Most exposure interviews should thus be conducted by the department of health. Nevertheless, an emergency department exposure interview may establish sufficient evidence to implicate a specific food item and allow a rapid response to limit the size of an evolving outbreak. When the number of exposed persons is small as may occur when a single family is involved, a complete exposure interview may be feasible in the emergency department.

Warning Others

The patient in the emergency department with a food- or water-related illness may represent the index case of an epidemic. Early recognition and correction of the problem combined with public warnings may avert or minimize the outbreak.[27] Public education may also prevent the next outbreak. Emergency department staff must work in cooperation with local health departments to achieve these goals. The decision to urgently notify the health department is made based on the population deemed to be at risk and on the severity of illness.

Family members and others sharing the same food should be warned that they could also be at risk for developing the same symptoms. It is difficult to know with certainty which food item was responsible, but educated guesses can be made based on the exposure history and symptomatology. Patient education sheets which describe the common food-borne disease stereotypes, list foodstuffs most commonly found to be at fault, and describe methods of proper food handling will facilitate the task of patient education.

Urgent notification of the health department is required for all suspected cases of botulism and other food-borne illnesses with high morbidity and mortality. Whenever a commercial food product or restaurant is the suspected source the health department must be urgently involved since many persons may be at risk. The management of the restaurant should also be informed at once so that they do not serve the suspect food to other patrons. Saving a refrigerated sample of the suspect food item will help in future diagnosis of the causative chemical or microorganism.

Suspicion of a water-borne pathogen also mandates urgent involvement of the health department since everyone in the community dependent on that water supply is at risk.[28–29] Once such an outbreak is recognized; *all patients* coming to the emergency department should be warned that the water is unsafe and given the steps required to treat tap water before consumption. This may include boiling water before use or avoiding tap water altogether until the problem is rectified. Instruction sheets and notices in waiting areas will help to convey this information.

Occasionally the source will be a private well or improperly treated surface water affecting only several persons. In this situation, all persons involved can be warned to avoid or treat the contaminated water and the health department can be involved on a nonurgent basis.

Data Collection and Reporting

Reporting suspected cases of food- or water-borne illness to the department of health is an important emergency department responsibility. This allows earlier recognition of statewide or national trends that may not be apparent from the perspective of a single emergency department. Maintaining an accurate database of food- or water-borne illnesses allows insight into the magnitude of the problem and permits rational decisions concerning allocation of funds for education, prevention and treatment on a departmental, city, state, or national level. Assessing regulations governing food and water safety also requires an accurate database.

At the community level, emergency department data collection may allow earlier recognition of local disease outbreaks. The expense of such data bases is justified if this can be translated into prevention. A local disaster may be averted by early interventions to limit its size or by giving health care facilities time for preparation. Emergency department personnel can increase community awareness of a problem by notifying local health departments, by use of local news media and through notices posted in hospital waiting areas.

An emergency department database could range from a list of suspected cases based on discharge diagnoses to detailed data including symptomatology, eating habits, addresses, and place of work. Specific data collection sheets could be made in response to suspected disease outbreaks. This would require frequent chart review and communication between staff members to allow early recognition of such outbreaks.

Education

Patient education about food- and water-borne diseases is an important part of the emergency department management. Patients may be especially receptive to instructions about proper food and water preparation. Information sheets concerning home canning, water treatment when camping or food and water precautions when travelling could be part of a series of public health oriented information sheets available for patients in the waiting area. Emergency physicians should be able to answer patients' questions concerning symptoms and prevention of food- and water-borne illnesses. Instruction sheets specific to a current public health problem such as contamination of the community water supply may be rapidly prepared and distributed. Notices posted in hospital waiting areas also aid in disseminating important information.

Interested emergency physicians may give public health–oriented lectures on a wide range of topics including recognition, treatment, and prevention of food- and water-borne disease. These lectures would be of special interest to those who travel, camp, or preserve foods at home as well as to other health professionals. Besides the public health benefit, such lectures would increase the profile of the emergency department in the community.

CONCLUSION

Food- and water-borne illness is relatively common and usually benign. Nevertheless, there is potential for disastrous disease outbreaks on an epidemic scale. Furthermore, the spectrum of illness caused by food- or water-borne agents is vast, and the cause is not always immediately apparent. Beyond treating the patient, the emergency department management includes directly warning others who may be at risk, educating patients about future prevention, and notification of the department of health. Early recognition is the most important factor required to limit the extent of a disease outbreak. Definite determination of the cause will often require special investigations by the health department. The health department is able to take action to limit distribution and consumption of a suspect product. The health department should be notified for all suspected cases of food- or water-borne disease. Urgent involvement of the health department is indicated when such diseases are potentially life-threatening or when they threaten many persons.

NOTES

1. Goldfrank LR, Kristein RH. Food poisoning. In LR Goldfrank et al. (eds.). *Toxicologic Emergencies,* 4th ed. East Norwalk, CT: Appleton & Lange, 1990.

2. Okun DA. Water quality management. In Last LM, Wallace RB, Barrett-Connor E, et al. (eds.). *Public health and preventive medicine,* 13th ed. East Norwalk, CT: Appleton & Lange, 1992.

3. Blatherwick FJ, Peck SH, Morgan GB. UpDate: International outbreak of restaurant associated botulism—Vancouver, British Columbia, Canada. *MMWR* 1985; 34:643.

4. St Louis ME. Water-related disease outbreaks, 1985. *MMWR* 1988; 37:13–20.

5. Personal communication with Dr. James Welch, Royal Victoria Hospital, Montréal, Quebec.

6. Askew GL, Finelli L, Genese CA, et al. Boilerbaisse: An outbreak of methemoglobinemia in New Jersey in 1992. *Pediatrics* 1992; 94:381–4.

7. Personal Communication with Dr. Lyn Finelli, New Jersey Department of Health.

8. MacKenzie WR, Hoxie NJ, Proctor ME, et al. A massive outbreak of Cryptosporidium infection transmitted through the public water supply. *N Engl J Med* 1994; 331:161–7.

9. Gessner BD, Beller M, Middaugh JP, et al. Acute fluoride poisoning from a public water system. *N Engl J Med* 1994; 330:95–9.

10. Hargrett-Bean N, Griffin PM, Goulding JS. Food-borne disease outbreaks, 5-year summary, 1983–1987. *MMWR* 1990; 39:99–139.

11. Morgan JP. The jake walk blues. *Ann Intern Med* 1976; 85:804–8.

12. Morgan JP. The Jamaica ginger paralysis. *JAMA* 1982; 248:1864–7.

13. Smith HV, Spalding JMK. Outbreak of paralysis due to ortho-cresyl phosphate poisoning. *Lancet* 1959; 2:1019–21.

14. Tsuchiya K. Various effects of arsenic in Japan depending on type of exposure. *Env Health Perspect* 1977; 19:35–42.

15. Clarkson TW, Amin-Zaki L, Al-Tikriti SK. An outbreak of methylmercury poisoning due to consumption of contaminated grain. *Fed Proc* 1976; 35:2395–9.

16. Kilbourne EM, Rigau-Perez JG, Heath CW, et al. Clinical epidemiology of the toxic-oil syndrome. *New Engl J Med* 1983; 309:1408–14.

17. Swygert LA, Maes EF, Sewell LE, et al. Eosinophilia-myalgia syndrome: Results of national surveillance. *JAMA* 1990; 264:1698–1703.

18. Varga J, Uitto J, Jimenez SA. The cause and pathogenesis of the eosinophilia-myalgia syndrome. *Ann Int Med* 1992; 116:140–7.

19. Belognia EA, Hedberg CW, Gleich GJ, et al. An investigation of the cause of the eosinophilia-myalgia syndrome associated with tryptophan use. *N Eng J Med* 1990; 323:357–65.

20. Sidhu KS. Standard setting process and regulations for environmental contaminants in drinking: State versus federal needs and viewpoints. *Reg Tox Pharm* 1991; 13:293–308.

21. Moore AC, Herwaldt BL, Craun GF, et al. Surveillance for waterborne disease outbreaks—United States 1991–1992. *MMWR* 1993; 42:1–22.

22. Kolmos HJ, Thuesen B, Nielson SV, et al. Outbreak of infection in a burns unit due to Pseudomonas aeruginosa originating from contaminated tubing used for irrigation of patients. *J Hosp Inf* 1993; 24:11–21.

23. Memish ZA, Oxley C, Contant J, et al. Plumbing system shock absorbers as a source of Legionella pneumophila. *Am J Inf Con* 1992; 20:305–9.

24. Anonymous. Ethylene glycol intoxication due to contamination of water systems. *MMWR* 1987; 36: 61;1–614.

25. Arnow PM, Bland LA, Garcia-Houchins S, et al. An outbreak of fatal fluoride intoxication in a long term hemodialysis unit. *Ann Intern Med* 1994; 1121:339–44.

26. Berkelman RL. Emerging infectious diseases in the United States. *J Inf Dis* 1993; 170:272–7.

27. St Louis ME, Peck SHS, Bowering D, et al. Botulism from chopped garlic: Delayed recognition of a major outbreak. *Ann Intern Med* 1988; 108:363–8.

28. Levine WC, Stephenson WT. Waterborne disease outbreaks 1986–1988. *MMWR* 1990; 39:87–98.

29. Herwaldt BL, Craun GF, Stokes SL, et al. Waterborne disease outbreaks, 1989–1990. *MMWR* 1991; 40:1–21.

22

Airborne Environmental Exposures

E. MARTIN CARAVATI

CONTENTS

- Problem definition
- Illustrative cases
- Applications
- Sentinel health events

CHAPTER SUMMARY

Environmentally caused disease is the result of humans' interactions with their surroundings. It is ultimately preventable either through changes in behavior or via control of the source of exposure. Patients suffering from acute or chronic exposures to hazardous chemicals, toxic gases and fumes, heavy metals, and pesticides often present to the emergency department (ED) with nonspecific symptoms. The diagnosis may be elusive or incorrect unless an accurate environmental history is obtained by the physician. Once an environmentally caused illness or disease (i.e., carbon monoxide poisoning) is suspected or diagnosed, it is necessary for the emergency physician to identify the source and any other possible victims. The ill patient in the ED may be the "sentinel event" representing many more victims at large. Organizations such as the regional poison control center, state or local health departments, Agency for Toxic Substances and Disease Registry, Con-

sumer Products Safety Commission, and Environmental Protection Agency are important resources for managing and preventing further illness or injury from these exposures. Advocacy for public safety with respect to the home, community, and work environment can have an important impact on the prevention of these increasingly prevalent health problems.

Case #1

A 34-year-old female presents to the emergency department complaining of a throbbing bitemporal headache. She went to bed feeling well and awoke with a headache and nausea. She took acetaminophen but vomited shortly before coming to the ED. Her mother has a history of migraine headaches and the patient occasionally has "migraines," but this headache is very different. She admits to generalized malaise and blurry vision. She denies fever, chills, stiff neck, diplopia, numbness, tingling, and motor weakness. She is married with three children and typically stays at home with them during the day. She notes that it was more difficult than usual to arouse her children this morning and they all refused to eat breakfast. She wonders whether the family is coming down with the flu. Her husband remains at home asleep. He stayed up late last night working on the furnace because of a recent cold spell. Upon exam, she is alert and oriented with normal vital signs. Her pulse oximetry measurement is 96 percent on room air. Her physical exam is normal including a detailed neurologic exam. Your differential diagnosis includes influenza, viral syndrome, common migraine, subarachnoid hemorrhage, and carbon monoxide poisoning. You place her on 100% oxygen by non-rebreathing mask and order a CBC and carboxyhemoglobin saturation. Twenty minutes after the administration of oxygen she states her headache is much improved and the lab calls you with a carboxyhemoglobin saturation of 28 percent. You immediately request that the mother's children in the waiting room be admitted to your department for evaluation and that an ambulance be dispatched to her home because her husband does not answer the telephone when you call.

Q: Why is the diagnosis of mild to moderate carbon monoxide intoxication often difficult to make in the emergency department?

Carbon monoxide is a colorless and odorless gas, which renders it undetectable by its victims. This leads to increased morbidity and mortality associated with exposure because it is not detected early and exposure continues unabated. It is the most common single agent responsible for poisoning deaths in the United States and results in an estimated 10,000 emergency department visits per year. In 1993, almost 13,000 exposures to carbon monoxide were reported to the American Association of Poison Control Centers' Toxic Exposure Surveillance System.[1] Ninety-seven percent of these exposures were accidental, and 46 percent were treated in a health care facility. Death rates from carbon monoxide are higher in the northern states because there are more garages and greater heater use during cold weather. Death rates are 3 times higher in the winter months compared with the summer.[2] The incidence of mild to moderate carbon monoxide poisoning is probably underestimated because of its atypical clinical presentation consisting of flulike symptoms such as lethargy, malaise, dizziness, headache, nausea, and vomiting.

Q: What are the common environmental sources of carbon monoxide exposure?

Carbon monoxide is produced by the incomplete combustion of carbon. Potential sources include automobile exhaust, combustion of coal, kerosene, wood stoves and natural gas, smoke from fires and hibachi and charcoal briquette stoves. Methylene chloride, a solvent used to remove paint or varnish is metabolized in vivo to carbon monoxide and is a potential source for intoxication to those who use it in poorly ventilated environments. In addition to the home, other sites of multiple victims of occult CO poisoning include a motel,[3] the back of pickup trucks,[4] ice-skating rinks, poorly ventilated workplaces, and heating or cooking with "sterno" in camping tents.

Q: What questions can you ask a patient with headaches and nausea which will raise your index of suspicion for occult carbon monoxide poisoning?

Key points in the history which should raise the index of suspicion for carbon monoxide poisoning include the onset of headaches while in a poorly ventilated area, especially during the winter months, and more than one patient sharing similar symptoms and time of onset (i.e., symptomatic co-inhabitants). It has been shown that 3 to 5 percent of patients presenting to an urban emergency department during the winter months with complaints of headache or dizziness have unrecognized carbon monoxide poisoning.[5] During the winter months the use of space heaters, gas stoves, furnaces, and the sealing of windows increases the potential exposure to carbon monoxide in the home. Specific questions that follow this line of inquiry should be asked of patients who present with headache or dizziness in the emergency department. People who burn charcoal briquettes indoors are at risk for CO poisoning.[6] Many persons who are poisoned by charcoal briquettes cannot read the warning label on the package or are non-English-speaking. The indoor burning of charcoal is common in Korea, for example, and many first-generation immigrants may continue this practice without awareness of the risks involved in such activity. Patients who present with unexplained headache and constitutional symptoms associated with working around combustion engines in closed spaces also warrant evaluation for carbon monoxide intoxication.[7] The exposure may occur outside the usual setting of the home or work place, as in the case of motel guests who are exposed to carbon monoxide from a faulty furnace.[3]

Q: What specific actions and patient education should the emergency physician pursue in order to prevent further morbidity from this exposure?

Once the diagnosis of carbon monoxide intoxication is established and the patient(s) treated, the emergency physician must try to identify the source of exposure and take appropriate action. Removal of the patient from the source of exposure and proper ventilation of all combustion devices is essential in preventing further morbidity and mortality from these exposures.

The emergency physician must recognize that other victims may still exist and should make an effort to identify them. A telephone call to the home, hotel, local fire department, EMS system, or police will prevent further poisoning and perhaps death.[3]

Discharge instruction should include patient education regarding proper home ventilation and checking chimneys and flues for obstruction and defects. Preventive education of motor vehicle drivers includes information about the risks of running an engine in a closed garage or when parked for long periods of time, and the danger of driving vehicles with defective exhaust systems or with holes in the vehicle body. Excessive sleepiness or drowsiness while driving should be discussed as a possible warning signal for carbon monoxide intoxication.[2] If the exposure occurs in the work place, then notification of the health department is required so that the work environment may be inspected for compliance with the Environmental Protection Agency standards for ambient CO exposures in the work place.[7]

Improved technology has increased the effectiveness of CO detection devices. CO detectors for home use are now available and the Underwriters Laboratories has recently implemented a standard for certification (UL 2034).[8] Inexpensive card-type CO detectors are available for home use but their accuracy has been recently challenged and more testing is needed before recommending their use to patients and the public.[9] More sophisticated devices, which utilize semiconductor or enzyme sensors and audible alarms when the CO detection threshold is reached, are preferred for home and industrial use. These devices are more expensive, but they are reported to meet or exceed the standards set by Underwriters Laboratory for detection of CO gas (100 ppm over 5 min.). Since a large percentage of unintentional deaths from CO poisoning are associated with exposure in the home, the Consumer Products Safety Commission (CPSC) has suggested mandatory installation of CO detectors in all new residential construction beginning in 1995. The agency also recommends installation of these devices in all existing homes. The CPSC is an independent federal regulatory agency which is charged with protecting the public against unreasonable risks of injury associated with consumer products. It is also charged with maintaining an Injury Information Clearing House to collect, analyze, and disseminate data relating to causes and prevention of accidents involving consumer products. The commission has assumed responsibility for the Flammable Fabrics Act, the Poison Prevention Packaging Act of 1970, the Federal Hazardous Substances Act, and the Refrigerator Safety Act.

Diseases from toxic environmental exposures other than carbon monoxide can also masquerade as other medical disorders and are frequently misdiagnosed as viral illnesses, psychiatric disturbances, neurologic disease, and cardiovascular disease, when in fact they are caused by exposures to pesticides, hydrocarbons, polymer fumes, heavy metals, and other hazardous materials. In order to avoid misdiagnosis, the emergency physician needs to inquire about exposures at work or at home as a source of symptoms. Questions directed specifically toward recent exposure to fumes or chemicals or any temporal relationship between home or work activity and the chief complaint.[10] The physician should ask about current and past occupations and hobbies. Symptoms that resolve over the weekend or on vacation and return at the start of work suggest a job-related exposure. Inquiring about illness in other workers or household occupants may point to a common source of exposure. There are federal laws to control outdoor air quality and work place chemicals, but there is no regulation of the home's indoor environment. Certain hobbies are known to introduce hazardous substances into the household and have resulted in significant toxicity to the hobbyist and co-inhabitants. Recreational crafts such as painting, ceramics, welding, woodworking, and photography all involve toxic chemicals and when used in a poorly ventilated space can create a toxic environment.[10] Other elements in the environmental history may include asking about exposure to home cleaning agents, pesticide exposure, home insulation or renovations, home location, hazardous waste exposures, and occupations of household members.

Between 1979 and 1988, 100,000 years of potential productive life were saved as a result of a decrease in unintentional carbon monoxide poisoning. This decrease in deaths is attributed to a combination of environmental legislation, stricter regulatory standards, improved product safety, and preventive efforts such as public education by state and local health departments.[2]

In theory, all environmental disease is preventable since it results from exposures to toxins which should be containable or easily detectable. Emergency physicians can be important advocates for prevention of morbidity and mortality from these exposures. A specific example would be to work with your state legislature in order to enact a law which would minimize the risk of carbon monoxide poisoning to children who ride in the back of pickup trucks.[6] Physicians are encouraged to become involved in community awareness programs directed at the hazards associated with improperly ventilated furnaces, indoor use of charcoal briquettes, the dangers of methylene chloride, and the maintenance of proper exhaust systems for automobiles. Assistance for enhancing community awareness of potential environmental hazards can be obtained from hospital and university public relations officers who can facilitate the development of press releases, conferences and television and radio announcements which address important community issues. Advocacy will help improve public safety.

APPLICATIONS IN A BROADER CONTEXT: THE SENTINEL HEALTH EVENT AND ENVIRONMENTAL EXPOSURE

Q: What is a sentinel health event and what is its implication for the emergency physician?

The majority of environmental exposures are secondary to inhalation rather than ingestion. Fumes, gases, vapors, pesticides, and chemicals are among the most common causes of exposure. Patients with health effects from environmental exposure tend to have higher morbidity and mortality and have increased utilization of health care resources compared

to those with other types of poisonings reported to poison control centers.[11] The majority of these exposures are preventable and involve more than one potential victim. This type of health event is termed a "sentinel health event." It is defined as "an unnecessary disease, disability, or unnecessary, untimely death."[12] The rationale for selecting a particular condition as a sentinel event is that if the health care had gone well, the condition would have been prevented or managed. This concept has been fairly well developed and implemented in occupational and environmental health but is less well-known among emergency physicians. A list of conditions for use as sentinel events has been developed and includes "man-made diseases induced by toxic agents" and "physical hazards" as "clear-cut" sentinel events. Some of the conditions in this category include direct chemical hazards (carbon tetrachloride), pesticides, and contact sensitizers (nickel). Cases listed as "clear-cut sentinel events" justify an investigation into that event in order to prevent further morbidity or mortality.

On an individual level, the primary identifiers of sentinel events are primary health care providers such as physicians, nurses, dentists, and veterinarians. The alert clinician should be knowledgeable about disease epidemiology so that when an unusual event occurs, it will be detected.[13] After a sentinel event is observed, the case must be analyzed to determine the circumstance that led to its occurrence so that preventive strategies may be identified and implemented.

Case investigations will rely on the cooperation between the practitioner and a public health agency. The agency is needed for evaluation, confirmation, and preventive public health strategies for the events (see Figure 22-1). Uniform case definitions are essential for interpretation and reporting of sentinel event surveillance data. In 1989, a consensus panel met and developed a set of diagnoses clearly related to the environment.[14] These diagnoses signal the need to initiate actions in order to prevent illness or injury from related environmental exposures. They identified poisonings from environmental exposures as a prototypical sentinel event. Such exposures included pesticides, toxic gases, heavy metals, solvents, and chemical spills. Another clearly identifiable, environmentally caused sentinel event was methemoglobinemia. This may result from excessive nitrate levels in the drinking water and is usually manifested in infants.[15] For the emergency physician, toxic environmental exposures such as those listed above would qualify for reporting.

Q: What are the local and national resource organizations for environmental exposures?

Nationwide surveillance for environmental exposures is poor. The Agency for Toxic Substances and Disease Registry (ATSDR) maintains a registry for exposures related to hazardous waste sites, but this is very limited and has little impact on the emergency patient population.

In 1987, a sentinel event notification system for occupational risks (SENSOR) was developed to perform active surveillance on selected occupational conditions. This system was a health provider reporting system and was initially started in 10 states.[16] The first component was a network of individual practitioners, laboratories, or clinics which would operate as sentinel providers. The provider recognized and reported the case to a surveillance center. The center analyzed the data and directed intervention activities toward the case and the work site from which the case was reported. The center was also responsible for confidentiality and in determining the appropriateness and effectiveness of the intervention. It provided technical consultation on a wide variety of occupational health issues. In order to facilitate cooperation by the sentinel providers, the scope of the program was limited to 6 conditions that lent themselves to easy reporting. These conditions were silicosis, occupational asthma, pesticide poisoning, lead poisoning, carpal tunnel syndrome, and noise-induced hearing loss. The development of SENSOR was a significant milestone toward comprehensive surveillance for occupational disease and injury in the United States.[17] A similar system could be developed in emergency medicine using the emergency physician as the reporter and perhaps the Regional Poison Control Center as the surveillance center.[11] Regional Poison Control Centers open 24 hours a day are available for collecting exposure data from emergency departments. It is a simple and convenient process for the emergency physician to report possible sentinel health events that result from toxic environmental exposures. A unique advantage of using the poison center database is its unique focus on

Figure 22-1   Emergency Department Evaluation of a Sentinel Health Event

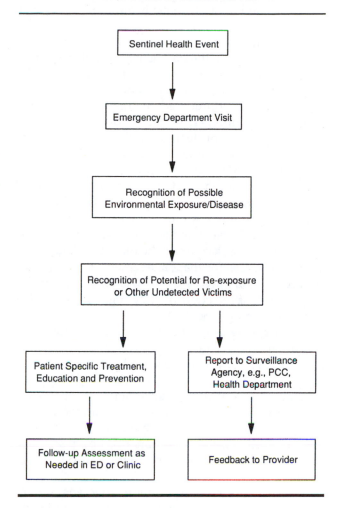

individual environmental exposures. The poison center can provide a mechanism for identifying additional victims and short term follow-up of exposures.

One of the major roles of poison centers is poisoning prevention. They often work closely with local and state public health departments. Poison centers may be able to analyze their data for temporal clusterings of poisonings[18] and identify outbreaks that may not be obvious to the individual practitioner. Patient outcomes and analysis of community exposures can be relayed back to the providers. Regional poison centers may vary in their interest and capability in acting as a surveillance center. Mutual interest in this function among primary health providers, poison centers, and health departments will foster further development and expertise in this much needed area of public health and emergency medicine.

If the environmental exposure involves a hazardous material, then the emergency physician should implement the hospital's disaster or mass casualty plan if necessary. Even one contaminated patient can overwhelm an unprepared emergency department. The most common chemicals reported to cause injury, evacuation, or death in accidental releases are pesticides, gases (chlorine, ammonia), corrosives (HCl, HF, NaOH) and fuels (gasoline, diesel oil). Toxin identification must be made early. HAZMAT teams are trained to identify unknown chemicals released in the environment. Material Safety Data Sheets (MSDS) can provide information for specific chemicals but lack complete health effect data. Additional resources for the management of site specific and community problems are available from the Environmental Protection Agency regional office and ATSDR for major incidents.

A list of agencies that provide information and consultation is included in Appendix 22-1.

The ATSDR is the lead federal public health agency for hazardous material incidents. The experts available for consultation include (1) an Emergency Response Coordinator within 10 minutes; (2) a Preliminary Assessment Team consisting of a toxicologist, a physician, and environmental health scientist; and (3) if the incident necessitates, an on-site response team.

The Chemical Transportation Emergency Center (CHEMTREC) also provides information to health care personnel regarding hazardous chemical spills and workplace chemicals. They provide information on the content of shipments and the MSDS but not management information. It is sponsored by the Chemical Manufacturers Association and is affiliated with approximately 13,000 companies. It maintains a large file of MSDSs.

The Radiation Emergency Assistance Center/Training Site (REAC/TS) can provide information for radioactive material accidents on an emergency basis.

Risk communication to the press and the public is an essential part of the hazardous materials incident plan. A credible spokesperson for the hospital must relay accurate information concerning the incident to the press in a timely manner. This can avoid

rumors and possible mass psychosocial stress which may precipitate many unnecessary visits to the emergency department.[19] The emergency physician may be called on to play such a role.

NOTES

1. Litovitz TL, Clark LR, Soloway RA. 1993 Annual Report of the American Association of Poison Control Centers' Toxic Exposure Surveillance System. *Am J Emerg Med* 1994; 12(5):546–84.
2. Cobb N, Etzel RA. Unintentional carbon monoxide-related deaths in the United States, 1979–1988. *JAMA* 1991; 266(5):659–63.
3. Wharton M, Bistowish JM, Hutcheson RH, Schaffner W. Fatal carbon monoxide poisoning at a motel. *JAMA* 1989; 261(8):1177–8.
4. Hampson NB, Norkool, DM. Carbon monoxide poisoning in children riding in the back of pickup trucks. *JAMA* 1992; 267(4):538–40.
5. Heckerling PS, Leikin JB, Maturen A. Occult carbon monoxide poisoning: Validation of a prediction model. *Am J Med* 1988; 84:251–6.
6. Hampson NB, Kramer CC, Dunford RG, Norkool BM. Carbon monoxide poisoning from indoor burning of charcoal briquettes. *JAMA* 1994; 271(1):52–3.
7. CDC: Unintentional deaths from carbon monoxide poisoning-Michigan, 1987–1989. *MMWR* 1992; 41(47):881–3.
8. Fawcett TA, Moon RE, Fracica PJ, Mebane GY, Theil DR, Piantadosi CA. Warehouse workers' headache: Carbon monoxide poisoning from propane-fueled forklifts. *J Occup Med* 1992; 34(1):12–15.
9. Woolf A, Softley LJ, Leek, Yanigasawa Y. Accuracy of card-type carbon monoxide detectors. *Vet Hun Toxicol* 1994; 36(4):344 (abstract).
10. Goldman RH, Peters JM. The Occupational and Environmental Health History. *JAMA* 1981; 246:2831–6.
11. Litovitz T, Oderda G, White JD, Sheridan MJ. Occupational and environmental exposures reported to poison centers. *Am J Pub Health* 1993; 83:739–43.
12. Rutstein DD, Berenberg W, Chalmers TC, Child CG, Fishman AP, Perrin EB. Measuring the quality of medical care: A clinical method. *N Eng J Med* 1976; 294:582–8.
13. Armenian HK. Case investigation in epidemiology. *Am J Epidem* 1991; 134:1067–72.
14. Rothwell CJ, Hamilton CB, Leaverton PE. Identification of sentinel health events as indicators of environmental contamination. *Environ Health Perspect* 1991; 94:261–3.
15. CDC. Methemoglobinemia in an infant—Wisconsin 1992. *MMWR* 1993; 42(12):217–19.

16. Freund E, Seligman PJ, Chorba TL, Safford SK, Drachman JG, Hull HF. Mandatory reporting of occupational diseases by clinicians. *JAMA* 1989; 262: 3041–4.

17. Baker EL. Sentinel event notification system for occupational risks (SENSOR): The concept. *Am J Pub Health* 1989; 79:18–20 (Supplement).

18. Hryhorczuk DO, Frateschi LJ, Lipscomb JW, Zhang R. Use of the scan statistic to detect temporal clustering of poisonings. *J Toxicol Clin Toxicol* 1992; 30(3):459–65.

19. Kirk MA, Cisek J, Rose SR. Emergency department response to hazardous materials incidents. *Emerg Med Clin North Am* 1994, 12:461–81.

Appendix 22-1 Resource Organizations for Environmental Exposures

---

Carbon Monoxide Information Bureau
Consumer Product Safety Commission,
Washington, DC 20207
CPSC Product Safety Hot Line 800-638-2772
  or 301-504-0220

Agency for Toxic Substances and Disease
  Registry (ATSDR):
Emergency Response and Consultation Branch
Division of Health Assessment and Consultation
The Agency for Toxic Substances and Disease Registry
1600 Clifton Road, NE (E32)Atlanta, GA 30333
Phone: 404-639-0615 FAX: 404-639-0655

Chemical Transportation Emergency Center
(CHEMTREC): 1-800-424-9300

Radiation Emergency Assistance Center/Training Site
REAC/TS: 615-481-1000

23

Occupational Health

L. KRISTIAN ARNOLD

CONTENTS

- Occupational health—elements of the history and physical exam
- Incidence of work-related injury and illness
- Economic consequences
- Role of the ED practitioner
- Sentinel health events
- Surveillance
- Rights of workers
- Referral, follow-up, and return to work
- Developing professional expertise and expanding the practitioner's role

CHAPTER SUMMARY

The discipline of emergency medicine (EM) sits in the crossroads between the community and the medical world, providing the EM practitioner with a more global view of the overall health of the community than can generally be appreciated by individual practitioners of other medical disciplines. This vantage point allows the EM practitioner to have a sense of many of the broad issues affecting the community's public health.

For many injured workers, the point of entry into the medical care system is through the emergency department (ED). The initial management of workplace injuries and illnesses can have a significant impact on the overall course and ultimate outcome. This is true from a sociopsychologic perspective as well as a strictly physiologic perspective.

Work-related "accidental" injuries generally have a fairly clear association with an occupational activity. For many work-related illnesses the relationship between work activities and the presenting complaint is not obvious. The practitioner who is sensitive to the possible contributions of a work setting and activity to an underlying condition can serve patients with a more efficient brand of health care. The following case will illustrate these points as well as serve as a focus for discussion of a number of other issues related to the role of the emergency medicine practitioner in relation to occupational health.

Case #1

A 55-year-old female presents to the emergency department complaining of unilateral headaches. Although she has had headaches on and off throughout her adult life, she now complains of daily headaches for the last 2 weeks. She characterizes the pain as a steady pressure in one or the other parietal area, with radiation to the occipital area and pressure behind the eye on the same side. She denies any nausea, vomiting or visual changes, trauma, weakness or sleep disturbance due to the headaches. However, she relates that she has awakened sometimes with tingling in the ring and fifth fingers of one hand or the other. This usually resolves after being awake for a few moments. She denies any fever, chills, malaise, or other symptoms of systemic infectious illness. She has been using acetaminophen with variable relief. She denies any other past medical history, tobacco, illicit drug, or excessive alcohol use.

She is a slightly overweight, healthy looking, neatly dressed woman appearing slightly distressed, rubbing her temples from time to time during the evaluation. Vital signs are normal. General physical exam with the patient seated on the side of the stretcher is normal. HEENT exam is unremarkable with no nasal congestion or sinus tenderness. Cranial nerve function and funduscopic exam are both normal. Strength testing of upper and lower extremities reveals 5/5 strength, equal bilaterally in major nerve root distributions. Sensory testing of upper and lower extremities is also normal and equal bilaterally to sharp and light touch in all root distributions.

The patient is told she has a tension headache. The physician advises ibuprofen 800mg TID, warm bath, and stress reduction. For further evaluation of the tingling sensations she is given a referral to a neurologist since she has no primary care physician.

Q: Why should the patient have this recent change in headache pattern? What would additional history contribute?

In many "tension headaches," the tension is physical as implied by an alternate term for the same syndrome: "muscle contraction headache." Recognition of this pathophysiologic correlation should lead to questioning as to the source of increased muscle tension in the upper back, shoulder girdle, neck, and head. As noted in the case presentation, this patient denied any trauma. Trauma is an important consideration since wrenching injuries of the upper back, neck, and shoulder girdle may all lead to persistent headaches due to resultant muscle spasm. Increased muscle tension may also be the result of inappropriate postural biomechanics while performing tasks.

In situations where the task duration is limited, such as suturing in an awkward position, resulting muscle-group-fatigue induced hypertonus or spasm is easily overcome with return to unstrained positioning and varied tasks. Increasingly in the workplace, complex tasks are being broken down into isolated tasks with workers spending the majority of a workday repeating the same task. If the worker is performing the tasks in a way that places excessive persistent or repetitive strain on certain muscle groups, these groups may fatigue. As a result of such

fatigue other muscle groups are recruited to aid in postural support and performance of the task.

Case Continuation

Further questioning of this patient would have revealed the following additional information: When job history was elicited, she described work as a telemarketing representative recording responses to a questionnaire. The actual task involved allowing a computer to constantly dial numbers, speaking with the first person to answer, entering data and moving on to the next call as quickly as possible, since there was an incentive pay package with monitoring of productivity in terms of numbers of calls completed and keystrokes per minute when inputing data.[1] She worked 12 hours per day, 6 days per week, since she was a single parent; her husband had been killed in a construction accident. During a typical 12-hour shift she would leave her workstation only for three bathroom breaks of 5 minutes and one 30-minute meal break. She related that the computer was a standard desktop model with the monitor sitting on top of it, placed on a long table at which there were eight stations. Her telephone was a headset type. There were eight such tables in two rows in a windowless cinderblock room. When asked to mimic sitting at her workstation, she demonstrated poor posture with her torso slightly slumped and her neck in extension to view the screen. She had been at this job for six weeks, having been unemployed for the prior 10 months. Previously she had been a secretary for a small business for 15 years. Since starting this job, she had taken one 4-day weekend during which she did note resolution of her headaches by the second day, and of the nocturnal parasthesias by the last night.

The discipline of ergonomics (from the Greek *ergon* = work + *nomos* = law) addresses the factors governing the performance of work. These factors include the characteristics of the worker (anthropometry and physiology), the work environment, the man-machine interface, biomechanics of the task. Ergonomic factors largely influence the musculoskeletal health of workers. For the patient in question a number of ergonomic principles come into play in the production of her symptom complex. The poor posture demonstrated relates both to the design of the workplace and to musculoskeletal conditioning and training of the worker. Poor posture maintained for extended periods of time leads to exertional imbalance of anterior and posterior truncal and neck erector musculature. The adverse biomechanical features of rapid, repetitive motion over prolonged periods of time without rest breaks leads to recruitment of secondary muscle groups to support muscles fatigued by the primary task, in this case keystrokes.

Q: How can the symptoms of intermittent tingling in the C8 distribution as presented be explained? Does the patient have more than one problem?

The symptom of parasthesias in the distribution of either a nerve root or peripheral nerve suggests probable compression of the involved nerve. The ulnar nerve sensory distribution correlates closely with that of the isolated C8 root. Irritation anywhere from the point of exit of the root from the cord (proximal to the neural foramen) to the mid-forearm may lead to symptoms in the hand.

Disorders affecting the ulnar nerves in this distribution can be grouped into three anatomically related segments. Lesions at or proximal to the neural foramen generally are anatomically fixed lesions such as tumors, herniated intervertebral disks, and osteophytic narrowing of the neural foramen. Lesions distal to the axilla are largely limited to local entrapment syndromes such as cubital canal entrapment at the elbow and Guyon's canal syndrome at the wrist. These should all be considered in the differential diagnosis. Plain radiographs of the cervical spine will rule out severe osteophyte formation. Absence of tingling in the distribution of the nerve with tapping over the suspected area of entrapment when the nerve is stretched by flexion of the elbow or extension of the wrist (Tinel's sign) decreases the likelihood of a local entrapment. The third anatomic grouping comprises the region of the thoracic outlet, the region defined by the clavicle anteriorly, the trapezius and scapula posteriorly and the cervical spine medially.

The region of the thoracic outlet has a complex array of bones, muscles, nerves, and vascular structures. A number of pathophysiologic processes in this region have been proposed to account for neuro muscular problems of the arm. The best known are cervical ribs, long transverse processes of C7, apical lung tumors (leading to Pancoast's syndrome), and congenital fibrous bands between muscle groups. All of these entities may compress both nerves and blood vessels traversing the region. An increasing appreciation of symptoms in the absence of any structural lesion has led to a number of diagnostic classifications such as cervicobrachial syndrome and scalenus anticus (anterior scalene) syndrome.[2] Plain radiography of the chest and cervical spine will rule out cervical ribs and long transverse processes of C7 as well as a large apical tumor. If there is further reason to be suspicious of a small apical tumor, more specific radiographic evaluations may be warranted. For purposes of the remainder of the discussion the term *thoracic outlet syndrome* (TOS) will be used to refer only to syndromes *not* associated with a fixed anatomic lesion.

The symptom complex of TOS can include pain in the neck, shoulder girdle, and arm. Patients may also report parasthesias and numbness, most commonly in the ulnar (C8) distribution. Subjective sensations of swelling of the hand may occur. Objective finding of significant swelling should lead to further investigation regarding anatomic lesions. Autonomically mediated symptoms of the hand such as sensations of cold and patchy skin blanching may be reported. Sensory symptoms of parasthesias and numbness are frequently intermittent. On careful questioning, though, the physician can often find specific positional or functional associations. Many patients will report symptoms only nocturnally or with positioning of the arms in anterior shoulder flexion (such as driving a car with the hand gripping the top of the steering wheel). Carrying items with the shoulder in adduction and the elbow in extension (briefcase, shopping bag, bucket) may reproduce or exacerbate symptoms.

Q: What might a more comprehensive neuromuscular examination reveal?

As with the patient presented here, the upper extremity neurovascular exam is frequently normal if the patient is early in the evolution of the syndrome. The classic TOS physical finding of obliteration of the pulse with elevation of the hand above the head may not be present in patients with myotendinous TOS. Examination will generally reveal tenderness of the muscle groups that comprise the neck-shoulder girdle complex. This region should be examined since patients do not always specifically complain of muscle pain, and may present, as in this case, with secondary symptoms of headache or upper extremity neurologic symptoms. The examiner should remember that the posterior shoulder girdle actually extends inferiorly at least to the lower trapezius attachments to T12 at the thoracolumbar junction (the transition point between the kyphotic thoracic curve and the lordotic lumbar curve). If one takes into consideration the latissmus dorsi as part of the support mechanism of the shoulder girdle, the inferior reaches of the shoulder girdle, in terms of direct muscular links, extend to the pelvic brim and the lumbo-sacral spine via the aponeurosis of the latissmus.[3] Superiorly the trapezius has its insertions along the occipital ridge of the skull.

Examination of the muscles of the back and neck is best done with the patient lying down as this puts the normal postural musculature at rest and facilitates palpation of deeper muscle groups. Examination of the neck and upper thoracic region is best done with the patient lying supine. Examination of the back below the level of the upper thoracic region is best accomplished with the patient lying prone. The examiner should stand at the head of the bed to examine the head, neck, shoulders, and upper back.

The examiner will better appreciate differences in general muscle tension as well as deep muscle spasm if the two sides are examined simultaneously. Palpation of the neck musculature should commence with the sternocleidomastoid muscles, progress to the trapezius and then to the cervical and upper thoracic paravertebral muscles. Palpation is most sensitive if the examiner has relaxed hands/fingers with the wrist held in a fixed position near neutral and uses motion of the forearm to modify the palpatory pressure. The point of finger contact should be on the palmar pads of the distal phalangeal segment, not on the tips of the fingers. Ideal initial pressure of the examining hand is between 3 and 5 pounds. At this level of pressure usually the patient does not suffer enough discomfort to voluntarily guard the tender muscles and the examiner is able to gain the confidence of the patient, thus allowing deeper palpation of underlying muscle groups.

The tissues are best surveyed initially with a stroking motion of the subcutaneous layers, i.e. the examining fingers do not slide on the skin, but rather move the skin with them sliding over the deeper

tissue planes. If asked for differential reporting of pain and if the exam is being done correctly, patients will frequently be able to lead the examiner to areas of deep muscle spasm. To the examiner, these areas have a palpatory consistency similar to lymph glands. Not infrequently, if the examiner identifies areas of deep, discrete muscle spasm particularly in the mid upper trapezius and levator scapula, direct firm pressure on these areas of spasm may either precipitate or aggravate pain and possibly paresthesias in the arm or hand. This phenomenon has been termed "trigger points."[4]

Case Continuation

A careful examination of this patient's posterior shoulder girdle and neck would have revealed diffuse tenderness. Additionally, she had several areas of discrete palpable tender "knots" in different muscles such as the upper trapezius, levator scapula, and upper and mid rhomboids. She had no obliteration of the radial pulse with elevation of the hand to 180°. She did have reproduction of ulnar parasthesias with holding her arms straight out in front. During this maneuver it was noted that she significantly elevated her scapulae (as in shrugging the shoulders). A diagnosis of myotendinous TOS was established.

Q: Were discharge plans and instructions adequate?

Since the initial evaluation of the patient did not lead to a correct understanding of the etiology and pathophysiology underlying her symptoms, it is highly likely that the therapeutic plan would be inadequate.

Treatment for myotendinous TOS is based largely around physical therapy. The general principles are to increase flexibility, strength, and endurance. More specifically, exercises are directed at correcting relative weakness of the posterior muscles of the shoulder girdle. Due to the degree of controversy existing around the exact origins of myotendinous TOS actual therapeutic regimes may vary. Inital treatment plans from the ED should involve gentle stretching exercises for those muscles found to be tight and tender. Gentle, firm massage and moist heat are also easily accomplished at home and effective. Overweight patients should be advised that weight loss may also help.

For the patient presented here, a more appropriate patient plan would include: timely referral to an occupational medicine facility; advice regarding gentle stretching exercises such as neck rolls, shoulder shrugs, torso stretches and forearm-hand stretches; a note for work advising time off until the follow-up appointment or modified duty to allow for rest/stretching breaks.

Q: What are the public health implications of this case?

An understanding of the etiology of this patient's symptoms should raise concern regarding the other employees of the same firm. In contrast to the situation with hazardous chemical substances in the workplace, no standards exist regarding ergonomic factors for many jobs. OSHA is currently planning to begin implementing worksite design standards based on ergonomic principles. Since there are no "standards," there is currently no regulatory agency with a specific role in regards to ergonomic factors. Some states have begun surveillance programs and are tracking certain workplace illnesses and injuries.[5]

In this case, the simplest public health intervention would be to inform the patient of the probable association and to indicate that others may have similar problems. Encouraging this patient to then let her coworkers know of the association may be beneficial. It is also possible that she may be hesitant to "stir up trouble" for the not unrealistic fear of losing her job. If there is no occupational medical practice in the community to which this patient can be reported, the interested emergency physician may take the inititive personally to contact the employer. A great deal of tact and discretion are necessary if this route is chosen to avoid violation of patient confidentiality or unnecessarily jeopardize the patient's employment. The patient should be informed of any intended direct contact with the employer. Most businesses are grateful, however, for feedback with constructive suggestions, particularly if it is presented as a means of saving on workers' compensation costs.

DISCUSSION

Incidence

Various surveys and studies have attempted to document the incidence of work related injuries and illness. The most widely quoted data comes from the Bureau of Labor Statistics, a division of the Department of Labor. The BLS surveys only private companies with greater than 11 employees. There is no organized data collection for government workers, farmers, or self employed persons. The data is derived by tabulating the data from OSHA 200 "Logs and Summary of Occupational Injuries and Illnesses" from those establishments surveyed by the BLS. OSHA requires maintenance and presentation on demand of the 200 logs. Data from 1990 indicated 332,000 new cases of occupational illness. Data from New York state was used to project national statistics in the late 1980s. Based on 5,000 to 7,000 deaths per year in New York attributable to occupationally related illness, projections indicated an estimated 50,000 to 70,000 deaths and 350,000 new cases of illness each year from occupational exposure.[6] National Safety Council data for 1990 indicate 1.8 million disabling injuries resulting in approximately 10,000 deaths. Ineffective data collection and uncoordinated efforts most probably lead to an underestimation of both incidence of injury and illness as well as an underestimate of the prevalence of occupational related medical conditions.[7]

Economic Consequences

Work-related injuries and illnesses are a major socioeconomic burden for society. Generally valid figures for medical costs and lost wages for injuries are $48 billion.[8] In most studies only the costs of medical care and lost wages are used with no consideration for "pain and suffering," which increases the average cost by 50%.[9] These costs figures refer only to injuries. Since many occupational illnesses go unreported, the true cost for both injuries and illnesses is grossly underestimated. Since these injuries and some of the illnesses are covered by workers' compensation insurance policies, the premiums for these policies represent additional indirect costs of each injury. The insurance industry administrative costs may amount to an additional 28% above the wage and medical costs themselves.[10]

Workers' Compensation

The current system of workers' compensation has developed over a number of years, generally having origins around the beginning of the twentieth century. At that time the workers' compensation system was developed as an alternative to having workers file suit to gain restitution for injuries suffered in the workplace.[11] Each state has its own laws governing workers' compensation. A basic understanding of some key elements of the local laws is helpful for the EM practitioner. Both physicians who care for injured workers and employers find the laws generally laborious and complex. It is not uncommon to find medical specialists who will not accept workers' compensation cases for a variety of reasons, among which is the relatively low compensation for services.

The relative contribution of an occupation to a medical condition that is required to qualify the condition as work-related varies among the states. Generally, it is not necessary that the work activities or exposures be even the primary factor, but only that they be contributing factors.[12] Stress-related issues represent an area of evolution in the workers' compensation law in terms of determining work-relatedness of a condition.

EM Practitioner Role

The practice of emergency medicine can be approached in two ways: (1) ruling out serious medical-surgical disease and treating only those entities that present a significant risk of mortality or acute morbidity; or (2) practicing more comprehensively as a member of a health care resource team for the individual patient and community. In the latter model, the emergency physician takes an active role not only in the overall therapeutic plan of every patient, but also in facilitating change to benefit the public health of the community.

In the case of the woman telemarketer with the headache, once the EM practitioner felt comfortable that this was not a subarachnoid bleed, tumor, or meningitis, for example, the patient could have been discharged with instructions on analgesia and fol-

low-up as originally planned. Alternatively, as presented in the case discussion, the physician could extend his concern beyond the patient at hand to the co-workers who are exposed to the same ergonomically unsound conditions, as part of a proactive, preventive approach to occupational illness and injury.

Occupational History

Since EM practitioners must make rapid, accurate diagnoses with a minimum of technologic support, our information gathering process becomes the embodiment of the ancient medical truth that 90+ % of the diagnosis lies in the history. Additionally, as the initial caregivers we often have the best chance to capture history accurately while it is fresh in the mind of the patient. Both of these concepts are crucial to delivering effective emergency medicine for workers. Hence, it is extremely important for emergency physicians to incorporate a brief occupational history in the patient interview.

The emergency medicine practitioner learns in many settings not to accept a "situation" at face value, but to approach certain cases with a heightened index of suspicion of the *unoffered history* (for example with child abuse or drug use) However, in many other presentations the underlying diagnosis is accepted without question. Asthma is a prime example in which (particularly in a busy ED) patients may be assessed for the acute episode without any questioning regarding possible exposure to other inhaled irritants that may have precipitated the immediate episode or been a factor in the initial onset of the disease process. A brief occupational history combined with even rudimentary familiarity with the concept of occupational exposure-induced asthma[13] could quickly lead to a much more satisfactory outcome from the same health care encounter. A simple model has been proposed in which there are four basic steps: (1) routine screening questions on environmental etiologies [current and past longest-held jobs; present or past known exposures; factors affecting the chief complaint]; (2) consideration of sources of exposure [jobs and duties; ill coworkers, home environment]; (3) identification of toxic substance used in the workplace [chemical name, handling procedures, route of entry into the body]; and

(4) follow-up [consultation sources, resolution of the initial exposure problem].[14] Obtaining a brief occupational history may open the door to the diagnosis for the individual patient as well as alert the physician to risks for other workers or the community at large.

Sentinel Health Event

Occupationally related diseases and injuries, once identified, are theoretically some of the most readily preventable adverse health events. Presentation for evaluation of a disease or injury related to occupation is an "occupational sentinel health event." Rutstein defined the original concept of a generic "sentinel health event" (SHE) as

> a preventable disease, disability or untimely death whose occurrence serves as a warning signal that the quality of preventive and/or therapeutic medical care may need to be improved[15]

Rutstein et al modified this concept for occupational health (SHE(O))

> a disease, disability, or untimely death which is occupationally related and whose occurrence may: 1) provide the impetus for epidemiologic or industrial hygiene studies; or 2) serve as a warning signal that materials substitution, engineering control, personal protection, or medical care may be required.[16]

With the publication of the concept of a SHE(O), a listing of diagnoses was also proposed that was meant to serve as a surveillance tool *and* as a reference tool for individual practitioners. This list was formulated around the World Health Organization's International Classification of Diseases (ICD) codes. Although the original listing of 50 ICD codable diagnoses was expanded to 64 in the 1991 update,[16] some conditions do not appear in the listing because of the methodology utilized in analyzing the supporting documentation for each condition.

The National Institute for Occupational Safety and Health, Centers for Disease Control (NIOSH) developed the concept of SHE(O) and continually updates the list of diagnoses to be considered. Another notable feature of these listings is that they do not include accident-injury events ascribable to

external events, as these are covered by a separate set of ICD codes commonly known as "E" codes. Such a listing is available from NIOSH on request.

Familiarity with Occupational Diseases

The general EM practitioner population undoubtedly has an awareness of the relation to occupation of a number of medical conditions such as carpal tunnel syndrome and asbestosis. The link for many other conditions is less well known to the medical population largely due to lack of education.[17] Some cause and effect relations are less well established because of a lack of epidemiologic evidence. An improved understanding of the NIOSH listing of occupationally related diseases and its shortcomings will help the EM practitioner to recognize potentially removable worksite hazards as well as diagnose work-related illnesses. Some of the NIOSH listed non-injury diagnoses that may initially present to the ED are

> Contact and allergic dermatitis
> Mononeuritis of upper limb
> Acute renal failure
> Agranulocytosis
> Asthma
> Methemaglobinemia
> Bronchitis
> Hepatitis
> Carpal tunnel syndrome
> Raynaud's phenomenon

The EM practitioner should realize that the list is constantly expanding, and hence is not necessarily inclusive of all work-related conditions. Through identification of the sentinel case and effective recording and reporting, further injuries or illness may be prevented. As the individual EM practitioner gains an understanding of the public health methodologies used in surveillance, an appreciation for the relevance of using ICD codable discharge diagnoses will become evident. Reporting of cases that the practitioner feels might need follow-up may be done through one of several routes. NIOSH may conduct a health hazard evaluation of a work site in response to an ED contact through the emergency reporting number. The Occupational Safety and Health Administration (OSHA) can also be called, although their involvement is primarily limited to situations that violate one or more of their codes. Additional resources for follow-up include local or regional occupational health programs and state departments of public health.

Surveillance

Even in the emergency medicine setting, it may be difficult for any one practitioner to notice trends in injury patterns given the changing hours of presence on duty. Hence, it is vitally important for emergency department directors to advocate for a computerized log system. This allows searching by diagnosis as well as by demographic information (employer, insuror), and identifies work related injuries, provided the information is accurately captured by the registration system and the physician uses discharge diagnoses that facilitate ICD coding. A method for applying ICD-E codes to ED patients has been described.[18]

For more complete and useful data for epidemiologic and intervention oriented surveillance the American National Standards Institute ANSI Z16.l2 method of recording information regarding work injuries has been used as the basis for reporting by the National Electronic Injury Surveillance System (NEISS). The full ANI+SI Z16.r method is very detailed in terms of type of activity in which the victim was engaged at the time of the injury and is not directly transferrable to medical conditions. Approximately 60 hospitals participate in the NEISS reporting.[19]

Injury and illness surveillance data has immediate relevance to the EM practitioner to heighten sensitivity for diagnostics. For example, realization that welding can lead to metal fume fever, which mimics a viral syndrome, may tip off the astute practitioner to the diagnosis in a patient who works in an enclosed construction project. Population research on particular industrial hygiene issues is equally important, but this information is of relatively less value if it is not integrated into the personal database and practice patterns of practitioners seeing patients in the primary care setting. Not all persons with work related injuries or illness will be referred directly from the work site.

Understanding of Community Work Site Risks

The construct "mechanism of injury" describes the relationships of job factors to disease processes. In the broadest sense of the term, work site factors that may lead to illness or injury are another form of "mechanism of injury" to a worker. In emergency medicine, this concept can be used effectively to broaden diagnostic thinking and to activate protocols.

If the EM practitioner elicits a work history and understands the processes involved a patient's industrial setting (the potential "mechanisms of injury"), the speed and accuracy of diagnosis will be improved. ED representatives should be in constant contact with the business community to become aware of new installations or major changes in processes involving worker risk. With many of the changes in the industrial demographics that are occurring in the last decade of the twentieth century, there may be sudden changes in the job descriptions of large numbers of workers to tasks with little or no oversight regulation.[20] One particularly notable sector is the poultry processing industry which has expanded at a phenomenal rate, and lacks the regulation that has been applied to the beef slaughter and packing industry ever since attention was first drawn to it by Upton Sinclair in his 1906 publication of "The Jungle." The Bureau of Labor Statistics predictions for the 10 fastest-growing occupations from 1990 to 2005 includes largely medical and other service sector jobs, which are presently not scrutinized as closely as is the manufacturing sector.[21]

The training of emergency medicine physicians is structured to give a broad competency in the diagnosis and management of the majority of medical entities. Depending on the types of industry present, a community may have a much higher incidence of certain illnesses and injuries, and practitioners may not be adequately prepared to assess these particular manifestations. Two examples that may not be included in training in general emergency medicine include fish fanciers finger caused by *mycobacterium marinum* (found in longshoremen as well as tropical fish handlers) and occupational asthma in detergent formulators (secondary to bacillus-derived exoenzymes).[22] There exists a real risk of missing a number of cases if the physician new to a community is not oriented to these community-specific issues or, if the physician does not have a practice of obtaining an occupational history as a part of the exam. As a service to the community it is advisable that the director of any emergency department, or an EM practitioner with occupational medicine interest, become familiar with such community-specific disease and risk patterns. This information should be passed on to the rest of the ED staff and included in orientation material for new or temporary staff, including housestaff who may rotate to the hospital.

Knowing the Rights of Workers

Workers' compensation statutes require the employer to know what illnesses and injuries have occurred in direct relation to their business. Hence, employers can have access to the diagnosis of a work-related illness or injury, but *not* generally to the full medical record without a release provided by the patient. The American College of Occupational and Environmental Medicine Code of Ethical Conduct states that physicians should not convey any information to the employer regarding non-work-related conditions that do not have an effect on the patient's ability to do work. If conditions have an effect on the worker's ability to perform, then a statement of limitations of activity is the limit of information to which the employer is entitled. The emergency medicine medical record in an industrial injury should be recorded appropriately for the incident. The treating physician should be attentive to potential problems that may be created for the worker/patient if other non-work-related information is included in the record and ultimately the record is requested by the employer. One good solution is to review with the patient what has been written.

Follow-Up Referral/Return to Work

In recommending follow-up care for injured or ill workers the treating physician should, in addition to or, in some settings, in place of other medically appropriate referrals, make a referral either directly to the occupational health service that covers the worker/patient, or refer the patient back to a worksite supervisor with a recommendation for employee health follow-up. Pursuant to workers' compensation statutes in most states, workers have the right to choose their treating physicians. At the same time

most data on the topic have shown that case management rehabilitates workers faster and at less cost.[23] The case management concept involves some form of oversight of the rehabilitation process of injured or ill workers to assure that they are receiving the maximum benefit from medical care and are integrated back into the workforce at the earliest medically appropriate time. Case management is usually coordinated through the employer's employee health service or contracted provider.

As noted above, at the time of the ED visit health care practitioners have the opportunity to capture the best history. At the same time, EM practitioners have a major opportunity to start the rehabilitation process immediately and on the best course possible. No matter how badly a patient may have been "wronged" by the unintentional or intentional negligence of the employer, in the long run all three parties share one common goal: a speedy return to as great a functional capacity as possible. Each party has different reasons for wanting this outcome, but, if the tone can be focused on the attainment of maximum recovery at the outset, a service will have been performed for all honorable parties.

The concept of early return to the workforce, even if in a modified, "light," duty status has become increasingly accepted as a facilitating factor in rehabilitation. In at least one study on low back injuries a significant reduction in absenteeism and disability occurred with the use of light duty.[24] When appropriate, light duty should be prescribed as a set of limitations on activities—a statement of impairment. It is then the responsibility of the employer to decide whether there is a job available that fits the impairment. This has greatest significance when workers have minor injuries that preclude performance of usual work activity, but the expected duration of impairment is short enough that they might not qualify for workers' compensation benefits (typically less than 5 to 6 days).

Government Agencies

In order to have an effective impact on workplace hazards, the EM practitioner would benefit from an understanding of the role of several government agencies. The Occupational Safety and Health Administration (OSHA) is mandated in a regulatory capacity to assure workplace safety. This is done through a series of "rulings" that are published in the Code of Federal Regulations, Title 29, Chapter XVII. These regulations are updated regularly with new rulings published first in the Federal Register and incorporated into the Code annually. The rulings and regulations of OSHA are interpretations of laws passed in Congress.

The National Institute for Occupational Safety and Health (NIOSH) is intended to function as an agency for research and education in issues related to workplace safety and health. NIOSH is administratively a part of the Centers for Disease Control (CDC) located in Atlanta. In the late 1980s NIOSH developed a surveillance system known as the Sentinel Event Notification System for Occupational Risks (SENSOR).[25] The SENSOR system is meant to serve as a monitoring and follow-up system to give practitioners a single point of reporting possible SHE(O)s. Unfortunately, to date the SENSOR system does not fully cover the country, nor does it track all of the conditions listed in the most recent NIOSH update of the SHE(O) list. When NIOSH established the SENSOR program it decided to leave each state the options of which and how many SHE(O) conditions to monitor since occupational demographics will vary among states.

The Environmental Protection Agency (EPA) is largely concerned with protection of the environment, but, not rarely, occupational exposures represent possible environmental contamination as well. The Agency for Toxic Substances and Disease Registry (ATSDR) is primarily devoted to activities designed to protect the public from exposure to toxic substances. In addition to developing a registry of health effects of toxic substances, the agency has developed medical management guidelines for treatment of some chemical exposures.[26]

Opportunities for Personal Professional Involvement

Opportunities abound for interested and qualified practitioners in the various aspects of delivering quality health services to workers. In 1991, the Institute of Medicine estimated a shortage of 3,100 to 5,500 physicians with special competence in occupational and environmental medicine. All occupational health services, whether corporate-sponsored, hospital-based, or private need nursing staff versed in the issues particular to occupational medicine.

Most emergency medicine physicians will have a sense of kinship with the field of occupational medicine. As a medical specialty with board certification, occupational medicine is young. Many of the physicians delivering occupational medical services have developed their expertise through postresidency learning experiences. The board certification is administered by the Board of Preventive Medicine. Some practitioners make a slight distinction between the concept of occupational health as being more focused on preventive services and occupational medicine as being more focused on the care of the ill or injured worker. Another distinction that is sometimes made is between occupational medicine and industrial medicine. In this case the former is thought of as being more focused in epidemiologic and preventive activities and the latter referring to the primary care for occupational illness and injury. These distinction are by no means official, though the division of labor forces does exist largely based on where practitioners develop an expertise. For EM practitioners there are several routes by which they can increase their expertise and involvement in occupational and environmental medicine.

The interested emergency medicine practitioner can seek involvement at any degree from passing information back to the worksite, as proposed in the case presented above, to consulting with businesses, to political advocacy, to splitting professional time between the two roles. Offering feedback to local businesses is an excellent starting point for any ED practitioner. Once some experience and expertise has been gained from going to CME courses the practitioner may find formal consulting interesting. The politically interested physician will find ample opportunities to share expertise with lawmakers either directly or by testifying, particularly on topics that may impact the ED operations, such as right-to-know legislation (legislation requiring information on hazardous chemicals be given to employees and be available for emergency workers).

Personal Knowledge and Expertise Building

Increasing attention has been given to the need to educate medical students and residents about the

Figure 23-1 Application of Haddon's Matrix to the Case Study

	Host	Agent/Vehicle	Environment
Pre-event	Training on proper posture at the computer	Ergonomically correct construction of workstation	Installation of safety posters
Event	Regular exercises and good posture	Equipment maintenance	Supportive management
Postevent	Accurate diagnosis, appropriate therapy and reeducation	Reassessment of workstation design	Legislative advocacy to have regulations for workstations

SOURCE: Adapted from Haddon W. Advances in epidemiology as a basis for public policy. *Public Health Reports* 1980; 95:411.

importance of occupational associations with various diseases.[27] Family practice residency programs have begun to offer some degree of training in occupational and environmental health.[28] A number of review articles have been published in attempts to improve the general medical awareness of occupational health issues.[29–31] In addition to the articles referenced above, the interested practitioner will find several handbooks and reference works that will either treat the subject in question or lead to more detailed reading.[32–34]

Mini-residencies (1 to 4 nonconsecutive weeks) have been established at several institutions nationally.[35] The American College of Occupational and Environmental Medicine conducts a three-part "Basic Curriculum" in conjunction with semiannual meetings. The University of Wisconsin School of Public Health offers a correspondence course Masters in Public Health degree.[36]

In a response to the need for more qualified physicians, NIOSH established 14 Educational Resource Centers in the late 1970s. These continue to regularly offer CME courses in various aspects of occupational and environmental health. They also offer courses directed to nurses and industrial hygienists.

Approach to a Problem Issue

For the practitioner interested in pursuing involvement beyond the doors of the emergency department, there are several ways in which to get started.

In order to address an issue around an occupational injury it may be helpful to apply Haddon's epidemiologic model of the interactions between the host, environment, and agent/vehicle to cases like the telemarketer's. This model facilitates breaking the situation down into more manageable components (see Figure 23-1).[37]

The easiest place for most EM practitioners to enter the field might be through educational ventures. These can take several forms. One might create a hospital based committee of consultants to assist local industries. Individual case follow-up can provide an excellent service for the individual worker, the employer and the emergency department. Most businesses are very happy to have follow-up contact and will welcome a worksite visit by an interested physician and be willing to discuss solutions for a particular health related problem. Community service clubs and business clubs are generally delighted to have an EM physician speak to their groups. One does not have to be presented as an expert in occupational and environmental health, but rather as what the ED practitioner truly is: a health care professional with a unique perspective from the crossroads of the community and the medical establishment. A health care professional who develops specific interests in direct lay teaching, knows the topic and makes it interesting can even keep the attention of a group of urban police when teaching stress management.[38]

As time permits and interest prods, the EM practitioner may develop more and more interest in the areas of surveillance and research to better define the problem and improve pre and post event health interventions. This may span the spectrum from devising improved methods to electronically linking various tracking systems to studying specific work site interventions.

As was mentioned earlier, with changing industrial demographics a number of poorly regulated segments of industry are growing rapidly. Herein lies an opportunity for involvement at the public policy level. Policy makers need input from health practitioners who see the direct effect of health policies both good and bad.

Across the wide spectrum from individual patient care to broader issues of occupational risk surveillance, practitioners of emergency medicine can expand the realm of overlap between fields to have far reaching influence in the improvement of public health.

NOTES

1. Horwitz, T. Nine to nowhere: These six growth jobs are dull, dead-end, sometimes dangerous. *Wall Street Journal* 1994; 224(104):1.

2. Leffert, RD. Disorders of the neck and shoulder in workers. In Millender, LH. (ed.). *Occupational Disorders of the Upper Extremity*. New York: Churchill Livingston, 1992.

3. Clemente, CD. *Anatomy: A Regional Atlas of the Human Body*, 3rd ed., Baltimore: Urban & Schwarzenberg, 1987, fig. 524.

4. Travell, J, Rinzler, SH. The myofascial genesis of pain. *Postgrad Med* 1952; 11:425.

5. Freund, E, et al. Mandatory reporting of occupational diseases by clinicians. *JAMA* 1989; 262(21):3041.

6. Landrigan, PJ, Markowitz, S. Current magnitude of occupational disease in the United States: Estimates from New York State. *Ann NY Acad Sci* 1989; 572:27.

7. Hanrahan, LP, Moll, MB. Injury surveillance. *Am J Pub Health* 1989; 79(supp.):38.

8. Baker, SP, Conroy, C. Occupational injury prevention. In CDC: *Setting the National Agenda for Injury Control Conference*. Atlanta: Centers for Disease Control, 1992, p. 327.

9. French, MT. Estimating the full cost of workplace injuries. *Am J Pub Health* 1990; 80(9):1118.

10. Etter, IB. The National Safety Council's Estimates of injury costs. The 1987 Conference on Injury in America. *Pub Health Rep* 1987; 102(6):665.

11. Felton, JS. 200 Years of Occupational Medicine in the U.S. *JOM* 1976; 18:809.

12. McElveen, JC, Jr., Beck, T. Legal and ethical issues. In McCunney, RJ (ed.). *A Practical Approach to Occupational and Environmental Medicine*, 2nd ed. Boston: Little, Brown, 1994.

13. Mullan, RJ, Murthy, LI. Occupational sentinel health events: An updated list for physician recognition and public health surveillance. *Am J Ind Med* 1991; 19:775.

14. Goldman, RH, Peters, JH. The occupational and environmental health history. *JAMA* 1981; 246:2831.

15. Rutstein, DD, et al. Measuring the quality of medical care: A clinical method. *NEJM* 1976; 294(11):582–8.

16. Rutstein, DD, et al. Sentinel health events (occupational): A basis for physician recognition and public health surveillance. *Am J Pub Health* 1983; 73(9):1054–62.

17. Levy, BS. The teaching of occupational health in United States medical schools: 5 year follow-up of an initial survey. *Am J Pub Health* 1985; 75:79.

18. Ribbick, BM, Runge, JW, et al. Injury surveillance: A method for recording E-codes for injured emergency department patients. *Ann Emerg Med* 1992; 21:37.

19. Hanrahan, LP, Moll, MB. Injury surveillance.

20. Horwitz, T. Nine to nowhere.

21. Table 630. *Statistical Abstracts of the United States*. Washington, DC: U.S. Government Printing Office, 1992.

22. Mullan, RJ, Murthy, LI. Occupational sentinel health events.

23. Harris, J. Economics of occupational medicine. In McCunney RJ (ed.). *A Practical Approach to Occupational and Environmental Medicine*, 2nd ed. Boston: Little, Brown, 1994.

24. Wiesel, SW, et al. Industrial low back pain: A prospective evaluation of a standardized diagnostic and treatment protocol. *Spine* 1984; 9:199.

25. Baker, EL. Sentinel Event Notification System for Occupational Risks (SENSOR) *Am J Pub Health* 1989; 79(Supp):18–20.

26. ATSDR, 1600 Clifton Rd. E-28, Atlanta, GA 30333. Office of Regional Operations: (404) 639-0707 to obtain regional center. Emergency Response and Consultation Branch: (404) 639-0615.

27. Levy, BS. The teaching of occupational health.

28. American Medical Association. *Directory of Graduate Medical Education Programs*. Chicago: AMA, 1992.

29. Cullen, MR, Cherniack, MG, Rosenstock, L. Occupational medicine, I. *NEJM* 1990; 3332:594.

30. Cullen, MR, Cherniack, MG, Rosenstock, L. Occupational medicine, II. *NEJM* 1990; 332:675.

31. Landrigan, PJ, Baker, DB. The recognition and control of occupational disease. *JAMA* 1991; 266:676.

32. McCunney, RJ (ed.). *A Practical Approach to Occupational and Environmental Medicine,* 2nd ed. Boston: Little, Brown, 1994.

33. Zenz, C. *Occupational Medicine: Principles and Practical Applications,* 3rd ed. St. Louis: Mosby, 1994.

34. Hadler, NM. *Occupational Musculoskeletal Disorders.* New York: Raven Press, 1993.

35. University of California at San Francisco contact Division of Occupational and Environmental Medicine University of Cincinnati; contact the Department of Occupational Medicine, Joseph LaDou, MD, Director.

36. Academic Program in Occupational Medicine, Medical College of Wisconsin.

37. Haddon, W. Advances in the epidemiology of injuries as a basis for public policy. *Pub Health Rep* 1980; 95:411.

38. Personal experience.

24

Injuries in the Emergency Department: An Opportunity for Treatment and Prevention

STEPHEN W. HARGARTEN

You know, sometimes it feels like this. There I am standing by the shore of a swiftly flowing river, and I hear the cry of a drowning man. So I jump into the river, put my arms around him, pull him to shore, and apply artificial respiration. Just when he begins to breath, there is another cry for help. So I jump into the river, reach him, pull him to shore, apply artificial respiration, and just as he begins to breath, another cry for help. So back in the river again, reaching, pulling, applying, breathing, and then another yell. Again and again, without end, goes the sequence. You know, I am so busy jumping in, pulling them to shore, and applying artificial respiration that I have no time to see who the hell is upstream pushing them all in.

—*Irving Zola**

CONTENTS

- Epidemiology of injury
- Prevention
- Rehabilitation

*From McKinley JB. A case for refocusing upstream: The political economy of illness. In Enelow AJ, Henderson JB (eds.). *Applying Behavioral Science to Cardiovascular Risks*. Chicago: American Heart Association 1984, pg. 7.

- Advocacy role
- Surveillance

CHAPTER SUMMARY

Every year, an estimated 140,000 people in the United States (U.S.) die from injuries: motor vehicle drivers, firearms, drownings, poisonings, house fires and others.[1] In 1993, there were 40,115 deaths in the United States from motor vehicle crashes.[2] In 1992, the latest year available, there were 37,776 firearm deaths.[3]

In 1992, about 40% of Emergency Department (ED) visits were injury related (34 million) or 13.1 injury related visits per 100 members of the population.[4] An estimated 3,125,000 motor-vehicle related injuries were treated in EDs in the U.S. during 1992.[1] An estimated $9.2 billion was spent on injury-related ED visits in 1992.[4]

Emergency medicine is in an important leadership role for the prevention, acute care, and rehabilitation of the injured patient.[5-8] Emergency physicians treat injured patients on a daily basis. They are also involved in research and advocacy efforts to reduce the frequency and severity of these injuries.[9] Emergency physicians and other health care professionals are crucial for increasing seat belt and helmet usage through advocacy efforts as well as addressing other strategies for prevention such as fire-safe cigarettes and safe handguns.[6]

This chapter addresses the injury problem in a general fashion and introduces a framework for

240

emergency medicine health care professionals to develop clinically oriented prevention strategies.

Case #1

The patient is a 9-year-old female who was riding a bicycle on a city street. She was not wearing a helmet. An automobile pulled out of a driveway and crashed into the patient and her bicycle. She fell off the bicycle, struck her head on concrete, and became unconscious.

The prehospital BLS unit transported the patient with C-spine precautions and oral airway to the ED. Upon arrival to the ED the patient was unconscious with a Glasgow Coma Scale (GCS) score of 8. She had a blood pressure of 90/60, a pulse of 100, and a respiratory rate of 28. The remainder of the examination was unremarkable except for abrasions to the forehead and upper extremities.

The patient was intubated, hyperventilated, and was sent for a CT scan. The CT scan was positive for a small subdural hematoma that did not require surgery. The patient was comatose for 6 days, then gradually became conscious, and was discharged from the hospital after 30 days.

The patient has experienced significant difficulty in school with memory and cognitive deficits, and was required to repeat the school year. After 1 year, the patient is still experiencing recurrent headaches.

Q: What protection do helmets provide with patients who are involved in bicycle-related crashes?

Helmets reduce the severity of head injuries in bicyclists by 85%.[10] About 30% of bicycle-related injuries treated in U.S. EDs involve injuries to the head or face.[11] About 62% of bicycle-related deaths are due to severe head injury.[12] However, only 27% of bicycle riders own or use a helmet.[13] Increased efforts by health professionals are needed to increase helmet ownership and usage for bicyclists, motorcyclists, ATV riders, and horseback riders.

Q: What are the unique issues regarding rehabilitation of patients who are head injured?

It is crucial that patients who are head injured receive ongoing comprehensive rehabilitation. These patients have cognitive problems, concentration diffi-

culties, and attention deficit disorders. They require special attention, particularly school-aged kids, while they attempt to resume and continue their school work.

Q: What environmental approaches should be considered to reduce the incidence of bicycle crashes?

A crucial area for prevention of bicycle injuries is the environment itself. Every effort must be made to separate bicycle riders from automobiles and trucks. Designated bike lanes and bike paths are examples of this injury prevention strategy. When separation is not possible, increasing the visibility of the rider and bike is important. Reflectors (for night riding) and flags on the bicycle are helpful for increasing the visibility of the bicycle and rider and reducing the risk of motor vehicle crashes.

Case #2

This case involves a 26-year-old male who came home after working for 18 hours, began smoking a cigarette on his couch, fell asleep, and dropped the lighted cigarette. The couch began to smolder and burn. Approximately 1 and 1/2 hours later, the apartment was filled with smoke. The patient's neighbor noticed smoke and called 911. The patient was found unconscious by EMS personnel and was transported to the nearest emergency department.

On arrival in the ED, the patient had a blood pressure of 130/80, a pulse of 110 and a respiratory rate of 24. His GCS score was 8. Other findings included: PERRL, chest clear, abdomen soft. Neuro: The patient was decerebrate. There were no signs of burns. Arterial blood gasses revealed a PO_2 94, CO level 55. Hyperbaric treatment was initiated, but the patient never regained consciousness and was later discharged to a rehabilitation center for ongoing chronic care.

Q: What is the most common cause of house fires? What is the most common cause of fatal house fires?

The most common cause of house fires is ignition of cooking materials. However, the most common cause of *fatal* house fires is a cigarette (28% of deaths).[1] Every year, approximately 1,500 people die in house fires caused by cigarettes.[14] Fire-safe ciga-

Figure 24-1 Haddon's Matrix: Fires and Burns

	Host	Agent/Vehicle	Environment
Pre-event	Reduce fatigue and at-risk alcohol usage.	Fire-safe cigarettes, child-proof lighters, matches.	Fire-safe furniture. Fuses in homes.
Event	Reduce disabilities.	Pilot lights on stoves.	Smoke detector. Sprinkler system.
Post-event	Special care of the elderly.	Redesign gas tanks in cars and trucks.	911, Fire extinguisher, EMS

rettes are technically feasible and cost no more than regular cigarettes.[15] Fire-safe cigarettes are a classic example of a "passive" injury control strategy that could have prevented this tragedy.[16] Passive injury control strategies do not require human behavior to achieve their effects. An example is an automobile airbag. The airbag does not require any action by the motor vehicle driver or passenger to prevent or reduce injuries during automobile crashes. Fire-safe cigarettes do not require any human behavior to achieve injury prevention.

Q: Could a smoke detector or sprinkler system have prevented this house fire injury?

Yes. The value of smoke detectors and sprinkler systems is widely recognized. Five out of six houses in the United States had smoke detectors by 1988. However, only two-thirds had working batteries.[1] Sprinkler systems automatically extinguish fires and require little maintenance. Sprinkling systems are another "passive" prevention strategy to reduce house fire deaths and injuries.

DISCUSSION

Injuries occur to organ systems when energy is exchanged which exceeds the body's (organ's) ability to absorb it. Injuries such as motor vehicle crashes, bicycle crashes, falls from heights, and firearms involve kinetic energy exchanges. Thermal energy is involved in house fires and hot water burns. Addi-

tional sources of energy which can result in injuries to organs include chemical, electrical, and radiation energy.

These energy exchanges take place over milliseconds during the injury event. This is in contrast to repetitive lower energy exchanges, which result in a different spectrum of injuries, including carpal tunnel syndrome and chronic low back pain.

Haddon's Matrix is the best descriptor-diagram of the complex interactions of an injury event (see Figure 24-1). Originally described in the 1960s, Haddon's Matrix is useful for developing multiple complementary strategies that can prevent and/or reduce the severity of injury events. Emergency physicians along with EMS personnel have been active in the post-event environment phase: caring for injured patients. Educational strategies to change human behavior (pre-event human factor) have traditionally been emphasized and oftentimes are the only injury prevention strategies employed in communities. But as one can see from the matrix, there are several other areas for developing prevention strategies. For housefires and burns, there are nine areas to develop strategies instead of just one or two.

DISCUSSION

The public health approach to reducing injuries and deaths is a relatively new model. Traditionally injuries have been felt to be random events largely due to human behavior. They were "accidents." In the 1950s, a paradigm shift occurred. Scientists began to examine motor vehicle crashes in a different way. The public health model with equal attention to the host, agent/vehicle, and the environment was utilized and emphasized (see Figure 24-2). This public health paradigm shift culminated in the 1960s with Ralph Nader's publication of *Unsafe at Any Speed* and the subsequent congressional hearings on the safety design of the Corvair.[17] Instead of just concentrating on changing the behavior of the driver (host), Nader and physicians working with him began to apply equal emphasis on motor vehicle safety standards and the environment. The public health paradigm shift for injury prevention and control is still being applied in the 1990s. Attention is switching to the cigarette, the firearm, and other agent-vehicles that are part of the injury triad.

The first textbook on injuries was published in 1964 by Haddon.[18] Physicians increasingly became interested in part due to the National Academy of Sciences publication in 1966 on *Accidents: A Neglected Epidemic.*[19] In the 1980s and early 1990s, there has been an explosion of injury control texts.[1,20-22] Injury prevention and control is now a recognized science.[20-23]

Emergency medicine physicians have increasingly become interested in injuries as a public health issue, not only within the context of acute care but also in prevention of the injuries: going upstream. The application of multiple strategies (Haddon's Matrix) to injuries, especially to motor-vehicle crashes, has begun to pay dividends. With the advent and usage of seat belts, airbags, helmets, crashworthy-designed cars, reduced speed limits, seat-belt laws, better roadways, and improved emergency medical services; motor-vehicle crash injuries, deaths, and disabilities are being reduced.[2] Motorcycle helmets, for example, reduce the risk of fatal injury by 30%. Raising the minimum drinking age to 21 is credited with saving $1.7 billion and nearly 1,000 lives every year. As a result of the new laws aimed at young drivers, the proportion of those 15 to 20 years old who were involved in a fatal accident while intoxicated dropped from 31% in 1982 to 15.8% in 1993. Airbags reduce driver deaths by an additional 14% over conventional seatbelt use.[24]

Emergency medicine physicians are critical in being advocates for reducing injuries and deaths. They know the high-risk groups since they are treating these patients in the emergency department. They know the environment since they interface with

Figure 24-2 The Public Health Model

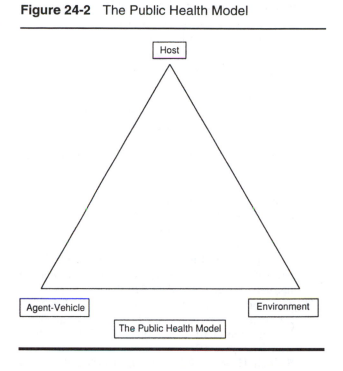

emergency medical services. They are important research advocates for seeking solutions on a local, regional, and national level. (Ralph Nader was quoted: "And when we finally get out of school and join the work force, we're taught how to make a buck and not how to make a difference." By going upstream, physicians and EMS professionals can make a difference.)

Continued involvement of emergency physicians is critical, especially in the areas of high-risk groups (teenagers and elderly), high-risk vehicles such as ATVs, bicycles, and pickup trucks, and high-risk behavior such as at-risk alcohol use. Legislation and advocacy must be based on community data and targeted with discrete measurable outcomes such as decreasing head injuries with bicycle helmet legislation. Emergency physicians must become active in injury surveillance.[25]

NOTES

1. Baker SP, O'Neill B, Ginsburg MJ, et al. *Injury Fact Book.* New York: Oxford University Press, 1992.
2. *Traffic Safety Facts 1993.* U.S. Department of Transportation, National Highway Traffic Administration. DOT HS 808(169), 1994.

3. Centers for Disease Control. *Advance Report of Final Mortality Statistics—1992;* 43(6)1994.

4. National Center for Health Statistics. *National Ambulatory Medical Care Survey: 1992 Summary #253,* Centers for Disease Control, August 18, 1994.

5. Martinez R. Injury Control: A Primer for Physicians. *Ann Emerg Med* 1990; 19:72–7.

6. Hargarten SW, Karlson T. Injury Control: A Crucial Aspect of Emergency Medicine. *Emerg Clin N Amer* 1993; 11(1):255–62.

7. Hargarten SW. Injury Control. *Acad Emerg Med* 1994; 1(2):168–71.

8. Waxweiler RJ. Public Health, Injury Control, and Emergency Medicine. *Acad Emerg Med* 1994; 1(3):204.

9. Kellermann AL, Reay DT. Protection or Peril? An analysis of firearm deaths in the home. *N Engl J Med* 1986; 314:1557–60.

10. Thompson RS, Rivera FP, Thompson DC. A case control study of the effectiveness of bicycle safety helmets. *N Eng J Med* 1989; 320:1361–7.

11. Tinsworth DK, Polen C, Cesidy S. *Bicycle-Related Injuries: Injury Hazard and Risk Patterns Technical Report.* Washington, DC: U.S. Consumer Product Safety Commission, 1993.

12. Sacks JJ, Holgreen P, Smith SM, Sosin DM. Bicycle-associated head injuries and deaths in the U.S. from 1994–1988: How many are preventable? *JAMA* 1991; 266:3016–33.

13. Rodgers GB. Bicycle helmet use patterns in the U.S.: A description and analysis of nation survey data. *Accid Anal Prev* 1995; 27(1):43–56.

14. Botkin JR. The fire-safe cigarette. *JAMA* 1988; 260(2): 226–9.

15. Technical Study Group. Toward a Less Fireprone Cigarette. *Final report of the technical study group on cigarette and little cigar fire safety.* Washington, DC: U.S. Consumer Product Safety Committee, 1987.

16. McLoughlin E, McGuire A. The Causes, Cost, and Prevention of Childhood Burn Injuries. *Amer J Dis Child* 1990; 144:677–83.

17. Nader R. *Unsafe at Any Speed.* New York: Grossman, 1965.

18. Haddon W, Suchman EA, Klein D. *Accident Research, Methods, Approaches.* New York: Harper & Row, 1964.

19. National Academy of Science. *Accidents: The Neglected Epidemic,* 1966.

20. Wilson MH, Baker SP, Teret SP, et al. *Saving Children: A Guide to Injury Prevention.* New York: Oxford University Press, 1991.

21. Robertson LS. *Injury Epidemiology.* New York: Oxford University Press, 1992.

22. Waller JA. Injury Control: A Guide to the Causes and Prevention of Trauma. Lexington, MA: Lexington Books, 1985.

23. Christoffel T, Teret SP. *Protecting the Public: Legal Issues in Injury Prevention.* New York: Oxford University Press, 1993.

24. Airbags save lives. *Insurance Institute for Highway Safety* 1995; 30:1–10.

25. Garrison HG, Runyan CW, Tintinalli JE, et al. Emergency department surveillance: An examination of issues and a proposal for a national strategy. *Ann Emerg Med* 1994; 24(5):849–56.

Unit III

The Emergency Physician's Role in Public Health, Education, and Public Policy

25

Firearm-Related Injuries

ARTHUR L. KELLERMANN
ELIZABETH HOLLIGER

CONTENTS

CHAPTER SUMMARY

Epidemiological research has revealed that many deaths and injuries due to firearms affect identifiable high-risk groups, follow an often predictable chain of events and are therefore preventable. By viewing firearm injuries as the product of a complex interaction between the victim, the assailant, the firearm and the environment, we can more readily understand how these injuries occur and formulate strategies for their prevention. Options to prevent firearm injuries and/or mitigate their severity may be grouped into one of three broad categories:

Education. Violence prevention curricula have been developed in recent years, but evidence for their impact is scant. Education of homeowners and would-be purchasers of firearms about the risks of keeping an unsecured weapon in the home may decrease rates of ownership and unsafe storage, but this strategy has not been evaluated in a prospective manner. Firearm safety training may improve weapon-handling skills, but current evidence of the effectiveness of these curricula is lacking.

Enforcement. The traditional criminal justice approaches of deterrence (crime control through the threat of punishment), incapacitation (isolation of violent individuals from society at large), and rehabilitation are costly but essential components to an overall approach to violence control. Most gun control laws attempt to regulate the use of firearms after they have been purchased, often with little effect. In the United States, few restrictions are placed on firearm sale or ownership.

Engineering. Many unintentional firearm injuries could be prevented if all guns were required to have an automatic trigger arrestor and a loading indicator. User specific firearms are also under development. Modifying high-risk environments (such as cabs and all-night gas stations) to make them safer is costly but effective.

Emergency physicians can support firearm injury prevention by conducting population based surveillance of rates and patterns of firearm injury, supporting community-based violence prevention efforts, identifying and treating associated risk factors (e.g., alcohol and drug abuse), referring victims of violence for protective services, and supporting policies aimed at reducing the incidence and impact of firearm-related injuries.

Case #1

Five days before the Christmas of 1993, JC, a 9-year-old male, was rushed to the emergency department of Grady Memorial Hospital in Atlanta, Georgia. A few moments before, he had sustained a gunshot wound to his head. Grady paramedics found the child comatose and unresponsive with decerebrate posturing. Because his jaws were clenched, they were unable to intubate him prior to arrival in the ED. Instead, respiratory support was provided by bag-valve-mask.

According to the paramedics, JC was shot by his older brother after the boys found his mother's handgun under her bed and began playing with it. Although JC's brother removed the magazine of bullets from the .25 caliber semiautomatic, one round was retained in the chamber. Thinking that the gun was empty, the boy pointed the weapon at JC and pulled the trigger.

The initial examination in the emergency department revealed a young male in acute distress with decerebrate posturing. A single gunshot wound to the right fronto-temporal region was identified, and the patient was noted to have epistaxis. No exit wound was found. The boy's airway was patent, and spontaneous respirations were noted at a rate of 26. His initial blood pressure was 197/121 mm of mercury. JC had no verbal or eye opening response to painful stimuli, yielding a Glasgow coma score of 4. His pupils were noted to be equal at 3 mm and bilaterally reactive, and his toes were down going bilaterally. His rectal exam revealed diminished tone and no gross blood. No other injuries were noted, and the remainder of his examination was unremarkable.

Initial management included immediate endotracheal intubation with midline immobilization following rapid sequence induction. Proper placement of the ET tube was confirmed by auscultation, capnography and a portable chest x-ray. Hyperventilation was initiated. A portable skull film in the ED revealed a defect in the right superolateral region of JC's skull and a bullet projecting into the left temporal region. A stat CT scan confirmed the entry site in the right frontal lobe and the bullet in the left occipital lobe, just posterior and superior to the petrous bone. Multiple bony fragments were noted at the entry site, and intraparenchymal hemorrhage was evident throughout the bullet track. Both the right basal ganglion and the left thalamus appeared to be severely damaged. Diffuse cerebral edema, subarachnoid bleeding and intraventicular hemorrhage were evident.

Shortly after admission to the pediatric intensive care unit, JC sustained a cardiac arrest. Although he was initially resuscitated, his condition steadily deteriorated. After two detailed neurologic exams indicated brain death, his family agreed with the decision to remove life support.

A follow-up call to the investigating law enforcement agency confirmed the facts noted above. The firearm involved in the shooting was a .25 caliber semiautomatic pistol, manufactured by Raven Arms.

Case #2

Six months after JC's death, EMS was called to the scene of another critically injured child. GJ, a 10-year-old boy, was shot by his 8-year-old cousin as the two played with a small caliber handgun they had smuggled into GJ's home. While their mothers cooked dinner downstairs, the children removed the pistol's magazine. Thinking that the weapon was unloaded, the 8-year-old pointed the pistol at his cousin and fired.

The bullet struck GJ in the center of his back and exited just above his heart. Upon hearing the gunshot, the adults rushed upstairs and found GJ apneic and pulseless. An uncle initiated CPR. He continued his efforts until EMS arrived.

Following endotracheal intubation on the scene, the child was rushed to Grady Memorial Hospital. Despite determined efforts in the emergency department, including an ED thoracotomy, a pulse could not be reestablished. GJ was pronounced dead.

A follow-up call to law enforcement confirmed the weapon was a Raven .25 caliber semiautomatic pistol. A magazine of bullets was also recovered at the scene. Evidently one round had been retained in the chamber. The source of the firearm could not be immediately determined.

Q: Could better emergency care have made a difference in the outcome of either of these patients?

No. Both children had nonsurvivable injuries. Both received aggressive prehospital and emergency department care, and one survived to the intensive care unit. However, neither would have benefited from additional treatment. Everything that could be done was done, at great cost to both families and the health care system.

Q: Aren't deaths like these rare?

Although unintentional shooting deaths of children are relatively uncommon, they account for a substantial degree of morbidity and mortality in this age group. The rate of unintentional firearm injuries has slowly declined throughout most of this century, but it remains a substantial problem among children. Unintentional shootings account for 43% of gunshot deaths among children aged 5 to 9, and 31% of firearm fatalities involving children aged 10 to 14.[1] Furthermore, unintentional shooting deaths are only the tip of the iceberg. The number of serious but nonfatal injuries caused by unintentional discharge of a firearm is many times greater than the number of deaths. Published estimates range from 16 to more than 100 times greater.[2,3]

Intentional firearm injuries (suicides, homicides, and assaults with a firearm) are a far more serious problem. After gradually declining during the first half of the 1980s, firearm related deaths rose 14% between 1985 and 1991. Initially, this rise was gradual, but it accelerated between 1988 and 1991. During the latter period, the rate of firearm related deaths increased by more than 3% each year. Ironically, during this 6-year time interval, the death rate due to motor vehicle crashes in the United States declined 10%. As a result of these changes, firearms will soon overtake motor-vehicle crashes as the leading cause of injury-related death in the United States.[4] Guns already kill more citizens than motor vehicles in seven states and the District of Columbia.[4] The rest of the nation is not far behind.

Much of the growth in firearm related mortality has been due to a sharp increase in the rate of firearm homicide. Between 1985 and 1991, the rate of firearm homicides in the United States increased 50 percent, from an overall, age-adjusted rate of 5.07 per 100,000 to 7.60 per 100,000. The rate of homicide among adolescents and young adults grew even faster than it did among the general population. Homicide among the 20-to-24-year-old males increased 104%, from 9.87 to 20.14 per 100,000. Among 15-to-19-year-old males, firearm homicides increased 187 percent, from 5.8 per 100,000 in 1985 to 16.62 in 1991 (Source: National Center for Health Statistics).

Homicide strikes particularly hard within the African American community. Although rates of homicide among African Americans have always been higher than among whites of comparable age, the gap widened even further between 1985 and 1991.[5] In 1985, the rate of firearm homicide among African American men aged 15 to 19 years old (37.4 per 100,000 person years) was more than seven times higher than the rate of firearm homicide among whites of the same age (5.0 per 100,000 person years). During the next 6 years, the rate of homicide among African Americans in this age group *tripled* to 124.23 per 100,000, while the homicide rate among whites *doubled* to 11.84 per 100,000. As a result, the ratio of deaths widened to more than ten to one (source: National Center for Health Statistics). Today, more U.S. teenagers die from gunfire wounds than from all natural causes of disease combined. Firearm-related mortality accounts for almost *half* of all deaths among African American teens.[6]

Q: Aren't firearm injuries and deaths an inevitable part of modern American life?

Many people consider injuries the consequence of unpreventable "accidents" or the result of simply being "in the wrong place at the wrong time." However, epidemiological research has shown that injuries disproportionately affect identifiable high-risk groups, follow a predictable chain of events, and are therefore *preventable*.[7] In biological terms, injury occurs when energy (the *agent* of injury) is transferred to the victim (or *host*) at a rate or amount that exceeds the body's ability to tolerate this transfer without damage.[8] Kinetic energy, the primary agent of trauma, is usually transferred through an inanimate object, or *vehicle*. Examples include a speeding car, a knife or a bullet. Biologic organisms, such as animals that sting, bite, or kick, are considered *vectors* of injury. Since most cases of penetrating trauma involve acts of violence, the nature and characteristics of the *assailant* must also be taken into consideration when analyzing these injuries.[9] Finally, each injury producing event takes place in a physical or social *environment*, the characteristics of which can influence the risk or severity of injury. By viewing gunshot injuries as the product of a complex interaction between the victim, his assailant, the weapon and the immediate environment, we can more readily understand how these tragedies occur and formulate strategies for their prevention.[9]

Q: What can be done to prevent firearm-related injuries?

Substantial reductions in the rate and severity of gunshot wounds can be achieved by employing a complementary mix of strategies to target various points in the chain of injury causation. In general, options to prevent or mitigate firearm injuries can be grouped into one of three broad categories: *education* of citizens about the dangers of unsecured firearms in the home and education of gun owners about proper gun handling and storage practices, *enforcement* of existing gun control regulations, and better *engineering* of firearms to make them less prone to unintentional discharge. Modification of high-risk environments has also been tried with some success.

BROADER PUBLIC HEALTH CONTEXT

Education

Violence prevention curricula.   In light of society's traditional focus on safety education, it is not surprising that interventions aimed at modifying the behavior of the offender or victim have received a lot of attention in recent years. Since most firearm injuries are the result of intentional acts by one or more individuals, many people feel that educational programs to teach conflict resolution skills may prevent deaths and injuries due to violence.[10–12]

Programs such as these are popular because they stress individual responsibility and target the behavior most proximately associated with crime and violence. Unfortunately, there is little evidence that they work. Despite great interest in implementing these programs across the United States, little effort has been made to evaluate their effectiveness. Webster[13] recently reviewed the literature published to date and found scant evidence of impact beyond minor, short term changes in knowledge and attitudes. Only one pilot program achieved significant changes in behavior, and the number of students involved was far too small to support a firm conclusion about its effectiveness.[14] No study has followed a substantial number of students over a sufficient interval of time to document long term benefits.

Firearm safety training.   Little is known about the value of programs that promote responsible use and handling of firearms. Not surprisingly, groups like the National Rifle Association strongly favor gun safety training over regulatory approaches to firearm injury prevention. In highly structured and rigorously supervised settings like firing ranges, training probably has beneficial effects. Unfortunately, the effectiveness of safety training in less structured settings is unclear.[9] Although "safe storage" of firearms is explicitly endorsed by the National Rifle Association and the Firearms Manufacturer's Association, research has shown that gun owners who have received firearm safety training are *less* likely to store their weapons locked and unloaded than owners who have not been trained.[15] However, the nature of the training these individuals received and the appropriateness of the instruction was not specified.

Data on the value of other types of safety training is not encouraging. Robertson and colleagues measured the impact of saturation advertising to promote voluntary use of seat belts in one city served by two cable television systems. One system aired over 1,000 high-quality promotional spots; the other aired none. No differences in the rate of seat-belt usage were noted among subscribers to either system.[16] Although driver education is a fixture in many high schools, it has not been shown to decrease crash related fatalities among teenagers. In fact, by encouraging teens to drive, these programs may have the opposite effect. Elimination of driver education programs in one school district was followed by a *decrease* in crash fatalities involving 16- and 17-year-old drivers.[17]

Parent and homeowner education.   Little effort has been made to educate consumers about the true balance of benefits and risks associated with keeping a gun in the home. Although firearms are kept for many reasons, "self defense" is cited more often than any other by owners of handguns.[18] Ironically, a study of firearm-related deaths in King County, Washington, found that a gun in the home was 18 times more likely to be involved in the death of a member of the household than it was to be used to kill an intruder in self defense.[19] Case control research has revealed that homes with guns are substantially more likely to be the scene of a suicide or a homicide than comparable homes without guns.[20–23] Family or intimate assaults with a gun are far more likely to end in death than assaults with knives or other weapons.[24]

As many as half of all unintentional shooting deaths among children occur when kids play with a loaded gun they have found.[25] Unfortunately, many parents have an unrealistic understanding of their children's cognitive and motor abilities around firearms.[26] As a result, firearms are often improperly stored, even in homes with small children.[1,27,28]

Many gun owners are unaware of these findings. One recent poll found that 40% of gun owners believe that owning a gun makes them safer. Only 3% stated that they felt that owning a gun makes them less safe. Twenty-three percent stated that they keep their gun loaded and ready for use.[28] In an effort to provide the public with a clearer understanding of these risks, the Commission of Fulton County, Georgia, recently passed an ordinance that requires all gun shops in the county to post a notice and attach hang tags to each firearm advising the purchaser of the danger of keeping a gun in the home.[29] The impact of efforts like these is unknown.

Enforcement

Deterrence. Criminal justice relies on the effects of deterrence, incapacitation and rehabilitation to control violent crime. Unfortunately, the impact of criminal justice sanctions on firearm violence is limited.[30] The Federal Bureau of Investigation maintains that homicide is a "societal problem over which law enforcement has little or no control."[31] Despite calls for swift and sure punishment of violent offenders, it is often difficult to identify, apprehend and convict perpetrators of violent crime. Wright and colleagues have reported that a burglar's chances of being shot by a homeowner during a burglary are greater than his chances of being arrested.[18] Evidently, deterrence—crime control through fear of criminal justice sanctions—has a limited effect on crime and violence.[30]

Incapacitation. In contrast to the limited impact of deterrence, the strategy of incapacitation (i.e., locking violent criminals away for prolonged periods of time) has proven to be more effective. Unfortunately, it is also very expensive.[30,32] The National Research Council Panel on the Understanding and Control of Violent Behavior recently reviewed the available

data on the impact of increases in sentencing.[30] They concluded that tripling prison sentences (and the prison population) between 1975 and 1989 decreased violent crime in the United States by no more than 15%.

Rehabilitation. Data on the value of rehabilitation appears to be even more discouraging. Critics note that jail has become a "finishing school" for many youthful violent offenders. The glamorization of prison attire and those who have "done time" is particularly disturbing. New approaches are being tried, such as alternative programs for juveniles and boot camps for less dangerous offenders.[33] Comprehensive evaluation of these programs is urgently needed.[30]

Proactive law enforcement. Many law enforcement agencies are beginning to realize that a broad based approach to crime prevention can enhance traditional police strategies. Community policing represents an attempt to restore contact with neighborhoods and the citizens who live there to identify and head off problems before they occur. Proactive efforts to identify and remove illegal firearms from circulation before they are used in violent crime have also shown promise. In Kansas City, a pilot program that targeted illegal guns reduced violent crime in the intervention neighborhood by 50 percent.[34]

Gun control. Since firearms are the principal instrument of fatal interpersonal and self-directed violence in the United States, many people feel that regulations are needed to limit rates of violent crime. Unfortunately, most gun control laws in the United States are not particularly effective.[35] This is because most of these regulations seek to restrict individual *use* of firearms rather than regulate the manufacture or sale of particularly dangerous weapons.[36] Measures to regulate the supply or distribution of particularly dangerous weapons would probably be more effective, but they are difficult to implement in the face of spirited opposition.[35–37]

Zimring has offered a useful typology to classify existing approaches to gun control.[36] In general, regulatory efforts are based on one of three strategies: prohibit high-risk uses of firearms, keep guns out of the hands of high-risk users, or ban high-risk firearms. Most gun laws in the U.S. seek to restrict the place or manner in which guns are used. Examples include laws which ban the discharge of a firearm in a populated area, the carrying of a concealed weapon without a permit or transporting a loaded firearm in a motor vehicle. Unfortunately, place and manner laws are difficult, if not impossible, to enforce. Their effect on preventing gun violence is unclear.[36]

Sentence enhancement statutes seek to deter criminal use of firearms by mandating stiffer penalties for crimes committed with a gun. This approach is popular with gun owners because it is directed towards discouraging gun crime without restricting individual gun ownership. Unfortunately, the penalties associated with serious crimes such as robbery and aggravated assault are already so high that adding more time to these sentences has little deterrent effect.[36] Loftin and colleagues have studied the effect of sentence enhancement statutes in several jurisdictions and found that their overall impact is small.[38]

Efforts to prevent high-risk users from obtaining guns generally fall into one of two strategies: "permissive" licensing systems, which presume that the buyer is eligible to purchase the firearm unless proven otherwise, and "restrictive" licensing systems, which presume that the buyer is *ineligible* to purchase the firearm unless he can prove that he is a member of a particular occupational group (such as the military or the police) or provide documentation of special need.[36] Canada has taken a restrictive approach to handgun purchases, but U.S. gun control has been far more permissive in nature. The relative ease with which handguns can be acquired in the United States has been associated with a higher level of firearm homicide.[39]

Keeping guns out of the hands of "bad guys" while allowing "good guys" to buy millions of them is no simple task.[36] The current federal approach relies on the purchaser to volunteer that he is a convicted felon, an alcoholic or adjudicated mentally ill to be disqualified at the point of sale.[35] Mandatory waiting periods and aggressive background checks in states like California and New Jersey have identified thousands of ineligible buyers, but violent offenders who plea bargain to misdemeanors remain eligible to buy guns.[40] Unfortunately, waiting periods are vehemently opposed by the NRA and other groups who consider them an unreasonable infringe-

ment on the rights of gun owners.[41] Also, federal licensing requirements do not address private transactions. Secondary transfers comprise at least one third of all legitimate firearm sales.[40,42]

Restrictive gun licensing is more effective, but it is also more burdensome to the average gun owner.[36] Loftin and colleagues evaluated the impact of Washington DC's restrictive handgun law on that city's rate of suicides and homicides. Shortly after the law went into effect, firearm homicides declined 25% and firearm suicides dropped by 23%. These declines were not mirrored in neighboring jurisdictions that did not enact the law.[43] Although these reductions were sustained for approximately 10 years, the effects of the law were eventually drowned by the rise in drug and gun smuggling that swamped the District of Columbia in the late 1980s.

The ease with which guns can be transported from a jurisdiction with lax gun control laws to another with tougher laws has blunted or negated the effect of restrictive legislation. Law enforcement agencies in New York City report that 80% or more of the guns they seize were purchased elsewhere.[40] Ironically, the MaClure-Volkmer amendments to the Gun Control Act of 1968 eased federal restrictions on interstate sale of long guns, although existing restrictions on the purchase of handguns were preserved.[41] Virginia was once the leading supplier of guns smuggled up the East Coast, but the state sharply reduced interstate gun trafficking by placing a "one handgun per month" limit on firearm purchases in the state. Other jurisdictions which do not limit gun sales have since taken Virginia's place as major source sites for gun running (R. Browning, Bureau of Alcohol Tobacco and Firearms, personal communication).

Could a national approach to restricting particularly dangerous firearms work? Studies by the Bureau of Alcohol, Tobacco and Firearms indicate that handguns are most likely to be misused in the first few years after their sale. In four U.S. cities, handguns 3 years old or younger constituted half of all weapons confiscated on the streets but only one fourth of firearms owned by civilians.[40] Cook has studied the relationship between community rates of gun ownership and the rate of robbery, armed robbery, and robbery murder. He found that higher rates of gun ownership had no effect on the overall rate of robbery, but rates of gun robbery and robbery murder were directly related to the prevalence of firearm ownership in a community.[44] This suggests that widespread ownership of guns does not deter crime, but simply makes it easier for criminals to acquire and use firearms. A National Research Council panel recently reviewed the data on the connection between guns and violent crime and concluded that greater gun availablity does not affect general violence levels, but it does appear to increase rates of murder and felony gun use.[45]

Enhance oversight of gun dealers. Federally licensed gun dealers serve as gatekeepers to the nation's supply of firearms. By law, they are supposed to screen potential buyers and keep records of their transactions. However, a minority of the more than 200,000 federally licensed dealers actually operate a legitimate retail business. Most obtained their license to purchase firearms through the mail—a privilege withheld from nondealers. Under the current system, almost anyone can become a licensed gun dealer by completing a two-page form and paying a small annual fee. Cook[42] has suggested that state governments could impose stiff state licensing fees and earmark these proceeds to finance dealer monitoring systems to discourage abuses of the system. Since several states have embraced the concept of "instantaneous background checks" at the point of sale, the need for careful screening and oversight of gun dealers is more important than ever.[41,42]

Raise the price of guns. Guns are a commodity. Therefore, any measure that significantly increases their price could discourage sales.[42] Ironically, the federal excise tax on handguns is less than the tax on shotguns and rifles. Increasing the tax on handguns and earmarking this revenue for law enforcement could blunt the sale of handguns and finance efforts to fight gun-related crime. Imposition of a "trauma center" surtax on 9-millimeter ammunition and other calibers that are specific to handguns could achieve the same goal while raising critically needed revenue for the hospitals that treat large numbers of gunshot victims.

Successful lawsuits against irresponsible manufacturers could increase the price of cheap handguns and other dangerous weapons. A single verdict against RG Industries (an importer of Saturday night specials) put that company out of business. Teret and colleagues have proposed that product liability suits should be brought against manufacturers who profit from the sale of poorly made or particularly hazardous firearms.[35,40]

Engineering

Build safer guns. In contrast to the contentious battle over gun control, little attention has been given to the idea of redesigning the weapons themselves. With few exceptions, no state or federal standards for firearm quality, accuracy, or performance exist. Although the Consumer Product Safety Commission has regulatory authority over almost all consumer products sold in America, firearms are specifically excluded from the jurisdiction of the CPSC.[46]

The General Accounting office has estimated that 30% of the unintentional firearm injuries could be prevented if all firearms sold in the United States had an automatic trigger arrestor (i.e., a "safety") and a loading indicator.[3] A "magazine safety" (which locks the trigger when the magazine is removed) would have prevented both of the fatal injuries described at the beginning of this chapter. Unfortunately, the likelihood that safety regulations of this sort will be adopted any time soon is small.[41] This is unfortunate, because improvements in the design of firearms could save the lives of far more children than laws which punish "careless" parents after a tragedy has occurred.

In the absence of better firearm designs, several companies have introduced trigger locks and other mechanical devices to render firearms difficult or impossible to fire by children. These products are better than nothing, but they are not likely to prevent as many injuries as automatic features built into the weapons themselves.[47] *Active* countermeasures, such as manual trigger locks, require the conscious cooperation of the gun owner each and every time they are used to be effective. In contrast, *passive* countermeasures (like automatic trigger arrestors and magazine safeties) exert their protective effects at all times.[9,37]

There is growing interest in the idea of developing technological options to make firearms user-specific. Incorporation of tamper-proof switches or electronic microchips that recognize a user-specific signal could substantially reduce the incidence of unintentional gunshot injures. Firearms of this sort would be useless if stolen. This kind of technology could save lives. Between 1981 and 1990, 16% of the 696 U.S. law enforcement officers killed in the line of duty were shot by their own gun.[48]

Some may argue that any effort to redesign guns or limit their intrinsic capacity to cause harm is pointless in a nation with 200 million guns. However, introduction of modified designs could begin to pay off faster than many people realize. New guns are disproportionately involved in violent crime. Studies suggest that the average life span of a handgun is substantially less than commonly believed, especially if the weapon is diverted into the criminal market.[2] Injury prevention measures introduced today could yield measurable dividends in a short amount of time.[9]

Modify high-risk environments.   In the face of a rising tide of firearm violence, many employers have implemented measures to physically protect their employees.[9] Bullet-proof vests made of Kevlar® have saved the lives of literally hundreds of police officers since they were first introduced.[30] A number of high-risk retail establishments have installed bulletproof booths for their clerks. In response to a growing number of robberies and murders of cab drivers, many cab companies have installed knife and bullet-proof partitions between the driver and the passenger compartment.[9,37]

Although the idea of modifying high-risk environments to prevent intentional injuries is a relatively new concept for public health, criminologists have been writing about "situational crime prevention" for years.[49] Redesigning neighborhoods to create "defensible space" has been advocated as a strategy to discourage crime.[50] Other researchers have identified characteristics that appear to increase a household's risk of burglary.[51] The Southland Corporation has identified specific aspects of the design and operation of convenience stores that can decrease their risk of robbery.[30] These include limiting cash on hand, installing security cameras, and improving visibility of the interior of the store from the parking lot.

Detect weapons.   Enforcement of laws which prohibit the carrying of firearms in high-risk settings can be strengthened by the widespread use of metal detectors and other devices in environments where this equipment can be consistently employed. "Skyjacking" was virtually eliminated in the United States after airports adopted an aggressive weapons screening program. In recent years, use of metal detectors has spread from airport concourses to federal courthouses, hospital emergency departments and a growing number of schools.[52,53] Although magnetometers can be effective, they are expensive and difficult to use.

Promote nonlethal alternatives to guns. Promotion of nonlethal alternatives to firearms could save lives. Introduction of the Taser and similar devices gave law enforcement officers a relatively safe and effective alternative to shooting a violent or disturbed individual.[54,55] Mace, tear gas, pepper spray, and other disabling aerosols are marketed to the public as useful adjuncts for personal protection, but their effectiveness is unclear.

In light of evidence that guns increase rather than decrease the risk of violent death in the home, research is needed to determine if *nonlethal* home security measures (such as electronic security systems, dead-bolt locks and exterior floodlights) are more effective for personal protection. If consumers could be offered safe and effective alternatives to keeping a gun in the home, the demand for "self-protection" firearms could be substantially reduced.

EMERGENCY PHYSICIAN'S ROLE

Public Health Surveillance

Emergency physicians, nurses, and prehospital personnel can play a key role in the prevention of firearm related injuries. Emergency department directors should require that their departments assign external cause of injury codes (E-codes) to all ED visits. This would allow them to track patterns and trends in the incidence of firearm-related trauma. Clinical information could be combined with data abstracted from police offense reports, medical examiner investigations and court proceedings to give a detailed picture of the epidemiology of penetrating trauma in the community. Quantitative data of this sort could help mobilize community resources and justify expenditures for trauma care. After sizing up the extent of the problem, ED based injury surveillance data could be used to evaluate the impact of community-based interventions to reduce firearm injuries and combat violent crime.[30,56]

Primary and Secondary Prevention

In addition to promoting community based primary prevention programs, emergency physicians must also become more aggressive at promoting secondary prevention. Studies have shown that patients admitted to trauma centers have high rates of recurrent injury and violent death.[57] The prevalence of concurrent problems such as alcoholism, drug dependence, and mental illness is also high. Unfortunately, few hospitals attempt to address these issues in a systematic way. Discharge planning is often limited to meeting the patient's immediate physical needs.[9]

Implementing a comprehensive program of care for victims of violence can be extraordinarily difficult. Youthful victims of assault are often unwilling to identify their assailant out of fear of retaliation or a desire for revenge. Proper planning for follow-up is impossible when a patient leaves suddenly against medical advice. Sometimes, it is even difficult to establish the true nature of the injury.

Victims of battering are particularly reluctant to divulge how their injuries occurred. One research team found that hospital emergency department staff fail to identify three out of every four victims of domestic violence.[58] It is essential that trauma care providers make every effort to identify victims of violence and offer them assistance. Battering tends to increase in frequency and severity over time.[59,60] If nothing is done to break the cycle of violence, battering can escalate and eventually lead to a homicide.[61,62]

Advocacy

Emergency physicians and other trauma care professionals can be influential advocates for injury prevention and control. Organizations like the American Public Health Association, the American Trauma Society, the Society for Academic Emergency Medicine, the Committee on Trauma for the American College of Surgeons, the American College of Emergency Physicians, the Eastern Association for the Surgery of Trauma, and the American Nurse's Association have helped shape public policy through public education and support of specific legislation. The testimony of individual emergency physicians, trauma surgeons, EMTs, and emergency nurses has added compelling relevance to otherwise dry statistics. Effective strategies to prevent trauma should not be blocked by accusations that a specific initiative is "pro" or "anti" gun. Emergency physicians and other professionals can play a key role in reshaping the terms of this debate.

CONCLUSION

The toll of firearm related violence and injuries in the United States is unacceptably high. Historically, both the police and emergency department personnel have reacted to these incidents after they occur. At this point, little is being done to prevent these tragedies. However, there is growing evidence that a proactive approach that stresses the value of prevention may enhance and compliment the traditional strategies of law enforcement and acute care. Options to prevent firearm-related injuries include education of the public and gun owners, enforcement of existing gun control laws, and engineering to build safer guns and reduce the threat of injury in high-risk environments. Effective reduction of firearm-related violence must involve the entire community. Emergency department staff can play a key role in this effort.

NOTES

1. Lee RK, Harris MJ. Unintentional firearm injuries: The price of protection. In Zwerling C, McMillan D. Firearm injuries: a public health approach. *Am J Preventive Med* 1993; 9 (3)(suppl):16–20.
2. Cook PJ. The technology of personal violence. In Tonry M (ed.). *Crime and justice: A review of research.* Chicago: University of Chicago Press, 1991:14:1–71.
3. U.S. General Accounting Office. *Accidental shootings: Many deaths and injuries caused by firearms could be prevented.* Gaithersburg, MD: U.S. General Accounting Office (Doc no. GAO/PEMD-91-9); March 1991.

4. Fingerhut LA, Jones C, Makuc DM. *Firearm and motor vehicle injury mortality—Variations by state, race, and ethnicity: United States, 1990–1991. Advance data from the vital and health statistics; no. 242.* Hyattsville MD: National Center for Health Statistics, 1994.

5. Zahn M. Homicide in the twentieth century: Trends, types, and causes. In Gurr, TR (ed.). *Violence in America, vol 1: The History of Crime.* Newbury Park, CA: Sage Publications, 1989.

6. Fingerhut LA. *Firearm mortality among children, youth, and young adults 1–34 years of age, trends and current status: United States, 1985–1990. Advance data from vital and health statistics; no. 231.* Hyattsville, MD: National Center for Health Statistics, 1993.

7. Committee on Trauma Research. *Injury in America: A continuing public health problem.* Washington, DC, National Academy Press, 1985.

8. Haddon W. Advances in the epidemiology of injuries as a basis for public policy. *Pub Health Rep* 1980; 95:411–21.

9. Kellermann AL, Lee RK, Mercy JA, Banton JG. The epidemiologic basis for the prevention of firearm injuries. *Ann Rev Pub Health* 1991; 12:17–40.

10. Prothrow-Stith D. Interventions, intentional injuries, groups at the greatest risk, violence prevention. *Pub Health Rep* 1987; 102:615–16.

11. Rosenberg ML, Mercy JA. Assaultive violence. In Rosenberg ML, Fenley MA (eds.). *Violence in America: A public health approach.* New York: Oxford University Press, 1991. pp. 14–50.

12. Slaby RG, Guerra NG. Cognitive mediators of aggression in adolescent offenders. *Develop Psychol* 1988; 24:580–8.

13. Webster DW. The unconvincing case for school-based conflict resolution programs for adolescents. *Health Affairs* Spring, 1995.

14. Hammond WR, Young BR. Preventing violence in at risk African American youth. *J Health Care Poor Underserved* 1991; 2:359–73.

15. Weil DS, Hemenway D. Loaded guns in the home: Analysis of a national random survey of gun owners. *JAMA* 1992; 267:3033–7.

16. Robertson LS, Kelly AB, O'Neill B, et al. A controlled study of the effect of television messages on safety belt use. *Am J Pub Health* 1974; 64:1071–80.

17. Robertson LS. Crash involvement of teenage drivers when driver education is eliminated from high school. *Am J Pub Health* 1980; 70:599–601.

18. Wright JD, Rossi PH, Daly K, Weber-Burdin E. *Weapons, crime and violence in America: A literature review and research agenda.* U.S. Department of Justice, National Institute of Justice. Washington, DC, U.S. Government Printing Office, 1981, pp 239–44.

19. Kellermann AL, Reay DT. Protection or peril? An analysis of firearm related deaths in the home. *N Engl J Med* 1986; 314:1557–60.

20. Kellermann AL, Rivara FP, Somes G, Reay DT, et al. Suicide in the home in relation to gun ownership. *N Engl J Med* 1992; 327:467–72.

21. Brent DA, Perper JA, Allman CJ, Moritz GM, Wartella ME, Zelenak JP. The presence and accessability of firearms in the home of adolescent suicides: A case-control study. *JAMA* 1992; 266:2989–95.

22. Brent DA, Perper JA, Goldstein CE, et al. Risk factors for adolescent suicide: a comparison of adolescent suicide victims with suicidal inpatients. *Arch Gen Psychiat* 1988; 45:581–8.

23. Kellermann AL, Rivara FP, Rushforth N et al. Gun ownership as a risk factor for homicide in the home. *N Engl J Med* 1993; 329:1084–91.

24. Saltzman LE, Mercy JA, O'Carroll P, Rosenberg M, Rhodes P. Weapon involvement and injury outcomes in family and intimate assaults. *JAMA* 1992; 267:3043–7.

25. Wintemute GJ, Teret SP, Kraus JF, Wright MA, Bradfield G. When children shoot children: 88 unintended deaths in California. *JAMA* 1987; 257:3107–9.

26. Webster DW, Wilson MEH, Duggan AK, Pakula LC. Parents' beliefs about preventing gun injuries in children. *Pediatr* 1992; 89:908–14.

27. Patterson PJ, Smith L. Firearms in the home and child safety. *Am J Dis Child* 1987; 141:221–3.

28. Hemenway D, Solnick SJ, Azrael DR. Firearm training and storage. *JAMA* 1995; 273:46–50.

29. Pendered D. Guns get warning label Nov. 1: Tags are required on all weapons sold in Fulton. *Atlanta Constitution,* October 6, 1994, p. 1.

30. Panel on the Understanding and Control of Violent Behavior. Reiss A, Roth J (eds.). *Understanding and Controlling Violence.* Washington, DC, National Academy Press, 1993.

31. U.S. Department of Justice. *Crime in the United States, 1986: Uniform Crime Reports for the United States.* Washington, DC, Federal Bureau of Investigation, 1987.

32. Langan, PA. America's soaring prison population. *Science* 1991; 251:1568–73.

33. Wilson JJ, Howell JC. *Comprehensive Strategy for Serious, Violent, and Chronic Juvenile Offenders: Program Summary,* 2nd ed. Office of Juvenile Justice and Delinquency Prevention, Washington, DC: U.S. Department of Justice, June 1994.

34. Butterfield F. Novel attack on gunmen: Get the guns. *The New York Times* Sunday, November 20, 1994, p. 22.

35. Webster DE, Chaulk CP, Teret SP, Wintemute GJ. Reducing firearm injuries. *Iss Science Technol* Spring 1991:73–9.

36. Zimring FE. Firearms, violence and public policy. *Scientific Am* 1991; 11:48–54.

37. Baker SP, Teret SP, Dietz PE. Firearms and the Public's Health. *J Pub Health Pol* 1980; 1:224–9.

38. Loftin C, McDowall D, Wiersema B. Evaluating effects of changes in gun laws. In Zwerling C, McMillan D. Firearm injuries: A public health approach. *Am J Preventive Med* 1993; 9(3):Suppl: 39–43.

39. Sloan JH, Kellermann AL, Reay DT, et al. Handgun regulations, crime, assault and homicide: A tale of two cities. *N Engl J Med* 1988; 319:1256–62.

40. Wintemute GJ, Hancock M, Loftin C, McGuire A, Pertschuk M, Teret S. Policy options in firearm violence. In Samuels SE, Smith MD (eds.). *Improving the Health of the Poor.* Menlo Park, CA: The Henry Kaiser Foundation, 1992.

41. Davidson OG. *Under Fire: The NRA and the Battle for Gun Control.* New York: Henry Holt, 1993.

42. Cook PJ. Notes on the availability and prevalence of firearms. In Zwerling C, McMillan D. Firearm injuries: A public health approach. *Am J Preventive Med* 1993; 9(3):Suppl: 33–8.

43. Loftin C, McDowall D, Wiersema B, Cottey TJ. Effects of restrictive licensing of handguns on homicide and suicide in the District of Columbia. *N Engl J Med* 1991; 325:1615–20.

44. Cook PJ. The effect of gun availability on robbery and robbery murder: A cross section study of fifty cities. In Haveman RH, Zellner BB (eds.). *Pol Stud Rev Ann* 1979; 3:743–81.

45. Roth JA. *Firearms and violence: National Institute of Justice research in brief.* Washington DC: National Institute of Justice, Office of Justice Programs, U.S. Department of Justice, NCJ 145533, February 1994, pp. 1–7.

46. Robertson L, Stallones L, Branche-Dorsey C, et al. Home and leisure injury prevention. In *Position papers from the third national injury control conference.* Atlanta: U.S. Department of Health and Human Services, Public Health Service, Centers for Disease Control and Prevention, 1992, pp. 253–319.

47. Kellermann AL, Hutson HR. Injury Control. In Schwartz GR (ed.). *Principles and Practice of Emergency Medicine.* Philadelphia: Lea and Febiger, 1992.

48. *Law enforcement officers killed and assaulted. Uniform Crime Reports.* Washington, DC: U.S. Department of Justice, Federal Bureau of Investigation, 1991.

49. Clarke RV. Situational crime prevention: Its theoretical basis and practical scope in crime and justice. In Tonry M., *Crime and justice: A review of research.* Chicago: University of Chicago Press, 1986

50. Newman O. *Defensible space: Crime prevention through urban design.* New York: Macmillan, 1972.

51. McDonald J, Clifford B. Territorial cues and defensible space theory: The burglar's point of view. *J of Environ Psychol* 1989; 9:193–205.

52. Donahue, T. *Weapons in schools. OJJDP Juvenile Justice Bulletin.* Washington, DC: U.S. Department of Justice, Office of Justice Programs, October, 1989.

53. Thompson B. Incidence and type of hazardous objects found among patients and visitors screened by magnetometer in an urban emergency center. *Ann Emerg Med* 1992; 21:618–19.

54. Ordog GJ. Electronic gun (Taser)injuries. *Ann Emerg Med* 1987; 16:73–8.

55. O'Brien DJ. Electronic weaponry—A question of safety. *Ann Emerg Med* 1991; 20:583–7.

56. National Committee for Injury Prevention and Control. Program design and evaluation. In Injury control: meeting the challenge. *Am J Prev Med* 1989; 5:Suppl:63–88.

57. Sims DW, Bivins BA, Farouck NO, Horst FM, Sorensen VJ, Fath JJ. Urban trauma: A chronic recurrent disease. *J Trauma* 1989; 29:940–7.

58. McCleer SV, Anwar RAH, Herman S, Maquiling K. Education is not enough: A systems failure in protecting battered women. *Ann Emerg Med* 1989; 18: 651–3.

59. American Medical Association. Violence against women: Relevance for medical practitioners. *J Am Med Assoc* 1992; 267:3184–9.

60. National Committee for Injury Prevention and Control. Domestic Violence. In Injury control: Meeting the challenge. *Am J Prev Med* 1989; 5:Suppl:223–32.

61. Mercy JA, Saltzman LE. Fatal violence among spouses in the United States, 1976–1985. *Am J Pub Health* 1989; 79:595–9.

62. Kellermann AL, Mercy JA. Men, women, and murder: Gender-specific differences in rates of fatal violence and victimization. *J Trauma* 1992; 33:1–5.

26

Safety Restraint Legislation

MARK D. PEARLMUTTER

CONTENTS

- The historical perspective
- The Massachusetts experience
- The role of the emergency physician in patient care, data collection, and research and advocacy

CHAPTER SUMMARY

Using the Massachusetts experience with seat-belt legislation as an example, this chapter illustrates how the emergency physician can have a significant impact on public health policy. Through surveillance, data collection, research, education, or community involvement, the emergency physician can play a vital role in injury prevention. A multifaceted, integrative approach to passage and retention of a seat-belt law is described.

Case #1

A 36-year-old black female presented to the ED after being involved in a car crash. As the patient described it, because she was driving her van within a mile of her home she didn't feel that a seat belt was necessary. Suddenly, and without warning, her left rear tire blew out while she was traveling around a curve at approximately 30 mph. She tried to maintain control, but her vehicle pulled to the left and struck a telephone pole head on. She recalls very little of what ensued.

Comment: "It's such a nuisance to wear a seat belt when I'm doing errands in and around my neighborhood where I almost never travel faster than 35 mph. However, I always wear my seat belt when I'm on the highway."

Three out of four crashes occur within 25 miles of the driver's or victim's home and on roads with posted speed limits of 45 mph or less. Hitting the windshield at 30 mph is like falling from the third story of a building.[1] Seat belts keep the head from making contact with the steering wheel, windshield, and dashboard.

Case Continuation

The paramedic report described moderate front-end damage with spidering of the windshield and an intact steering column. The patient was initially found conscious yet confused with multiple glass fragments embedded in her forehead and a 2 cm laceration to her nose. She was fully immobilized and transported to our ED where a head CT, chest x-ray, and facial and C-spine films were significant only for a nasal fracture. Her laceration was repaired and glass fragments removed from her forehead. Because of persistent confusion, she was hospitalized and discharged the following day in good condition. During her follow-up visit and over the next few months she complained of frequent dizzy spells and daily headaches. Her forehead injury eventually required dermabrasion for satisfactory cosmesis.

The author wishes to acknowledge the contribution of Jonathan Fischer, MS II, Tufts University Medical School, who assisted in the preparation of this manuscript.

Q: Is there any evidence that clearly demonstrates the injury reduction afforded by seat belts?

Seat belts allow the force of sudden deceleration to be transmitted to other portions of the body where the impact is better tolerated.[2] An emergency department study in New Mexico looked at the incidence of soft-tissue injuries to the head, face, and neck before and after the 1986 New Mexico Safety Restraint Law, and showed a 38% reduction in these injuries.[3] During a short-lived mandatory seat belt law in Massachusetts, usage rates increased from 20% to 37%, while occupant injuries were reduced by 20%.[4] In other studies it has been shown that belted patients have anywhere between a 20 to 50% reduction in facial and other moderate to severe injuries, when compared to the unrestrained crash victim.[5–7] This is not to say that seat belts are not associated with injury. Subtle and frequently overlooked injuries may occur, often as a result of an improperly worn seat belt or shoulder harness.[8] Overall however, injury severity scores, hospitalization rates, and acute medical care costs are significantly reduced.[5–9]

Case #2

A 15-year-old female presented to the ED on a Sunday holiday for evaluation of a knee injury sustained in a motor-vehicle crash. According to the patient, she and four of her friends were riding along a Massachusetts interstate when they were suddenly cut off by a car attempting to pass them on the left. The vehicle in which she was traveling at a speed of 60 mph swerved to the right and spun wildly out of control. The patient, who was sitting in the right front passenger seat, was the only occupant wearing a seat belt. Their vehicle rolled over twice, throwing her four friends 15 to 30 feet from the car. All except the patient were killed instantly. Her ED evaluation revealed only two deep lacerations to her right leg. She was treated and released the same day.

Q: How do you compare the overall risks of not wearing a seat belt with the risk of literally being trapped in your seat belt when your car catches on fire or becomes submerged in water?

This frequently heard statement, a scenario seen all too frequently on television, is a common misconcep-

tion. In fact, one is 25 times more likely to be killed if thrown free of a vehicle after a crash.[1] The incidence of crashes resulting in fire or water immersion are well under one-half of one percent. To put this in perspective, according to the Fatality Accident Reporting System (FARS), of the 365,000 occupant deaths in the last 10 years, only 9,200 people (2.5%) have been killed in crashes involving fire or water immersion.[10] Of these, it is felt that seat-belt usage was actually protective overall, since it secured the crash victim firmly in the seat, reducing head and body injury severity and allowing for more rapid exit from a burning or submerged vehicle. Overall, it is conservatively estimated that lap and shoulder belts reduce the risk of fatal injury to passenger occupants by 45%.[11] Moreover, unbelted occupants in a motor-vehicle crash are twice as likely to be injured. Simply stated, if everyone wore seat belts, nearly 9,000 lives would be saved in just 1 year.

Q: Whether or not seat belts are associated with an increased likelihood of injury or even death, isn't it my personal right to choose?

As emergency physicians, we can attest to the price we all pay in the name of personal freedom. Whether one considers the nation's collective health care costs, the pain and suffering of family and friends, or the utilization of precious prehospital and hospital resources, the issue goes well beyond individual freedom. It is the public health of society that is at stake.

HISTORICAL PERSPECTIVE

When automobiles first arrived on scene at the turn of the century, many were equipped with seat belts. In those days, seat belts were used primarily to prevent passengers from being literally bounced out of cars as they rode along bumpy unpaved roads. As roads improved and cars became enclosed, seat belts disappeared from most cars. In 1950, the Nash became the first car to offer factory-installed seat belts. It wasn't until January 1968 that the federal government required automobile manufacturers to install both lap and shoulder belts in all new cars.[12] Passengers soon complained that seat belts were too restrictive and uncomfortable to wear. Manufacturers responded in 1974 by introducing the automatic

Figure 26-1 Usage Increases with Enactment of Laws

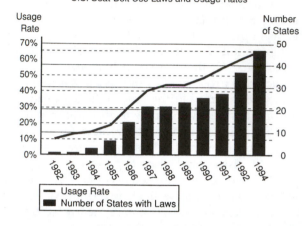

U.S. Seat-Belt Use Laws and Usage Rates

three-point seat-belt system that locks only when the car rapidly decelerates.[13] This technology made seat belts somewhat more comfortable and a bit more popular. Since 1990, lap-and-shoulder-type belts are also required for rear seats.

During the 1970s and early 1980s, it was estimated that between 10 and 20% of Americans were buckling up.[14] It wasn't until 1984 that New York became the first state to pass a mandatory seat-belt usage law that usage rates climbed to greater than 50%. Over the next 10 years, 48 of 50 states followed New York's lead by passing some form of mandatory seat-belt legislation. By 1994, the national seat-belt usage rate was 66%. (see Figure 26-1).

THE MASSACHUSETTS EXPERIENCE

The Massachusetts experience with seat-belt laws provides an example of how a multifaceted integrated team approach can favorably affect public health legislation. In 1985, Massachusetts' seat-belt usage rate was 20%. One year later, Massachusetts joined a growing list of states with a seat-belt law. Within several months of its enactment, seat-belt usage rates rose to 37%, a 17% increase. Generally, seat-belt usage increases anywhere between 10 and 20% following passage of seat-belt legislation. How-

ever, in the cradle of the American Revolution, civil libertarians raised objections. Spearheaded by a popular radio talk show host, they cited the personal right to choose. As a result, the seat-belt law was placed on a statewide referendum, where it was narrowly defeated 11 months later by a 53% to 47% vote. Unfortunately, immediately following repeal of the 1986 mandatory seat-belt law, seat-belt usage rates dropped to 24%, a 13% decrease.[15]

Without a seat-belt law, Massachusetts's traffic safety advocates shifted their focus to seat-belt education and awareness programs. This push was strengthened by passage of the Federal Intermodal Surface Transportation Efficiency Act of 1991 (ISTEA), which provided economic incentives to States which have enacted mandatory seat-belt use laws. Under section 153 of this act, states that have not passed mandatory seat-belt laws must set aside a certain amount of their federal highway dollars to support highway safety education. Despite this and other state and local efforts, seat-belt usage rates increased slightly over an 8-year period peaking at 32% in 1994. At that time, Massachusetts ranked forty-ninth in the nation in seat-belt usage rates (less than half the national average) and was only one of five states without a seat-belt law. It was clear that a mandatory seat-belt law was the only way to increase Massachusetts' usage rates to levels approximating the national average.

ROLE OF THE EMERGENCY PHYSICIAN

Patient Care

Motor-vehicle crashes are the leading cause of trauma and the leading cause of death in the 1 through 44 age group.[1,11] Each year, almost 40,000 people die in motor-vehicle crashes and an additional 5 million people are injured. Nationwide, over 2 million people per year visit our nation's emergency departments for injuries related to motor-vehicle crashes.[11] Nearly 80,000 of these total emergency department visits per year are in Massachusetts alone. As a result, the emergency physician has become highly proficient in the recognition of injury patterns and the acute management of the trauma patient. Beyond our expertise in patient care, the emergency encounter also provides us with a profoundly teachable moment to modify our patients' behavior patterns. In Massachusetts, for example, through individual patient counseling and placing of instructional brochures, posters, and even videos in our waiting areas, emergency physicians demonstrated their sense of community responsibility by educating patients and family about traffic safety and injury prevention.

Data Collection and Research

In 1986, during the 11 months the law was in effect, Massachusetts witnessed a 5% decline in death rates compared to a 1% increase in neighboring states that did not pass seat-belt laws.[15] Furthermore, while seat-belt usage rates increased 17%, data obtained from the Massachusetts Registry of Motor Vehicles and emergency department surveillance studies indicated that occupant injuries fell 20%, the equivalent of 10,000 prevented injuries. Conversely, when usage rates dropped 13% shortly after repeal of the law, motor-vehicle occupant injuries increased 11%.[4] Thus, the short lived 1986 mandatory seat-belt law provided Massachusetts emergency physicians with valuable pre- and post-seat-belt injury surveillance data.

Taking advantage of the changing climate in our health care system from a treatment to prevention model, emergency department studies focused on health care cost analyses. One of the first of such studies demonstrated that seat-belt use reduced one particular hospital's charges by 30% compared to unbelted car crash victims, a difference that could save their community hospital $100,000 in yearly treatment costs.[16] A Boston City Hospital Emergency Department study compared the relative ED and overall hospital charges of motor-vehicle crash injuries to belted versus unbelted occupants. They found that ED charges alone averaged 65% less for belted patients ($545 versus $331), a $500,000 yearly savings.[17] Total hospital charges amounted to an additional $1.5 million spent annually treating the unbelted crash victim. Similarly, a Massachusetts General Hospital trauma registry study found that total inpatient hospital days averaged 92% less for patients who wore their seat belts. This was equivalent to a cost difference of $2.7 million yearly.[18] With this data, it was estimated that bodily injury claims, the main component of high auto insurance premi-

ums, could be reduced by $186 million. So convincing were these studies that insurance companies offered a 5% reduction in bodily injury premiums if a mandatory seat-belt law was passed.

Attention also focused on the human side of injury reduction afforded by seat-belt use. Results of studies demonstrating reductions in potentially disfiguring facial and neck injuries by 38% were circulated.[3]

This research in emergency medicine clearly demonstrated the public health benefits of a mandatory seat-belt law. Through prevention of human suffering, injury reduction, and cost savings, seat-belt advocates in Massachusetts were able to build a strong case for reinstatement of the mandatory seat-belt law. The door was now opened wide for the emergency medicine community to enter into a statewide partnership as a convincing and influential advocate for public health policy.

Advocacy

It is well known that emergency physicians see firsthand the human pain and suffering of injuries related to motor-vehicle trauma. As a result, we are in a key position to effectively speak out on and lead injury prevention and public safety campaigns. One such grassroots coalition—the Massachusetts Advocates for Traffic Safety (MATS), formed in 1991—consisted of members representing the fields of health care, public safety, local government, business, civic and public health agencies, and advocacy groups. Because of its membership's broad base, MATS was able to marshal its various resources effectively to convince the legislature, media, and community at large to support reinstatement of a mandatory seat-belt law.

Although the seat-belt bill was again introduced, it was not until 1993 that it survived the legislative gamut and eventually made its way to the governor's desk. The bill was initially assigned to the public safety committee, where emergency physicians were among many who provided compelling personal testimony during public hearings. MATS worked closely with the bill's sponsor and members of the public safety committee to ensure a favorable report out of committee. As the bill worked its way through floor debates and various readings, the emergency medicine community assumed a leadership role

Figure 26-2

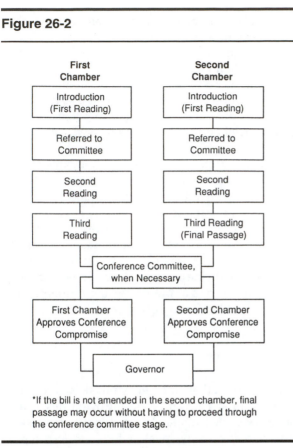

First Chamber / Second Chamber

Introduction (First Reading) / Introduction (First Reading)

Referred to Committee / Referred to Committee

Second Reading / Second Reading

Third Reading / Third Reading (Final Passage)

Conference Committee, when Necessary

First Chamber Approves Conference Compromise / Second Chamber Approves Conference Compromise

Governor

*If the bill is not amended in the second chamber, final passage may occur without having to proceed through the conference committee stage.

within MATS through its influential voice in the community, its lobbying efforts, and its interactions with the print, radio, and television media. Throughout Massachusetts' year-long legislative session, MATS continuously brought attention to the bill by collecting and compiling statistics, circulating fact sheets, collecting survivors stories, contacting media, writing editorials, promoting a speakers forum, and sponsoring a seat-belt survivor conference. Late in the legislative session, the bill finally made its way intact through both chambers as well as through the conference committee, only to be vetoed by the governor. (See Figure 26-2.) In response, MATS's entire membership was mobilized to override the veto. The Massachusetts College of Emergency Physicians sent a legislative alert to its total membership urging them to immediately call and write their state legislators requesting their support on this issue. As a result of these efforts, the legislature overrode the governor's veto and the law took effect in February 1994. Predictably, civil libertarians once again organized and

put the seat-belt law and the right to choose back on the November referendum.

The future of the seat-belt law was once again threatened by repeal. This time, however, libertarian zealots were not to be successful. Observational studies of seat-belt compliance during the first 6 months of the new law recorded an increase in usage from 32% to 47%.[19] Although a 12% drop in traffic fatalities was found during this time period it was not necessarily felt to be related to enhanced seat-belt compliance. What proved quite timely, however, was a study of medical costs related to motor-vehicle crashes conducted at Boston City Hospital Emergency Department which revealed a 39% drop in actual costs during the first 5 months of the new seat-belt law and a concomitant 42% relative reduction in soft-tissue injuries of the head, face and neck.[20] This finding corroborated earlier studies and provided further concrete evidence that seat-belt laws positively impact public health. The voters responded favorably to the new seat-belt law by a margin of 59% to 41%.

CONCLUSION

Using the Massachusetts seat-belt experience, this chapter seeks to assist and encourage the emergency physician to look beyond the acute treatment and management of the injured patient. Educational, surveillance, and research activities of emergency physicians are described. A traffic safety partnership model is presented to demonstrate how a well-integrated multidisciplinary injury prevention effort can successfully change public policy and societal beliefs toward injuries resulting from non-seat-belt use. By playing an advocacy role in the community, the emergency physician can assume a leadership position in other public health and injury reduction campaigns.

NOTES

1. U.S. Department of Transportation, National Highway Transportation Safety Administration. *1991 Occupant Protection Facts.* Washington, DC: NHTSA, 1992.
2. Sato TB. Effects of seat belts and injuries resulting from improper seat belt use. *J Trauma* 1957; 27:754–8.

3. Bernstein E, Pathek D, et al. New Mexico safety restraint law: Changing patterns of motor vehicle injury, severity and cost. *Am J Emerg Med* 1989; 7:221–7.

4. Hingson R, Levenson S, et al. Repeal of the Massachusetts seat belt law. *Am J Pub Health* 1988; 78:548–52.

5. Nakhegevany KB. Facial trauma in motor vehicle accidents: Etiological factors. *Am J Emerg Med* 1994; 12;160–3.

6. Hendey OW, Votey SR. Injuries in restrained motor vehicle accident victims. *Ann Emerg Med* 1994; 24: 77–84.

7. Lessino PC, Williams AP, et al: Motor vehicle crash injury patterns and the Virginia seat belt law. *JAMA* 1991; 165:1409–13.

8. Reath DR, Kirby J, Lynch M, et al: Injury and cost comparison of restrained and unrestrained motor vehicle crash victims. *J Trauma* 1989; 29:1173.

9. Marine, WM, Kerwin EM, et al. Mandatory seatbelts: Epidemiologic, financial, and medical rationale from the Colorado matched pairs study. *J Trauma* 1994; 36:96–100.

10. National Highway Transportation Safety Administration. *Fatality Accident Report System.* Washington DC: US Department of Transportation, 1993.

11. National Safety Council: *Accident Facts.* Itasca, IL: National Safety Council, 1993.

12. National Highway Transportation Safety Administration. *Occupant Protection Idea Sampler.* Washington, DC: U.S. Department of Transportation, 1994.

13. *About Cars: When will we learn to buckle up? The New York Times,* December 19, 1993.

14. National Highway Transportation Safety Administration. *Safety Belts: A history lesson for adults.* Washington, DC: U.S. Department of Transportation, 1992.

15. Hingson R, Levenson S, et al. *Safety Belt Use, and Motor Vehicle Occupant Injuries and Deaths in Massachusetts.* A report prepared for the Massachusetts Governor's Highway Safety Bureau, 1993.

16. Yeh C. New England Medical Center, unpublished data.

17. Bernstein E. Boston City Hospital, unpublished data.

18. Massachusetts General Hospital Trauma Service, unpublished data.

19. Hingson R. *Trends in driver behaviors, belief and traffic crashes: Massachusetts 1980–1993.* Boston: Massachusetts Governor's Highway Safety Bureau, 1993.

20. Bernstein E, Weikovich B, Hingson R, Heeren T, Accera K. Safety restraint law reduces soft tissue injuries and ED/hospital charges (abs). *Acad Emerg Med* 1995; 2:341.

Adolescent Social Action Program (ASAP)

ROBERT M. GOUGELET
LILY DOW
NINA B. WALLERSTEIN

Reflection without action is mere verbalism.
Action without reflection is pure activism.

—Training for Transformation

CONTENTS

- Epidemiology of substance abuse and violence among adolescents
- Prevention programs: description and theoretical basis
- Role of emergency department providers

CHAPTER SUMMARY

This chapter describes the New Mexico–based Adolescent Social Action Program (ASAP) and how an emergency medicine department is participating in prevention activities to address alcohol, substance abuse, violence, and other risky behaviors of adolescents. Through participation in this program, middle and high school students interview patients at the University Hospital Emergency Department and residents at the local detention center to become familiar with the consequences of alcohol and drug abuse. The chapter describes the role of the University, Hospital, Detention Center, and ASAP in preparing these students for the interviews, group discussions, and the follow-up process, which encourages the students to make healthy choices and to take an active role in promoting change within their lives and communities.

The chapter also presents case studies and defines the program in its broader public health context. The first case study is an account of an ED patient whose story of violence and the untimely death of a loved one contributed to her frequent visits to the ED. An emergency physician reflects on his role as a "facilitator" of the youth groups in ASAP and the relevance of this patient's story to emergency department operations and roles. The second case relays the consequences of a 17-year-old Native American woman's decision not to ride home with her inebriated brother after participating in ASAP. The third case involves an emergency department nurse whose 20 years of experience and commitment to working with young people is displayed daily in his job, at home, and in many other extracurricular activities dealing with youth. His dedication and conviction serve as a model to other hospital staff to become change agents and role models. The following three scenarios provide a brief glimpse of the program and its positive impact on the individuals involved, from the three perspectives of patient, adolescent participant, and health care provider. These vignettes are followed by a more detailed discussion of the problems of adolescent substance abuse and violence, the goals of prevention, a description of the ASAP program and a discussion of its broader implications.

Case #1

A 32-year-old female was brought into the emergency department (ED) by ambulance with a chief complaint of acute alcohol intoxication. The patient was triaged by the ED staff as "yellow," or noncritical, as the triage examination did not reveal any significant injury. On a Friday night, this meant a wait of at least 3 to 4 hours. The patient was introduced pejoratively by a cynical ED staff member as a "frequent flyer." A quick assessment of her medical chart revealed brief notes written by doctors and staff who had spent only minutes speaking with and evaluating her physical condition.

The ASAP participants were waiting in a nearby conference room when the charge nurse informed them the patient in cubicle 11 had volunteered to be interviewed. This was the group's first exposure to the emergency room environment and their first group encounter with a patient. The students were anxious to begin the interview. The patient, as is usually the case, displayed a sense of relief at having caring and interested people to talk with. She talked frankly with the group about how she got started drinking in her early teens, after her mother died. "I was so sad," she said, "and there was nobody to turn to. I'd be babysitting, and they'd give me a beer. I guess that was what I was worth. . . ." The students faces grew sad as they listened to her quiet voice, and expressed empathy for how hard her life had been.

Afterward, the patient told the preceptors that she appreciated being listened to, and she hoped these young people would learn something so they wouldn't have to do what she had done, and might have a chance to live a better life. The preceptor, who was an emergency physician, was acutely aware of the contrast between the stereotypical way the patient was perceived by ED staff and the depth and richness of experience she was able to share with the young people. Conversing with ASAP participants often results in a dialogue that is therapeutic for all parties involved. The debriefing and discussion period that followed the 45-minute interview was dominated by concern for the woman. The students expressed shock that this woman had suffered such horrible consequences to behaviors started so early in life. The discussion brought to life personal experiences from within the group, and facilitated both sharing and self-examination.

Case #2

Mary, a 17-year-old Native American from rural New Mexico, joined ASAP along with several other young people from her community. One Friday evening, the group, accompanied by an adult sponsor, drove 50 miles to Albuquerque's University Hospital Emergency Department with anticipation and excitement. This particular evening, several patients volunteered to share their personal experiences, hardships, and frustrations. Following the emotional interviews, the group met in the debriefing room. The intense dialogue among the youth reflected the dynamic process that was taking place among the ASAP participants.

The next day, Mary was invited to attend a party with her 19-year-old brother, Frank, and his friend. While at the party, Frank and his friend drank heavily. When the party ended, Frank tried to get Mary to ride home with them. Mary, recalling her experience in the emergency department the night before, refused to ride home with her inebriated brother and his friend. The group had role played how to say no, and she used the words that had been suggested by one of her peers. During the early morning hours, officers came to Mary's home. Frank and his friend had been involved in a serious automobile accident and both were taken to the University Hospital's Emergency Department. Frank suffered from severe closed head injuries and his friend suffered multiple internal injuries, lacerations, and contusions. Both men survived the accident that night, but Frank continues to have residual deficits which affect his daily activities.

Mary's decision not to ride home with Frank was clearly related to her participation in the ASAP program the night before. The program enabled Mary to make a positive decision for herself, which in this case may have saved her life.

Case #3

For over 20 years, Michael has worked as a trauma nurse specialist at the University Hospital's Trauma Center. The nature of his work continues to impress upon him the need for medical professionals to actively participate with young people in the community. Michael is currently facilitating an ASAP youth group from rural New Mexico, which is primarily composed of Hispanic high school students. Michael attempts to draw upon similarities between the patients' stories and those of many of the adolescent interviewers. He is often astounded at how hardened these young people have become to the psychosocial consequences of alcohol, tobacco and other drug use.

Michael states, "I've known about ASAP since its inception 12 years ago and my first impression was that it was much needed. In our emergency room, alcohol and drugs are the greatest contributor to the trauma that we see. It is my hope that ASAP and other prevention programs will cut down on the trauma related cases I've triaged. I'm convinced that I'm making a difference as a role model and as an adult interested in working with young people. It helps me to do a reality check with my own children and enables me to actively take part in prevention efforts outside the emergency department."

THE BROADER PUBLIC HEALTH CONTEXT

Drug- and alcohol-related morbidity and mortality, while affecting all segments of society, is having a devastating affect on our nation's youth. Unintentional injuries are the leading cause of death in U.S. citizens aged 13 to 18. Mortality related to alcohol and other substance abuse, as well as interpersonal violence, takes its greatest toll on those youth who live below the poverty line.[1]

According to the 1990 census, New Mexico was rated the second poorest state in the nation. One-fourth of its children live in poverty, compared to 20% nationwide. Twenty-eight percent of Hispanics, who comprise 39% of the population, live below poverty level, whereas 46% of Native Americans (9% of the population) and 28% of African Americans (2% of the population) are below poverty level.[2]

Mortality among New Mexican teenagers is 33% higher than the national average. The U.S. injury and mortality rate for all youth ages 15 to 24 is 51/100,000. Comparatively, New Mexican Native American and Hispanic youth have a rate of 169/100,000, and 88/100,000, respectively. Tragically, a huge proportion of these deaths involve drug and alcohol abuse. New Mexican youth, who represent only 8% of New Mexico's driving population, account for 65% of all alcohol related driving deaths.[2]

The Adolescent Social Action Program (ASAP), founded in 1982, is an attempt to prevent further ATOD (alcohol, tobacco, or other drugs)-related injuries and deaths. The program targets youth and operates in over 30 high-risk multiethnic (predominantly Hispanic and Native American) communities in New Mexico.[3] The program's two long-term goals are (1) to reduce morbidity and mortality from ATOD

violence and other risky behaviors among adolescents in high-risk communities, and (2) to empower program participants to become leaders capable of promoting change in their communities' norms and social values, such that ATOD use is unacceptable. Since 1982, the program has enrolled over 1,300 adolescents from over 30 middle and high schools in New Mexico and 300 volunteer "facilitators." The impact of this program has reached a much wider audience through peer education and social action activities. The peer education component of ASAP enables the adolescents to teach younger students about the risks of ATOD use. Social action projects encourage youth to interact with their respective communities by developing ATOD awareness campaigns.

ASAP is a multidisciplinary, experiential, student-centered, primary prevention program. The core of the program is the Hospital/Detention Center (H/DC) experience. This experience involves small groups of volunteer middle and high school students from "high-risk" communities. They participate in a series of visits to the University-affiliated hospital (three visits) and to the Bernalillo County Detention Center (one visit). During these visits, the students interview patients, the patient's families, hospital personnel, and jail residents who directly or indirectly experience ATOD related problems. Prior to the interviews, adolescents are trained by skilled facilitators (university students in medicine, public health, nursing, communications, sociology, psychology and health education) in active listening and questioning techniques. The interviews allow the adolescents to learn first-hand about the medical, legal, emotional, and social consequences of ATOD use and its relationship to interpersonal violence, sexual encounters, and other psychosocial constructs. Patients and their families are carefully screened by the facilitators and hospital staff for the suitability of the student interviews and to ensure confidentiality. The patients are deemed appropriate only when they are judged to be stable and willing to share their experience in a positive and helpful way. Detention center residents are screened in a similar fashion by the education coordinator of the county detention center. The structured dialogues enable the youth to empathize with the patients' and jail residents' experiences, to critically analyze the issues and influences that contribute to abuse, and to develop the belief that they, the students, can help prevent similar problems from escalating in their own lives and in the lives of those around them.

ASAP draws from the social dialogue theory of Brazilian educator Paulo Freire[4-6] and the protection-motivation theory of social psychologist Ron Rogers[7] for its philosophic basis.

Freire's approach uses structured listening and dialogue in which everyone participates as co-learners to identify problems and then uses critical thinking to analyze the societal context of these problems along with an action component to address the identified problem.[8] The protection-motivation theory of Rogers proposes that behavior is either adaptive or maladaptive based on the variables of personal vulnerability, severity, *response efficacy* (the belief that one's actions will make a desired difference), *self-efficacy* (the belief that one has the ability to complete a task), and a set of beliefs about the rewards and costs. One's *threat-appraisal* or personal sense of vulnerability is aroused by exposure to a stimulus. An adaptive behavior is more likely if one has a sense of self-efficacy and response efficacy.[8]

In practice, ASAP combines these two theories. The patients and jail residents arouse the students' threat appraisal to the consequences of substance abuse. Freirian dialogue helps to create an increased cognitive awareness of the precursors and consequences of abuse and this then allows for an increased coping appraisal with increased self and response efficacies.[8]

The critical thinking component generated by dialogue separates ASAP from programs such as "Scared Straight" that use fear to effect change. Fear alone has been proven to be ineffective or lead the helplessness.[9] Through additional curricular exercises in decision making, social skills training and resistance to social influences, the program strives to increase coping skills. Good coping skills are associated with healthy behaviors.[10,11]

The emphasis on both individual and socially responsible behaviors distinguishes ASAP from many other adolescent prevention programs. Many prevention programs have been developed for a culture that promotes personal assertiveness and decision-making strategies. ASAP places the emphasis on empathy, community and prosocial behavior coupled with personal skills which may be of more importance to minority or other high risk youth who experience alienation from the dominant society.[12] The combination of various prevention strategies,

public health issues, social action, adolescent, community and parental involvement, and cultural sensitivity allows for a comprehensive approach to prevention programming.

Upon completion of the H/DC experience, some of the students then participate in other components of the program, for example, Peer Education, Social Action, or Fotonovela (Storybook) Projects. The participants of these projects are trained at their school site to be peer educators, advocates of social change, and creators of health related educational materials for their schools, in feeder elementary schools, and in community settings.

As an educational program within an academic center, ASAP is offered as an elective university course for 2 to 3 credit hours, depending on departmental requirements. This course provides students at the University of New Mexico (UNM) with a unique hands-on approach to learning about primary prevention and public health issues of adolescents. There are four primary goals for the course: (1) to gain an understanding of adolescent primary prevention strategies; (2) to expose university students to experiential education methodologies in prevention; (3) to critically explore social action strategies which address the issues of ATOD abuse, violence, and sexuality; and (4) to enhance facilitation skills for working with youth and other adults.

The UNM students receive two days of intensive training as facilitators in the ASAP methodology. After the training, the facilitators attend 16 weekly seminars to discuss and present various health-, social-, and adolescent-related topics. The facilitators are then paired with participating adolescents. In the adolescent's community, the facilitators attend (prior to the first hospital session) a parent orientation and, after the last hospital session, they participate in a follow-up community session.

Both quantitative and qualitative research outcomes have been conducted on the program. Using a randomized quasi-experimental design, an early investigation found a statistically significant difference between a middle school intervention and control group on the perceptions of riskiness of driving under the influence of drugs or alcohol at the eight month follow-up.[13] The questionnaire has been expanded in a more recent demonstration grant to assess the program's impact on youths' self-efficacies to engage in self- and other protective behaviors, and intentions to engage in risky behaviors. While data analysis is not complete, several items at the immediate post test have shown preliminary encouraging results; the intervention youth are developing a statistically significant increase of socially responsible self-efficacies over the controls.

The qualitative research on ASAP high school students identified an interplay of personal and community change attitudes, with the youth initially developing an individual responsibility to protect themselves. Social responsibility came with an analysis of societal conditions and with a belief that group action could make a difference to change those conditions.[8] A recently received five-year National Institutes of Alcohol Abuse and Alcoholism (NIAAA) grant will allow ASAP's hypotheses of program effects on both personal and social behaviors to be measured.

THE ROLE OF EMERGENCY DEPARTMENT/PROVIDERS

The primary involvement of the emergency department and other departments within the hospital is to assist with the selection of appropriate patients and to discuss details of the interviewing process, specifically confidentiality issues. A conference room in close proximity to the ED provides a safe and quiet setting for pre- and postinterview discussions. The support of the Department in providing access to patients is essential to the program. The program does *not* enhance patient flow and may detract from normal duties in a routinely overburdened ED. Staff volunteer for the evening and generally continue their normal duties by making up the time after the shift is done.

The emergency physician is often involved in the initial selection of patients and usually provides additional information to program participants about the patient's disease process, severity, etiology, financial costs, potential outcomes and the possible effects on the patients' lives. Once again, in a busy ED, this role is dependent on the individual physician or ED staff and the events of the evening. The physical environment for the patient interviews, which the ED provides, sets a realistic tone and pace for the evening.

Through this commitment by the ED, community involvement becomes more than a buzz word. The ASAP program provides a direct link with com-

munity activists, students, their families, public school systems and other government agencies. The importance of this program to the University Hospital cannot be measured in dollars and cents; it is a major outreach resource for the community.

An emergency department physician in the major trauma referral center for the State of New Mexico stands witness to the seemingly endless carnage related to ATOD abuse. Intervening with youth within the confines of the ED before harm is done provides a very healthy outlet for an otherwise discouraging situation. Emergency medical personnel can transfer their frustration and anger at the daily tragedies they witness by participating in this program. When ED personnel function as "facilitators," they gain a new perspective on how patients are treated in the ED. This perspective can then be incorporated into positive behavior change.

The role of ASAP or similar programs can be particularly important in a teaching hospital. The importance of evaluating underlying psychosocial problems in ED patients should be emphasized to medical students, residents, and anxillary staff. Of equal importance is the need to spend sufficient time talking with patients. Early identification of the multiple problems inherent in alcohol, tobacco, and substance abuse such as underlying psychiatric disease, behavioral addictions, and violence within the family will lead to better care of the ED patient.

CONCLUSION

- The exposure of young students to individuals who are suffering the multiple consequences of alcohol and substance abuse in the ED or detention center, in conjunction with dialogue that fosters coping and enhances self-efficacies, provides a unique perspective that can stimulate positive behavior change.

- The involvement of emergency care professionals in ASAP allows them to look at their alcohol and substance abuse patients from a new perspective and explore other approaches to treatment. In addition, as providers become more actively involved with community groups, they discover healthier outlets for the frustration they experience on the ED battlefield.

- The use of the social dialogue theories of Paulo Friere in combination with the protection motivation theories of Ron Rogers shows promise for enhancing positive change in youth.

NOTES

1. National Center for Health Statistics. Advance report of final mortality statistics, 1988. Hyattsville, MD: U.S. Department of Health and Human Services, Public Health Service, *Monthly Vital Statistics Report*, 39: no. 7 (Suppl), 1990.

2. New Mexico Selected Health Statistics, *Annual Report*. Department of Health Division, Bureau of Vital Records and Health Statistics, 1992.

3. Wallerstein N, Bernstein E. Empowerment education: Freire's ideas adapted to health education. *Health Educ Q* 1988; 15, 379–94.

4. Freire P. *Pedagogy of the Oppressed*. New York: Seabury Press, 1970.

5. Freire P. *Education for Critical Consciousness*. New York: Seabury Press/Continuum Press, 1983.

6. Hope A, Timmel S. *Training for Transformation: A Handbook for Community Workers: Book #2*. Zimbabwe, Africa: Mambo Press, 1984.

7. Rogers RW, Mewborn CR. Fear appeals and attitude change: Effects of a threat's noxiousness, probability of occurrence, and the efficacy of coping responses. *J Personal Soc Psychol* 1976; 34, 54–61.

8. Wallerstein N, Sanchez-Merki V. *Health Educ Res* 1994; 9, 105–18.

9. Job RF. Effective and ineffective use of fear in health promotion campaigns. *Am J Pub Health* 1988; 78, 163–7.

10. O'Leary A. Self-efficacy and Health. *Behav Res Ther* 1988; 23, 437–51.

11. Strecher V, DeVellis B, Becker M, Rosenstock I. The role of self-efficacy in achieving health behavior change. *Health Educ Q* 1986; 13, 73–91.

12. Jessor R. Problem behavior and developmental transition in adolescence. *J School Health* 1982; 52, 295–300.

13. Bernstein E, Woodall G. Changing perceptions of riskiness in drinking, drugs, and driving: an emergency department-based alcohol and substance abuse prevention program. *Ann of Emerg Med* 1987; 16, 1350–4.

28

Project ASSERT

An ED Model of Health Promotion and Substance Abuse Detection, Intervention, and Referral to Treatment

EDWARD BERNSTEIN
GERALDINE BURTON
JUDITH BERNSTEIN
DIANE BARRY
JUDITH DYSON-MOUNDS
SUSAN PAYNE
KIM SEAWRIGHT
TODD STANLEY
BRENT STEVENSON

CONTENTS

CHAPTER SUMMARY

The rationale for an ED approach to health promotion and the barriers to health promotion efforts in the ED setting are described and illustrated by two case studies. These efforts include assessment of the health and safety needs of our patients, assessment of problem severity in the case of alcohol, tobacco and other drugs of abuse, intervention in the form of a brief negotiation interview, referral to appropriate treatment, and follow-up. At Boston City Hospital, ED health promotion is accomplished though Project ASSERT, a federally funded demonstration grant to improve **A**lcohol and **S**ubstance abuse **S**ervices, and **E**ducation of clinicians to increase **R**eferral to **T**reatment (Figure 28-1). Although the central focus of Project ASSERT is detection and referral to treatment for patients with substance abuse problems, its mission encompasses referrals to primary care, smoking cessation, breast screening, and other preventive services. Project ASSERT relies on paraprofessional community outreach workers (health promotion advocates) who function within the ED to provide health education to our patients and linkages to community service agencies. Three important elements of this program are described: (1) collaboration between health promotion advocates, emergency physicians, and nurses, (2) cultural competency, and (3) use of a brief negotiation technique based on a readiness to change concept that facilitates respect for patients and their right to choice.

CASE #1

Marie, a 37-year-old white female, was seen in the emergency department on August 11, for vaginal bleeding. She was very concerned about the possibility of losing her pregnancy. Because she was in tears at the time of triage, it was difficult at first to ascertain if she was experiencing pain. She stated that she thought she might be 5 months pregnant, but she had not sought prenatal care.

Q: What should be our approach to our patient?

The traditional approach to emergency medicine focuses on the patient's chief complaint. Priority is first given to assessment of Marie's potentially life-threatening condition of vaginal bleeding, ruling out a threatened or incomplete abortion. Since the patient's stated gestational dating of 20 weeks may not be accurate, and she is in the age range for increased risk of ectopic pregnancy, this diagnosis must also be considered.

Case Continuation

Fetal heart tones are detected in the left lower quadrant at a rate of 140. The pelvic exam shows some cervical erosion and bleeding with an associated trichomonas infection. Vaginal ultrasound demonstrates a normal 18-week intrauterine pregnancy with no evidence of placental separation or free fluid.

Q: Now that a life-threatening condition has been ruled out, what further assessment and treatment is indicated?

Trichomonas is a STD, and Marie should be tested for other sexually transmitted diseases, including gonorrhea, chlamydia, syphilis, and HIV. The physician might ask if there is a regular partner who might benefit from assessment and treatment. Flagyl®, the usual therapy for trichomonas, is contraindicated in the first trimester of pregnancy but may be used with

Figure 28-1 Project ASSERT

PROJECT ASSERT
To Improve. . . .

A	Alcohol and
S	Substance abuse
S	Services and
E	Education for Provider
R	Referral to
T	Treatment

A CSAT MODEL TREATMENT
IMPROVEMENT GRANT

---

caution in the last two trimesters, since no other pharmaceutical is proven effective. The patient should be referred to prenatal clinic. If there will be any delay in getting a first appointment, a Pap smear should be performed in the ED and results sent to the obstetrical service for follow-up care.

According to past models of medical care, no further evaluation is necessary, but a public health approach to emergency medicine suggests that there is much more to be learned here and much more to be done. Marie's story has just begun to unfold.

Case Continuation

While Marie was waiting for test results, one of the Boston City Hospital ED's health promotion advocates (HPAs) administered a health needs history to assess her general health and safety needs. From this interview, the ED staff learned that Marie had never had a regular primary care doctor but used the ED as her prime source of care. She had several significant risk factors. She smoked more than a pack of cigarettes daily, had been threatened and slapped by a partner in the last several months, and nearly always felt that she had nothing to look forward to. Several months ago, she was seen in the ED with a broken nose, and she was treated last year for pelvic inflammatory disease. She said she knew what safe sex was about but didn't feel able to ask her partners to use a condom. She also reported to the HPAs that she had been drinking within the last 24 hours, had more than 6 drinks on an occasion, and thought she might have a drinking problem. As trust developed during the interview, she also admitted to daily use of crack cocaine. She was living in a shelter and hoped to move to a new apartment, but the paperwork was held up because she needed proof of rental payments from a previous landlord in order to qualify.

Q: How common is the problem of illicit drug abuse and pregnancy and what are some barriers to treatment?

The critical question to address is Marie's crack cocaine use, especially during pregnancy, but it would be an error to address this problem independent of her many other issues. A National Institute on Drug Abuse (NIDA) National Pregnancy and Health Survey of 2,613 women at 52 hospitals estimated that 5% of the 4 million women who gave birth in 1992 used illicit drugs. An estimate of 221,000 women per year who used drugs while pregnant was projected from this data—45,000 women using cocaine and another 119,000 using marijuana. Of the total, 113,000 were white, 75,000 were African American, and 28,000 were Hispanic. In addition, 20.4% of pregnant women smoked, and 18.8% drank alcohol. Among the women who drank and smoked, the rate of illicit drug use was higher: 20.4% for marijuana use and 9.5% for cocaine.[1]

This survey reinforces the need to focus on women, who make up 37% of the drug using population. Nearly 70% of AIDS cases among women are related to injecting drugs or having sex with injecting users. Women seem to be more vulnerable and die of AIDS faster than do men, primarily because of delay in diagnosis and treatment for women. Stigmatization and the lack of treatment faculties capable of housing mothers and their children are fundamental barriers to drug abuse treatment for women. The pregnant user, who through her addiction behaviors may jeopardize the health of her offspring, often receives overt criticism and punitive reactions from providers. This response is a further impediment to prevention of this devastating problem. At the same time, concern for the unborn child can be a potent lever for bringing women into treatment.

Q: Is it sufficient to reassure Marie that she had a normal ultrasound and refer her to prenatal care? Why should the emergency department staff question patients about an array of health issues seemingly unrelated to the chief complaint?

The recent SAEM position paper, *A Public Health Approach to Emergency Medicine,* reprinted in this textbook, emphasizes the importance of integrating primary and secondary prevention into our clinical practice. It recommends that questions be added to our medical history to identify patients who may abuse alcohol, tobacco, and drugs or who are victims of violence. The article points out that

> . . . in the often-emotionally-charged environment of the ED, the impact of teaching by physicians, nurses, social workers, and counselors may be even greater [than in other settings]. Preventive patient education must be age, gender, culture, site and complaint specific, and should be incorporated into practice guidelines. The ED is often the only health care site for some people who seek care during crisis; it also may be the only site where the most disenfranchised persons can be reached.

More recently, a multisite ED study documented high rates of injury and chronic disease risk and concluded that "EDs should expand screening, counseling, and referral programs to prevent disease, disability, and premature death."[2]

Although Healthy People 2000 sets the objective that 75% of primary care providers screen, counsel, and refer,3 models that promote and develop this role in the emergency department are currently lacking. Providers base their responses to the addicted patient on negative experiences with recidivism and do not universally accept the relapsing chronic nature of addictive disease, or generally believe that treatment works.[4] There are major gaps in medical, nursing, and graduate education in substance abuse prevention and treatment. The critical role that physicians can play in the medical-clinical encounter needs to be explored, developed, piloted, and propagated.

Emergency department settings are often counterproductive for substance abuse case-finding, brief intervention, and referral because of a mismatch between patient needs and system needs and capacity. This mismatch "contributes to mutual frustration, treatment failure, repeated visits and wasted health care resources."[4] Emergency department design, understaffing, excessive patient load, physical and chemical restraints, stereotyping, racism, and blame-the-victim ideology often prevent the patient-provider relationship from being therapeutic. Because of these obstacles, the Emergency department is an unacceptably missing link in the survival chain that connects patients to treatment resources, primary care, and community reinforcement efforts. Emergency department protocols, practice guidelines, training, systems, and designs need to be altered and improved to identify people at risk, reduce morbidity, and decrease the enormous human and financial toll related to substance abuse. These changes can only be undertaken when providers grasp that case finding and brief, effective intervention can be easily integrated into their practice.

Case Continuation

The HPA who uncovered a serious alcohol and drug dependency asked the patient for permission to discuss her alcohol and drug use with her and talk about how it fit in with her present life situation. Marie consented and was asked at this point how ready she was to change her life. She was not sure. The HPA used the Brief Negotiation Interview to explore the pros and cons of drug use with Marie. Marie was very scared that her use of crack had caused her vaginal bleeding and feared that she would lose her baby. It was pointed out that she did have reason to fear, because cocaine is known to cause placenta abruption and fetal demise. Marie decided to enroll in Project ASSERT and accepted a referral to the MOMs Project, a program that provides an array of services and group therapy for pregnant women who use drugs. An appointment was made for prenatal care. At the 10-day follow-up interview, Marie was referred to a residential program and received assistance with her substance abuse and other problems. She was followed up after the delivery and reported that she had remained drug-free during the rest of her pregnancy and had taken her healthy baby girl to her well-baby clinic appointment that very day.

Q: How can health promotion and alcohol and other drug abuse detection be accomplished in the rushed and stressful ED environment?

Clearly, a team approach, insurance reimbursement, and federal support for ED interventions are necessary in order to provide comprehensive care for the millions of our patients with preventable conditions. The Carter Presidential Center, in a 1993 *JAMA* article,[5] attributed over 1 billion deaths annually (half of all deaths that occurred in 1990) to preventable conditions: tobacco (400,000), diet and activity patterns (300,000), alcohol (100,000), microbial agents (90,000), toxic agents (60,000), firearms (35,000), sexual behavior (30,000), motor-vehicle crashes (25,000), and illicit use of drugs (20,000). They also identified socioeconomic status and access to medical care as other contributors but were more difficult to measure.

The common aphorism "an ounce of prevention is worth a pound of cure" has not been appreciated adequately by those who make policy and law. Until there is equitable health care coverage for all Americans, society must either pay today for comprehensive preventive services in the ED or pay much more tomorrow. Yet, as 1995 SAEM President Lewis Goldfrank points out,

> We in emergency medicine care for all those denied access elsewhere. We in emergency medicine offer the only place where health care is a right. We are the foundation and safety net of the health care system in this country, but we have grave deficits. We are faced with the recurrent problem of our inability to achieve timely follow-up care for many patients, particularly the uninsured, who have been evaluated in the ED. We are inadequately financed and ill prepared to take advantage of the unique opportunity of the ED visit for health promotion and critical preventive intervention, as well as entry into a primary care health care system.[6]

Project ASSERT provides a model for integrating comprehensive care into the ED. Health Promotion Advocates are paraprofessionals with alcohol and substance abuse training, and community outreach and case management experience. They screen a large number of ED patients (over 7,600 in the first year of the project), identify health risks and empower patients to make lifestyle changes. Patient permission is elicited to share detected problems with providers (see Figure 28–2). Referrals are made to smoking cessation programs, to victim services, to STD Clinic for HIV testing, to breast screening clinic to arrange for mammography, to Primary Care Clinic, and to alcohol assessment and treatment services.

At present, the EDs of our country are under attack as centers of cost, and efforts are focused to manage patients away from the ED. But for many of the high-risk and vulnerable populations that use the ED, there is no other dependable source of care. In Chapter 33, Goldberg and colleagues propose a different type of team composed of social worker, nurse, and physicians to address these needs and provide a similar array of preventive services—immunizations, detection, and referral of patients with alcohol and substance abuse, identification and referral of victims of violence, and cancer detection (Pap smears and breast exams).

As programs are put into practice throughout the country, emergency medicine will have opportunities to research the major questions about site of delivery, the composition of the team, which services to offer, and criteria for reimbursement. Community involvement in program planning and evaluation is essential, since the majority of our patients' needs require outside resources, as the following case illustrates.

Case #2

Joseph, a 52-year-old homeless black male was seen in the ED for chest pain, his fourth visit that month. While he was waiting to be evaluated, the physician recognized his name and suggested that he be seen by one of the HPAs. During this interview with the health promotion advocate, it was detected that he had been abusing alcohol and cocaine for many years. He had no source of medical care and was without a job. He hesitated, as many do, about participating in Project ASSERT. He was assured it was his own choice and his care in the ED would not be jeopardized if he decided not to enroll. Project ASSERT, he was told, had a mission to empower ED patients to reduce their alcohol and other drug abuse and to provide referrals and information to help patients stay safe and healthy. He decided that maybe he was ready and wanted and needed to make changes in his

life. Arrangements were made for Joseph to stay overnight at a shelter across from the ED. He was transported by the BCH Alcohol and Drug Triage Program to Andrew House, a center that specializes in helping patients with dual diagnosis of both psychiatric illness and substance abuse. There he underwent detoxification. He completed the 10-day program and returned to keep his medical appointments and the initial follow-up with the Project ASSERT. He was placed by the HPA in the Pine Street Men's Transitional Program. At the 90-day follow-up, the HPA who had enrolled Joseph in Project ASSERT learned that at the Men's Transitional program this patient had received substance abuse counseling, room and board, educational training, and a job.

Q: What are some of the barriers to treatment for minority populations?

The obstacles for racial and ethnic minorities seeking treatment are numerous: social stigma, racism, language barriers, inadequate funding and marketing of available programs, and inadequate training of professionals in issues related to culture and communication.[7]

Watson, writing about barriers to treatment for African Americans, says that "the occurrence and maintenance of chemical dependency in the black community is a complex problem that involves political, economic, social and cultural elements."[8] Both the disease model and the genetic inheritance model that are widely accepted by therapists focus on the individual and the flaws that have predisposed that individual to illness. When models with this perspective are applied by those with power and the authority of majority status (the primarily white, middle-class therapeutic community) to those who are disenfranchised, lacking in power, and relegated to minority status (inner-city people of color with alcohol and drug abuse problems), there is enormous potential for bias, blame, stereotyping, and racist notions about inherent inferiority. A shame-and-blame approach promotes resistance and creates roadblocks to treatment; humiliation is part of the problem, not part of the solution.

With cultural competence comes an understanding that environmental influences and the effects of oppression—economic deprivation, racism and stress—carry as much weight as individual factors in the development of alcohol and drug depend-

Figure 28-2 PROJECT ASSERT—Provider Referral Form

Dear Provider: *This form is necessary for discharge planning. The Health Promotion Advocates detected the following health issues/risks on your patient, and made referrals. Please (1) reinforce and encourage follow-up, (2) sign this form, and (3) record referrals and phone numbers on the BCH ED Discharge Planning Form in the section marked "OTHER."*

Please Return This Form To Clerks With ED Record.
Clerks: Put in Project ASSERT folder. Call 534-4388 for questions.

Signature indicates appropriate referrals were made:

Please Circle: (1) RN   (2) RNP   (3) ATTENDING   (4) EMR PGY II   (5) PGY III   (6) PGY IV

(7) MED/SURG INTERN   (8) MED/SURG RESIDENT   (9) MED STUDENT

Patient consent to disclose HNH information to provider:

Print Name _____ Signature _____

Date:_____ Sequential # _____ MR# _____

	Detected	Discussed	Referred
No regular/primary care physician	____	____	____
Requests help in stopping smoking	____	____	____
Victim of violence, needs counseling	____	____	____
Counsel about regular seat belt use	____	____	____
Depressed/hopeless needs psych evaluation	____	____	____
No pap smear within two years (WHC)	____	____	____
≥50 years old—no mammogram last 2 yrs	____	____	____
Requests Immunodeficiency Information	____	____	____
Possible alcohol &/or drug issues	____	____	____

(Form valid from 1-23-95 to 6-19-95)

Primary Care Clinic 534-5951
Non-smoking clinic 534-4545
Latino and Young Male Clinic 534-4104
Breast Screening Program 534-4627
Drug Hotline 445-1500 (after hours)
Follow-up Nurse 534-7894
Social Worker 534-5895
Central Intake 1 (MGH) 742-4496

Women's Health Clinic 534-4893
Women's Advocate 534-5895
Project Direction Bp 230-0627
Room 5 Addiction Services 534-5554
Project Trust 534-3483
BCH Alcohol & Drug Clinic 534-4212
Acupuncture Services 534-5352
Central Intake 3/Dimock 442-2326

Figure 28-3   Principles of Project ASSERT

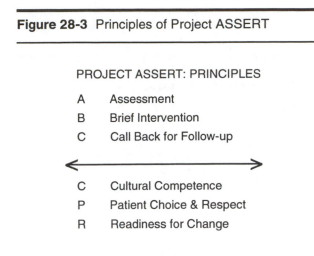

PROJECT ASSERT: PRINCIPLES

A   Assessment
B   Brief Intervention
C   Call Back for Follow-up

C   Cultural Competence
P   Patient Choice & Respect
R   Readiness for Change

ence. The detection and referral process must empower rather than detract from a person's sense of worth and efficacy, and enhance an individual's ability to participate in the life of a family, church, and community. "Successful programs work to create a positive environment and support system for a substance free community . . . a sense of the uniformity of spirituality among people."[9] Similarly, if a person's cultural heritage stresses the importance of family and community, programs that attempt to treat an individual in isolation from a community or insist on separating mothers from children have little hope of success. Among Hispanic people, a knowledge of and respect for how families operate is as important as language competency.[10] Project ASSERT is designed to reach out to the strengths within each individual, and develop the links to a support network. Project principles are described in Figure 28–3.

Q: What is Project ASSERT? How does it function?

Project ASSERT at Boston City Hospital provides an approach adapted to the multiracial and cultural setting in an inner-city Level I Trauma Center. Project ASSERT was funded to build linkages to improve emergency department "**A**lcohol and **S**ubstance Abuse **S**ervices and **E**ducate Providers about **R**eferral to **T**reatment." A 3-year grant from the U.S. Department of Health and Human Services' Center for

Substance Abuse Treatment provides funds for personnel, consultants, evaluation, training, travel, and materials and supplies to help serve patients presenting to BCH ED with alcohol and other drugs of abuse (ADOA)-related problems and to link ED patients with the Boston network of alcohol and drug treatment inpatient and outpatient services.

These original objectives were modified to provide detection, intervention, health education, and referral services for an array of other preventable conditions that include referrals to the primary care clinic, smoking cessation program, the battered women advocate and social worker, HIV testing, breast screening clinic, and women's health, black male, Latino, and homeless clinics. Initially, alcohol- and drug-screening questions were embedded in a health risk questionnaire to increase their acceptability to patients. Since the inception of the project, the team has come to realize the importance of reframing substance abuse as a part of the broader questions of the health and safety for all of our patients.

The program objectives are to (1) develop a total quality management team approach to administration and utilize a monthly continuous quality improvement meeting of staff that includes HPAs, nurses, physicians and management; (2) train project staff and providers in cultural competence, Brief Negotiation Interviewing (BNI), detection, and referral skills and resources; (3) apply the demonstration model in the BCH ED to increase the number of referrals to treatment and reduce the harmful consequences of alcohol and other drugs of abuse and other preventable conditions; (4) improve linkages between the ED and substance abuse treatment programs, primary care, and other preventive services; (5) evaluate the model; and (6) disseminate the results.

In March 1994, five HPAs were hired to work in the ED. They come from the minority communities which the BCH ED serves, and each of them has worked in a number of community agencies. They are experienced in community outreach, case management, and advocacy. They all have certificates from the BU School of Public Health's 6-week course in HIV and Substance Abuse Health Education. They began with 2 months of on-the-job training in how to function in the ED environment, how to administer the various screening, assessment and data collection instruments, and how to work collaboratively with

Figure 28-4 Project ASSERT

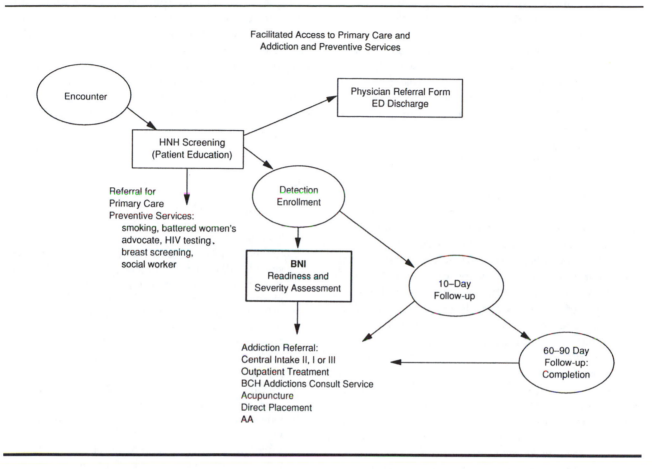

Facilitated Access to Primary Care and
Addiction and Preventive Services

the ED and ADOA treatment staff. They have been trained and supervised by one of our outstanding ED psychiatric nurses. The five HPAs work from 8 a.m. to 11 p.m. daily and weekends in the BCH ED, interviewing patients in the examining rooms on both the non acute and acute sides of the emergency department.

The HPAs, residents, and faculty had several training sessions in the technique of Brief Negotiation Interviewing (BNI), described in detail in Chapter 31, which is used in the enrollment process. It emphasizes respect for patients and for their right to choice and active participation in decision making. Enrollment consists of informed consent, the assessment of addiction severity using the AUDIT for alcohol dependency and the DAST for drug dependency, and an assessment of readiness to change, using an instrument that employs a scale of 1 to 10. Following

enrollment, further negotiation takes place around the appropriate referral to treatment. The patient is given a medical clearance, a referral form, and a follow-up appointment. Patients are followed up by HPAs at 10 and 60–90 days from their initial encounter. (See Figure 28–4). The follow-up allows an opportunity to discuss the patient's satisfaction and the efficacy of the referral, to learn about the barriers patients encountered, and to make another more appropriate referral if requested. It is also a time to learn about the accomplishments of patients like Marie, who worked so hard toward her recovery and improved quality of life with her new baby. The benefits derived from success stories like Marie's are passed on exponentially from the individual to the larger social circle, and from one generation to another. The benefits in health care cost reduction and resources now available for other needs are also enormous. The annual bill of almost $10 billion from substance abuse–complicated pregnancies is reduced by a conservative estimate of $5,000 for each individual.[11]

During a recent one year period, 7,600 patients were screened, 2,700 AODA problems were detected, and 1,100 patients were enrolled in Project ASSERT. The majority of the 900 referrals were made to an Alcohol and Drug Triage Program at our institution, where patients are matched to appropriate treatment modality and placed for treatment.

Project ASSERT's model of an ED brief intervention that assesses readiness to change and motivates patients to enter treatment had its origins in 1982 in the University of New Mexico School of Medicine's Adolescent Substance Abuse Prevention Program, later renamed the Adolescent Social Action Program.[12] This model, described by Gougelet and colleagues in Chapter 27, is based on the principles of active listening, authentic interchange or dialogue, reflective action, and a very democratic approach to change. It also relies on a theory of protective motivation that posits that behavior change comes about when people recognize the severity and likelihood of the consequences and take up a plan of action for change that is efficacious because it is likely to reduce the dangerous consequences.[13,14] This theory applies to our situation in the physician-patient encounter in the ED. Since patients present to us in crisis, often suffering serious consequences of their addictive behaviors, there is an opportunity to help them to look critically at the consequences of their actions and to plan jointly for an effective change strategy. It is also possible to create a user friendly system of referrals. Project ASSERT has adapted the work of Chavetz, Miller, and Rollnick[15,16] on brief intervention techniques to the ED setting.

CONCLUSION

Today more than ever, emergency medicine is in a respected and vital position in medicine and in society at large. We can serve to link our patients to the primary care system, preventive services, and community services. We do not have to play this role alone, however, but can collaborate, as we do every day in our work, with agencies and leaders outside of medicine. We can advocate for a broader perspective on the health of the public and for a deeper

appreciation of the need for major policy changes. Our goal is to improve the lives of our patients and the communities in which they live. Project ASSERT represents an important effort to bring a public health agenda of primary and secondary prevention into the practice of emergency medicine. Active listening, authentic dialog, and brief negotiated interviewing are skills that can help clinicians facilitate patient access to alcohol and drug treatment and other preventive services.

NOTES

1. Mathias R. NIDA survey provides first national data on drug use during pregnancy. *NIDA Notes* 1995; 10(1):6–7.
2. Lowenstein SR, Koziol-McLain J, Thompson M, Gerson LW, Blanda M, Buczynsky P, et al. Behavioral risks in emergency department patients: A multi-site study. *Acad Emerg Med* 1995; 2(5):341–2.2.
3. U.S. PHS. *Healthy people 2000: National health promotion and disease prevention objectives.* Washington, DC: HSSD, 1991.
4. Whitney R. Alcoholics in the emergency room. *Bull NY Acad Med* 1983; 59:216–21.
5. McGinnis MJ, Foege WH. Actual causes of death in the United States. *JAMA* 1993; 270:2207–12.
6. Goldfrank LR. Health care reform or a return to social Darwinism? *Ann Emerg Med* 1995; 25:692–4.
7. Brown L. Drug abuse treatment for African Americans. In: *National conference on drug abuse research and practice: An alliance for the 21st century.* Washington, DC: DHHS, 1991.
8. Watson D. Prevention, intervention and treatment of chemical dependency in the black community. In Braithwaite RL, Taylor SE (eds.). *Health issues in the black community.* San Francisco: Jossey-Bass, 1992.
9. Warfeld-Copeck N. Drug abuse treatment for African Americans. In: *National conference on drug abuse research and practice. An alliance for the 21st century.* Washington DC: DHHS, 1991.
10. Szapocznik J. Drug abuse treatment for Hispanic Americans. In: *National conference on drug abuse research and practice. An alliance for the 21st century.* Washington DC: DHHS, 1991.
11. Worner TM, Delgado IM. Women referred for treatment: Early versus traditional intervention. *Substance Abuse* 1995; 16:39–47.
12. Bernstein EB, Woodall, G. Changing perceptions of riskiness in drinking, drugs and driving: An emergency department based alcohol and substance abuse prevention program. *Ann Emerg Med* 1987; 16:1350–4.

13. Rogers R. A protection motivation theory of fear appeals and attitude change. *J Psych* 1975; 91:93–114.

14. May PA, Miller JH, Wallerstein N. Motivation and community prevention of substance abuse. *Exper Clin Psychopharmacol* 1993; 1:68–79.

15. Chavetz M, Blane HT, Abrams HS, Golner J, Lacy E, McCourt WF, et al. Establishing treatment relations with alcoholics. *J Nerv Ment Dis* 1962; 134:390–410.

16. Miller W, Rollnick S. *Motivational interviewing.* 1991. New York: Guilford Press.

29

One Emergency Department's Approach to Injury Prevention

ALISON LANE-RETICKER

CONTENTS

- ED based models for intentional and unintentional injury prevention
- Educational materials as part of the ED discharge process: firearm and car crash injuries; bicycle, motorcycle and pedestrian safety; fire hazards, choking

CHAPTER SUMMARY

A comprehensive emergency medicine response to injury prevention is described. Lessons are shared from several years of experience in ED based initiatives, from program development and funding to community outreach and outcome follow-up. In addition to interactive seminars, ED staff have developed an ongoing educational effort for a wide spectrum of injury prevention. Examples of teaching handouts for patients are provided.

Case #1

Four years ago, a young male was brought to our ED with a gunshot wound to the abdomen. The intial resuscitation went well, and the surgery was prompt. There was nothing special about the case. I had been asked to speak at a conference on violence, and I thought it would be helpful to learn as much about this seemingly ordinary young man as I could. His name was Kenneth.

On the day of the shooting, Kenneth had stopped after work for soda at a nearby convenience store. As he got out of his car, he was almost struck by a young man in a truck. He shouted an obscenity at the driver and continued on into the store. He heard footsteps behind him and turned as the driver asked, "What did you call me?" The driver did not wait for a response. He shot Kenneth in the abdomen.

Fortunately, the bullet missed his spinal cord and his lungs and liver, but it injured his small bowel and pancreas. He required a feeding jejeunostomy. After 40 days in the hospital, he went home on clear liquids, weighing 117 pounds, with the feeding jejeunostomy tube still in place.

One of the difficult things about being home was seeing the man who shot him, a friend of his father. The man had been charged in the assault but was out on bail awaiting trial. This was not the first violent encounter for this patient and his family. A brother had been shot and killed 4 years earlier when Kenneth and a friend had an argument. Bystanders cheered them on. Each boy had an older brother who took on the fight, and Kenneth's brother was shot in the chest. He died an hour later.

Kenneth had managed to pull himself together after his brother's death. He had finished high school. He got a job. He lived with both parents, and all three had jobs. A week after his trip to the trauma room, he had left no impression on the staff. There was nothing of note about his case, and I present it here because it is so ordinary.

Kenneth knew the man who shot him. The provocation was minimal. Kenneth said he did not know the man had a gun, and that if he had known, he would not have sworn. His brother's death illustrates the mundane nature of homicide, and the randomness of the victim-

perpetrator relationship. Kenneth's brother could as easily have been the perpetrator as the victim. The very fact that homicide seems so common, that it is hard to think of it as murder, prompted one of our department's injury prevention initiatives, Lives At Risk.

LET'S NOT MEET BY ACCIDENT

Several years ago, a driving instructor assigned his students the task of observing in an ED. Different nursing supervisors got several calls from students or their parents trying to make arrangements for the observation. The nurses got the idea of presenting a program for the students to encourage safe driving. They started with facts about drunk driving and stories about teenagers they had seen. They took the students to the trauma room and demonstrated what happens during a resuscitation. They showed *Staying Alive,* a film about teenagers who are killed because of drunk driving. The film also shows a girl in a vegetative state in a nursing home many months after a crash. They brought the students to the helipad and the family room. The program ended with a course evaluation and refreshments and a chance for students to mingle with staff and ask questions about what they had seen or about health care careers.

The program was very successful from the beginning. More and more people asked to bring students and sometimes their parents. Schools wanted to bring entire grades. A young man who had killed a woman in a drunk-driving incident became a part of the program for many months. He spoke about waking up and realizing what he had done and about living with this for the rest of his life. He talked about his trial, his jail term, and his desire to tell the victim's family how sorry he was. His presentation was very powerful, in part because he was such a normal, likable person. Eventually, it became too taxing for him to continue to participate.

In the course of this two-hour program, we stress the dangers of drinking and driving or riding with a driver who has been drinking. We stress the importance of seat-belt use. We mention motorcycles and the importance of helmets, which are not required in our state. We try to impress upon these students, most of whom are around 15 years old, that one bad decision, made in a moment of indiscretion, can change their lives, their parents' lives, their friends' lives, or strangers' lives forever.

As we try to break through the adolescents' wall of invulnerability, it helps to have them on our turf. For many students, the high point of the program is the trauma resuscitation room. The aura of the trauma center, the intensity of the huge operating lights in the ceiling, the practiced efficiency of the trauma team members, all make an impression. In the trauma room, one student lies collared on a backboard, while a nurse explains the sequence of events in a resuscitation. The students have an opportunity to see and touch the various tubes and catheters used in a resuscitation. Some of the students have to leave the room. We explain that if they come back as trauma patients, the three places they are likely to go from the trauma room are the operating room, the intensive care unit, or the morgue.

The program began in the fall of 1990 and has been staffed by emergency department nursing staff with help from the trauma nurse coordinator. We present the program approximately three times per month. We have reached approximately 5,000 students. The program has been widely acclaimed, but we know it is no panacea. We have had at least one participant return as a patient. We have received awards, including a Buckle Up award. The Insurance Association of Connecticut has supported this program with grants in 1992 and 1993.

LIVES AT RISK

The emergency department's second injury-prevention program, *Lives At Risk,* is a violence prevention program for teenagers closely modeled on *Let's Not Meet By Accident.* Starting in 1992, emergency nurses and physicians met with clergy, pediatricians, trauma surgeons, child psychologists, social workers, and others to discuss how a brief, hospital-based program could make a difference in the city's major injury problem, violence. The group concluded we should make the students aware of the scope of the problem, that we should stress the pain involved in violence, and we should teach some skills that would allow them to solve conflicts without fighting.

We piloted our first programs in 1992 and now are presenting as many as three sessions a month. The students meet in the amphitheater, where we begin with a word-association exercise based on the term *violence*. This gives us a chance to indicate that the word violence has many roots and many expressions. We discuss the interaction of drugs, poverty, and racism and the relationship between anger and aggression. We explain that injuries are rarely accidents, talk about common patterns for certain injuries, and then introduce the common pattern for homicide: friends having an argument, with one of them or both intoxicated and one or both carrying a weapon.

One of the trauma surgeons talks about growing up in a ghetto. He stresses the importance of education and of heroes. Then the students split into groups. Some go to the trauma room to see a film about young men with spinal cord injuries. The film is called "Wasted Dreams." Again we make the point that some changes are irreversible. Another group goes to the trauma room. As with *Let's Not Meet By Accident*, we have a student lie on the stretcher while a nurse explains the course of a resuscitation. She stresses that many of our patients are in severe pain, not just in the trauma room, but for many days and sometimes months and years. She explains why a colostomy may be needed. She stresses the lack of independence endured by patients with spinal cord injuries. The two groups switch and then the students return to the amphitheater for a presentation by The Looking In Theater. The teenaged actors present skits, bringing the action just to the brink of violence. Then the students ask questions of the actors in character. Eventually, the actors present the skits again with a nonviolent resolution. This program, too, ends with a critique. The students then join the staff and actors for refreshments before they leave.

Recently we have received funding from the Greater Hartford Urban League and a local charitable foundation. One of the emergency medicine residents has become interested in the program and has collated the results of the questionnaires we use to measure the success of the program. The questionnaire we use to evaluate the program is administered at the end of the program and asks the participants whether they are less likely to solve conflict violently than they were before the program. So far, we have not been able to look at attitude changes over time, nor have we found a measure that allows us to look at change in behavior.

One of the important outcomes of such a program is that it allows staff to respond to a problem that seems overwhelming to them. Lack of precise outcome measures is less important to the nurses and physicians than the feeling that they have finally found a way to save perhaps a few teenagers from this epidemic of violence.

Although we are booked a year in advancee, we have no plans to expand the program. Three presentations a month is about our maximum, especially considering we have two injury-prevention programs based in the emergency department. The Hartford police department is interested in working with us to see that all students in certain neighborhoods have the opportunity to attend the program.

In order to increase the impact of the program we hope to provide schools with some additional materials to be used before and after the visit. Some students need educational preparation for the field trip to the hospital. They are not familiar with words such as *bladder*. This applies particularly to children in modified classes, many of whom are judged by their teachers to particularly need violence prevention counseling. All the students would benefit from a continued discussion after the program. We would like to maximize the effect of their 2 hours with us by providing materials which can be used in specific classes to expand on issues raised in our discussion.

We hope to provide a package of graphs for use in math classes, a crossword puzzle for use in English classes (some teachers are already using the trip as a writing prompt), some trauma-related questions for biology classes and some discussion questions for use in history classes. We also hope to furnish materials to the parent-teacher organizations to facilitate home discussions of the issues raised by *Lives At Risk*. Some of our students come from church groups and others from neighborhood programs. A few have had experience with Deborah Prothrow-Stith's violence prevention curriculum. We hope to prepare a less academically oriented package of supplemental materials for church and community groups.

We also hope to develop a more meaningful evaluation tool. To do this, we will need cooperation from both the police and the schools and we will need to preserve confidentiality. Measurements over time are complex because our community is experiencing economic distress and an increase in gang activity. In this setting, progress may be simply no worsening in the present level of violence.

OTHER INITIATIVES

A major part of the department's injury-prevention initiative is patient education at the time of the ED visit. We have posters in our waiting room and in our fast track, and many of these have to do with injury prevention. In our waiting room, we have a videocassette player and a guest relations representative who can play tapes. These are aimed at both children and adults, and many deal with injury prevention. We have videos promoting seat-belt use, bicycle helmets, and safe boating. Other videos warn of the dangers of drunk driving. We use private areas such as rest rooms and examination rooms to display information for battered women, and we have pamphlets available on many injury-prevention subjects.

Both nurses and physicians make an effort to understand the context in which a given injury occurred and try to provide appropriate prevention strategies. This can require great tact when patients or family members are already feeling guilty or angry.

We have computerized discharge instructions for battered women just as we have instructions for people with lacerations. These instructions do not take the place of an interview with a social worker, but they can be helpful for women not yet willing to talk about the problem.

In an effort to reach a broader audience we have developed a calendar of injury-prevention messages which can be added to our computerized discharge instruction, one message for each month. Some of these patient education messages that are incorporated into the discharge process are included here as examples.

Preventing Firearms Injury

Evaluate the need for a gun in your home. Having a gun in the home increases the risk of homicide and suicide. Homes with guns are almost five times more likely to be the scene of a suicide than homes without a gun. When a gun kept in the home is used to kill someone, only 3% of the time that someone is a stranger. Usually the someone is a relative or acquaintance. You are probably safer without a gun. If you decide you must keep a gun in your home, empty it out and lock it up. Lock the ammunition in a separate place. Make sure that children do not have access to guns when they play in others' homes. Teach children to leave the area and tell an adult if they see a gun. Teach them never to touch a gun. Teach them that what looks like a toy gun may turn out to be real. Remember that guns and alcohol or drugs are a deadly combination. Connecticut law holds gun owners responsible for injuries caused by improperly stored guns.

Preventing Car-Crash Injuries

Obey the speed limit. You may need to drive more slowly in bad weather or lighting conditions. Drive expectantly. Watch for pedestrians, cars changing lanes, and sudden stops. Concentrate on your driving. Do not try to discipline children or read a map while driving. Keep the radio low enough so you can hear what is going on outside the car. Driving safely may mean that you cannot eat a snack or talk on the car phone. Never drive after drinking. The odds of crashing increase when your blood alcohol level is only half of what is considered legally intoxicated. Do not drive when you are taking medication that makes you drowsy. This includes over-the-counter medicines. If you are sleepy, stop at a rest area for a brisk walk and a snack. Illegal drugs such as marijuana and cocaine make driving unsafe.

Never ride with a driver impaired by drugs, alcohol, or fatigue. A socially awkward conversation is much better than being injured or killed. Practice how you would decline a ride if you found your companion impaired. Use a designated driver system. FRIENDS DON'T LET FRIENDS DRIVE DRUNK. Also, teach your children the skills that will keep them away from drunk drivers. Try role playing. Pick them up without question if they call asking for a ride home.

Some people should not drive at night. Those with night blindness and many elderly people should not drive after dark, and young drivers should avoid late night trips. Consider imposing a curfew on young drivers. The first year of driving is risky. Sixteen-year-olds have a higher death rate than older first-time drivers. Consider having your child wait a year before getting a license. Death rates are highest on Friday and Saturday nights.

Maintain your car in good repair. Choose safe cars. Death rates are lowest in big cars. Air bags offer additional protection for front-end collisions, the most common fatal collision. BUCKLE UP. Use a lap and shoulder belt every time you drive from the start of every trip. Properly used, they reduce the chance of occupant death by 45%. Restrain your children appropriately. Children under 1 year should be restrained facing the rear of the car. Children between one and four should be in a seat facing front. Make sure the car seat is properly secured to the car. The safest place in the car is the middle of the back seat.

Bicycle Safety

Ninety percent of all bicycle deaths involve collision with a motor vehicle. Most bicycle deaths are caused by an isolated head injury. *Always wear a safety helmet.* They are required by law in Connecticut to age 12, but most fatalities occur in the teenage years. Obey the rules of the road. Obey traffic signals. Ride single file, and with rather than against traffic. Look for places to ride away from cars. Search out cycling paths. Watch for "Rails to Trails" conversions. Wear light or reflective clothing for increased visibility.Be especially careful at night, or better yet, do not ride after dark. Maintain your bike carefully. Make sure it has the necessary reflectors and lights.

Motorcycles

Motorcycles have 35 times the death rate of passenger cars when you consider the number of miles driven. About half of all motorcycle deaths occur in young men in their twenties. Up to 60% of people dying in single-vehicle motorcycle crashes at night are legally intoxicated. Avoid drinking and driving. Motorcycles designed to look like racing models are associated with increased death rates. Avoid these. Fatal accidents are most common between 10:00 p.m. and 2:00 a.m., so try to avoid late-night driving. Using headlights improves visibility. Follow the rules of the road. *Wear a helmet.* The motorcycle death rate in states with motorcycle helmet laws is 30% lower than in states without laws.

Pedestrians

Young children and the elderly are particularly likely to be struck by cars. Deaths peak at age 6, with other peaks at age 20 and over 70.The hour right after sunset is the most dangerous time for pedestrians. It is safest to walk on a sidewalk. If there is no sidewalk, walk single-file facing traffic and well to side of the road. Cross streets at crosswalks.

Wait for walk lights. STOP, LOOK, AND LISTEN before crossing the street, even if the light is in your favor. Beware of cars turning right on red. Be especially careful when it is slippery underfoot.Do not allow children to play near the street. Teach them not to go after a ball that has gone into the street. Avoid walking along the road at night. If you walk or jog at night, wear bright and/or reflective clothing. Do not walk after drinking especially at night. Nearly half of all pedestrians killed at night have high blood alcohol levels. Avoid crossing from between parked cars.

Burns and Fires

Deaths rates from house fires are highest for children and the elderly. Most fatal fires occur at night. You need a working smoke detector to warn you to escape. Check the batteries in your smoke detectors once a month or at least when you change your clocks every April and October. Plan and practice an escape route in case of fire. The careless use or disposal of cigarettes is responsible for more than one-fourth of residential fire deaths. Consider making your home smoke-free.People living in a multifamily dwelling where other tenants smoke while intoxicated are at increased risk of being injured in a fire. Make sure you have working smoke detectors, fire extinguishers, and a well-rehearsed escape plan. Consider moving. Ten percent of fire deaths are caused by kids playing with matches or lighters. Keep these out of the reach of children and teach children not to play with them. Be alert to other places besides your home where your children might encounter matches or lighters.

The actual cause of death in many house fires is smoke inhalation. If you are caught in a house fire, crawl to the exit. Do not wear loose clothing around stoves and grills. Kerosene heaters can be dangerous. Do not use the stove to heat your home. If you catch on fire, STOP, DROP, AND ROLL.

Scalds are responsible for most major burns in Connecticut. Turn down the hot water heater so that water will not scald (120°F maximum). Be especially careful with infants and toddlers and the elderly. Of course, you should never leave them unattended in the bathtub.

Children can suffer disfiguring electrical burns when they chew on electric cords or play with electrical outlets. If you have young children of your own, or young visitors, use plug protectors, available in the hardware store.

Remember all private fireworks, even sparklers, are illegal in Connecticut. Even when used by professionals, fireworks can be dangerous. Keep your children away from fireworks. Set a good example and obey the law yourself.

Choking

Children and the elderly are most likely to choke. Children choke on food (pieces of hot dog, grapes, candies, and nuts). Children choke on pieces of toys, including building sets and balloons. Adults are most likely to choke on a large piece of meat, especially if they have been drinking. Babies and children can suffocate from plastic bags. Do not leave these near small children or use them to protect infant bedding.Make sure your toy box has a safety device to keep the lid from falling on the child's neck. Secure window blind cords so they cannot asphyxiate a child. Do not tie a pacifier around a child's neck.

CONCLUSION

The two models described in this chapter demonstrate that it is indeed possible, within the limits of a busy emergency department practice, to develop injury prevention programs. The educational materials used in these programs can easily be adapted to a variety of settings.

Unit IV

The Medical Interview
in the ED

30

The Physician-Patient Encounter: An Opportunity for Healing

STEVEN ROSENZWEIG

CONTENTS

CHAPTER SUMMARY

Episodes of illness or injury are not isolated events, amenable to hit-and-run treatment. The emergency physician has an obligation to solve the presenting problem and relate effectively to the total health context as well.

Case #1

It's Friday at 5:00 P.M. at the beginning of a holiday weekend. Outpatient clinics have all closed early and the emergency department (ED) census is burgeoning. With seven patients waiting to be seen, the emergency physician (EP) grabs the top chart, glancing at the following information while walking toward the exam room: 26-year-old male whose chief complaint is right leg pain for 1 1/2 months. She pulls aside the curtain to glimpse a young African American man lying still on the stretcher, eyes half-closed.

Q: What communication barriers exist between you and this patient?

An encounter of strangers. The defining feature of the physician-patient encounter in the ED is that it occurs between strangers. Each person brings to the encounter numerous preconceived notions about the other. Mistrust is bound to occur. Differences of race, culture, class, gender, sexual orientation, and life-style often engender miscommunication and negative stereotyping.

It's also important to recognize that there exists a medical culture which itself creates a distance between physician and patient, with its own rules, language, dress, and power distribution. Patients are stereotyped according to their illness or behavior.

The EP might wonder whether this patient is malingering and drug seeking: He looks comfortable. His problem is "old." He presents on a holiday weekend when medical offices are closed; drug seekers know they have an advantage when the EP is unable to contact other providers to verify information. The patient also makes assumptions about the EP. For instance, it is common for patients to negatively stereotype physicians as a result of unsatisfactory past experiences.

Multiple stressors. The ability to relate openly with one another is further impeded by the number of stressors present. The EP suffers from fatigue, biorhythm disruption, and continuous distractions. The patient is stressed not only by illness but also by a chaotic and frightening ED atmosphere, seemingly endless waits, physical exposure and other iatrogenic discomforts.

Conflicting agendas. Priorities, values, and concerns of patients differ from those of their physicians. EPs feel pressured to take charge, save time, get the facts, keep moving. Patients need to collaborate, talk, feel cared for, understand new information. Conflict ensues from the attempt to ignore either set of needs.

Q: What is your approach to this patient and what information do you need to know to diagnose the problem correctly?

Case Continuation

The physician introduces herself and assists the patient to a semireclining position that facilitates eye contact. Pulling up a stool, she sits beside him at eye level. She asks him why he is here. He tells her that a month and a half ago he was walking home from work at the post office when he was assaulted and shot multiple times in his chest, abdomen, and buttocks. He underwent emergency surgery at his neighborhood hospital. At discharge, he was suffering severe right lower extremity pain and loss of motor function. He was sent home with crutches and a prescription for Percocet. After finishing this prescription, he subsequently made a series of visits to the same hospital's ED; on these occasions, he was dispensed four Percocet tablets and referred to surgery clinic since he was on Medicaid. His postal service job was new, and he had not yet qualified for health benefits.

The patient made the earliest available appointment at the clinic which was still 1 month away. Yesterday he phoned the surgeon who operated on him. This physician told the patient that he was just the surgeon on call the night of the shooting, and that he was not his personal physician. He instructed the patient to follow up with the surgery clinic. In the meantime, the patient had no analgesics. Walking was difficult and the pain even kept him from sleeping. He said he was unable to use crutches in his neighborhood because people with disabilities were often targeted for assault and robbery. The EP asks what it is the patient hopes to accomplish with this visit. He says he wants to change his care over to her hospital. He requests a prescription for Percocet. Physical examination of the patient's leg confirms significant neuromuscular dysfunction. The patient winces

with pain upon minimal range of motion of his foot and leg.

Q: What are this patient's most urgent problems?

This patient presents with two significant problems. The first is his pain syndrome. Any prescription of analgesics from the ED is only a temporizing measure. This patient is going to require ongoing support along with evaluations by neurology and physical medicine.

The second problem is that he has no primary care physician to provide continuity of care and to help him negotiate the medical system to obtain the appropriate referrals. While he does have medical insurance, he does not have appropriate access to care and is forced to utilize the ED as an only option.

Q: What is the most appropriate disposition for this patient?

Case Continuation

The EP acknowledges the patient's pain, frustration, and the horror of his story. As a result, the conversation becomes more relaxed and spontaneous. She explains her reservation about prescribing opioids for what is evolving into a chronic pain syndrome. The patient is willing to try a prescription for naproxen. She tells him that he will likely need to be seen by various specialists and that this should be facilitated and coordinated by a primary care physician. A special appointment book for the hospital's primary care clinic is kept in the ED for the purpose of arranging outpatient follow-up. She makes the earliest appointment for him, which is in 3 days' time. He is appreciative.

Q: Has the EP now concluded her responsibilities toward this patient?

A traditional view has been to consider the EP-patient relationship concluded at the time of discharge. This is often unrealistic for a variety of reasons. First, both EP and patient rely on the potential for future contact: questions arise, new test results need to be conveyed. Second, significant barriers may prevent patients from complying with their prescribed treatment plan. Lacking money or health insurance, or not having a telephone or transportation, the patient may be unable to obtain medication or arrange for follow-up care. These obstacles may not have been recognized during the ED encounter.

While the ED cannot possibly provide true continuity of care, a key follow-up contact may dramatically impact on a patient's care. At times, key information can be provided. Unable to obtain timely follow-up at one outpatient setting, the patient may be unaware of other options. At other times, a phone call can be made on behalf of a patient who is having difficulty negotiating the system. Brief telephone follow-up may avoid the most time consuming alternative—that is, a return visit to the ED.

Case Conclusion

On the day of the patient's clinic appointment, the EP calls to speak with the primary care physician who saw the patient but finds out that the patient never showed. She calls the patient at home. He tells her that he had come back to the ED the day following the initial visit because the naproxen was ineffective. His prescription was changed to ketorolac and this was helping significantly. The EP who saw him on the return visit suggested he see a neurologist and the patient made the earliest appointment, which was 6 weeks away. He had been in too much pain to travel on the buses to the clinic today.

The EP explains again her suggestion for him to have primary care follow-up. She tells him that she does agree that he will require consultation with a specialist and suggests that he also call the rehabilitation medicine clinic, which generally has earlier openings. She makes sure that he has all the correct phone numbers. He thanks her and tells her that no one at the other hospital ever bothered to take the time to explain these things to him.

BROADER PUBLIC HEALTH CONTEXT

EDs serve as a medical safety net for those who have no alternative access to health care. Among this group are more than 30 million Americans who have no health insurance. Who are the uninsured? Nearly half of all those living near or below the poverty line do not qualify for Medicaid. Many who are recently employed, self-employed, or work part-time also have no coverage.

More difficult to define is an even larger population of those who are underinsured. Health insurance may be inadequate due to restrictions on where a patient is entitled to receive care, exclusions placed on particular illnesses such as pre-existing conditions, exclusions on certain treatments, waiting periods, or dollar limits.

Patients covered by Medicaid form a special subgroup of the underinsured. They often lack access because of physician reluctance to treat. It is extremely difficult for these patients to receive timely, ambulatory care; they are forced to rely upon a limited number of overcrowded public health centers and clinics staffed by medical trainees. Such was the situation of the patient in this case study.

Inadequate health insurance is not the only barrier to health care. Lack of transportation, lack of telephone, need for after-hours treatment, changing residence, and lack of understanding of how to utilize available resources, are all significant obstacles. These barriers to care are perpetuated by additional public health concerns such as poverty, homelessness and substance abuse.

EMERGENCY PHYSICIAN'S ROLE

Access to health care is only one public health issue that has transformed the practice of emergency medicine. EPs practice at the center of epidemics of infectious disease, substance abuse, violence, and poverty. Facing these issues necessitates a redefinition of the practice.

Identity shift for EPs. The role of the EP is changing. It is time to abandon the image of the lone practitioner whose job is to fix quickly and save lives and who has no ongoing relationship to patients once they have left the department.

Participating in a health care continuum. There has always been an important connection between health care provided in the ED and care given at other locations and times. The success of past treatment and prevention affects a patient's need for emergency care. Similarly, the quality of an ED intervention impacts on future health care needs. The EP is actually a member of an extended health care network, participating in each patient's lifelong care.

Ways to enhance communication and collaboration with other providers should therefore be sought.

Providing appropriate, "nonurgent" care. Framing the ED visit within the context of this continuum, it becomes meaningful to address health problems for which there is no quick-fix. For instance, counseling an ED patient about risk-taking behavior such as smoking or unprotected sex does have impact since it will be reinforced in other settings. The current reality of the American health system is that tens of millions of patients lack access to care. EDs provide indispensable ambulatory care for these patients.

Carrying patients into the future. The practice of disengaging from a patient's care simply by referring her or him back to a personal physician is senseless when there is no real access to follow-up. Strategies need to be developed for the ED to become a true bridge to continued care. The concept of "discharge instructions" should be supplanted by that of "discharge planning." Certain obstacles to compliance can be addressed during the ED visit. Appointments can be made for patients by ED staff. Opportunities for telephone follow-up with the patient can be created. By intervening at a critical hour, EPs have always served to carry their patients into the future. This ability to have an impact on patients' futures is extended further through prevention work and by collaborating with health care providers who will continue care.

Emphasis on interpersonal skills. A public health approach requires risk detection, education, and counseling. The patient encounter must create a space in which urgent psychosocial concerns may surface and that facilitates patient disclosure and receptivity. These goals can be accomplished within the time constraints of the typical ED encounter when effective strategies and techniques are used. It should be kept in mind that enhancing communication and minimizing conflict are extremely time efficient.

Building rapport. Establishing a working alliance has always been essential to each ED encounter. Rapport speeds diagnosis, increases compliance and enhances satisfaction. The realities of mistrust, negative stereotyping, multiple stressors, and conflicting agendas necessitate rapid stabilization of the physician-patient relationship. Just as an EP might walk into the room and immediately place an unstable patient on oxygen, so one must enter and initially perform a series of maneuvers that secure rapport.

Beginning an encounter involves much more than introducing oneself, and nonverbal communication is exceedingly important. The EP can immediately attend to a patient's comfort by adjusting the stretcher, improvising a pillow, dimming lights, tying the back of the gown. These actions speak clearly.

Body language can be put to work. The EP should get at eye level and assume a receptive posture with head and torso oriented toward the patient. Even more effective is a technique called "mirroring" in which the EP temporarily takes on the patient's nonverbal cues such as body positioning, rate of breathing, and speech pattern. Rapport affects both people, building on itself. A physician who utilizes these nonverbal techniques effectively will experience a positive shift in his or her own ability to listen and collaborate.

Listening. A sense of time pressure usually leads to the "high control style" of medical interviewing in which the EP asks all the questions and allows the patient to talk as little as possible. This interviewing strategy is seriously flawed.

- First, it is driven by the irrational fear that the patient will never stop talking. However, if not interrupted patients generally conclude their chief complaint within two minutes.
- Second, it actually wastes time. Patients frequently do not offer the most important piece of information first; interrupting the patient too early will lead the physician down the wrong diagnostic algorithm. Barraging the patient with too many questions squelches the spontaneous flow of information—patients stop volunteering additional history after being interrupted just a few times.
- Third, a "facts only" approach is untenable. Patients do not categorize information in the same way as physicians. Essential facts flow together with subjective feelings and minor details.
- Fourth, the intense search for objective data invariably excludes key psychosocial information that can illuminate diagnosis and guide rational therapy. The alternative is simply to get a patient to tell his or her story for a few minutes. The EP can use body language and an occasional open-

ended question to support the information flow. The history can then be completed with a handful of focused questions.

This approach has distinct advantages. It requires less effort to be given information than to extract it. Listening is itself a therapeutic intervention; patients have a legitimate need to express their concerns and have them acknowledged. The physician learns something about the person as well as the disease. Allowing a patient some opportunity to convey subjective experience first creates the possibility for the EP to respond empathically.

Collaborating. Patient passivity and powerlessness ultimately undermines the possibility of healing. The ED encounter provides numerous opportunities for empowering the patient. The EP can share information with the patient throughout the interaction. Working diagnoses can be conveyed. Physical findings can be vocalized ("Your lungs are clear and your heartbeat is normal.") Rather than having his body passively handled, a patient can participate actively during the physical examination ("We need to examine your abdomen together. I need you to guide my hands to the problem spot").

The agendas of both patient and physician need to be brought out into the open to avoid frustration. If the patient came in with certain expectations of a test being done or being admitted to the hospital, these need to be discovered and addressed early on. If the EP's fixed agenda is to avoid writing a narcotic prescription, this should be conveyed openly.

Crisis seen as opportunity. Medical crisis is a time of reaching out for help. Personal defenses drop, and the usual social barriers which separate people become fluid. This potential for immediacy and authenticity is built into each ED-patient encounter. When allowed to emerge it creates an intimacy between physician and patient that transcends personal and social barriers. Crisis also becomes opportunity for personal change. The patient who is facing danger is less capable of denying health risks, and this makes successful counseling much more likely.

System solutions. An expanded identity for EPs calls for strategies to improve the system in which they deliver care.

Patient interactions with ED staff. Before meeting the physician, the patient has encounters with staff during triage, registration, and upon being placed in an examination area. Negative interactions that have alienated patients already place the medical interview on shaky ground. It is crucial for departments to address the overall quality of staff communication.

Brief continuity of care. EDs have instituted a practice of telephone follow-ups for targeted patients. These may help to reinforce patient education and to facilitate follow-up with other physicians or social agencies.

Inevitably, patients do make repeat visits to the ED. It is imperative that information from one visit be readily available on the next. The EP should seek out and consult with other physicians who cared for a patient on previous encounters. Sharing information among different EDs, within the constraints of patient confidentiality, can also improve the quality of care.

Support materials. Pamphlets and posters can be used to convey important health messages. They also serve to open up topics for discussion during the physician-patient encounter. A bulletin board display on domestic violence, for example, may encourage disclosure by a victim. Questionnaires can be used to screen for a variety of health risks.

Coordination with other providers. Problems with patient follow-up can be avoided by instituting a system in the ED for making referral appointments. The full content of the ED evaluation, including the physician's assessment and plan, should be available at the follow-up visit. Necessary, additional testing, can be ordered by the EP on behalf of the next provider.

Integration with social service and community resources should occur. Patients can be educated about application for medical assistance. Some may qualify for home health or paratransit services. Volunteers from advocacy groups, such as Women Organized Against Rape, can play an important role in the ED.

Social action. EPs can bring changes to their community that promote a public health agenda through personal lobbying efforts, organizational activities, and coalition building.

CONCLUSION

Emergency physicians are an important link in the health care continuum and often are the only resource available to patients without access to traditional services. Specific communication/listening skills can be acquired that facilitate receptivity to verbal and nonverbal cues to diagnosis. Often the crisis of an emergency department visit is an opportunity to establish rapid rapport and deep and meaningful communication to fundamentally be of real service to our patients. A medical encounter based on a comprehensive view of the presenting problem, patient-physician collaboration and a team approach is more likely to result in a satisfactory outcome for both patient and physician.

31

Motivating Patients for Change: A Brief Strategy for Negotiation

GAIL D'ONOFRIO
EDWARD BERNSTEIN
STEPHEN ROLLNICK

CONTENTS

- Identification and referral of high risk behaviors
- Components of the Brief Negotiation Interview (BNI)
- Traps to avoid in the interviewing process
- Strategies for promoting readiness to change

CHAPTER SUMMARY

Significant health risks may be identified during an emergency department (ED) visit. This chapter describes a 10-minute intervention, the Brief Negotiation Interview (BNI), in which the provider assists the patient to express reasons for concern, and arguments for and against changing behavior. Strategies are then utilized depending on the patient's readiness to change. Information giving is patient-centered and collaborative, in contrast to a traditional physician interaction that involves persuasion and advice-giving. Appropriate plans for referral and intervention are discussed.

Case #1

A 24-year-old white male presented to the ED at 2:00 A.M. on Wednesday as an unrestrained driver involved in a single-car motor vehicle crash (MVC). His car had hit a utility pole and sustained moderate front-end damage and a spidered windshield. There was no loss of consciousness. The patient was found at the scene awake, rambling incoherently, with normal vital signs. He was C-spine–immobilized and transferred.

In the ED, he was uncooperative and abusive to the staff. He had a strong smell of alcohol on his breath. Physical exam revealed abrasions over forehead and upper extremities and a 2 cm laceration to his left eyebrow. He had a swollen, tender left knee. The remainder of the exam was unremarkable. C-spine and knee films were negative. His blood alcohol level was 190mg/dl. After several hours, the patient's laceration was sutured, and he was medically cleared. He denied any previous medical illnesses or surgeries. He was alert and oriented x 3, cooperative and ready for discharge. He was instructed not to drink and drive, and given follow-up for his suture removal.

Q: What responsibility does the physician have in the identification and referral of high-risk behaviors?

The emergency department is often the point of entry into the health care system for patients who have nonacute illnesses in addition to an acute presenting condition. During such a "crisis" visit, the physician or other health care worker may identify significant health risks such as substance abuse, smoking, obesity, and abusive relationships that are secondary diagnoses that need to be addressed. Emergency medicine specialists have a responsibility to the patient, to themselves, and to society to ask appropriate questions, to identify health risks, and to provide feedback to patients respectfully in the form of useful information. Even within the time limitations of a brief ED interview, it is possible to empower patients to begin the process of developing solutions for themselves.

Q: What further information should be obtained regarding past medical and social history?

In the case presented above, it is clear that the physician must do more than medically clear this patient. It would be easy just to clean and suture his external wounds, observe him until his alcohol level decreased, and discharge him with an admonishment not to drink and drive. Traditionally, physicians do not feel that negotiating behavior change is a high priority.[1] While assessing the extent of the crash, the patient's mental status and his physical wounds, the physician also has the opportunity to obtain valuable information about precipitating factors and begin to establish rapport. This information can often be obtained without an extra time investment—while suturing the patient or during a repeat exam once the patient is less intoxicated.

Case Continuation

With a few additional questions, the patient admitted that this was in fact the second car crash he had been involved in this year. He admitted to drinking with his friends earlier in the evening. He usually has six to eight beers on three or four occasions per week. Tonight he had a few shots of tequila as well. He works as a waiter in the evening and goes to school during the day.

Q: What would be the usual physician response to this information?

Interventions usually involving persuasive tactics or advice giving have resulted in limited success.[2–5] Patients also often have reservations about being told what to do by their doctors.[6] While some researchers have shown advice giving to be somewhat helpful in motivating behavior change with excessive drinking and smoking,[2] others suggest that a more patient-centered approach ensures better outcomes.[7–9]

Case Continuation

Before the patient was discharged, the ED physician had the following conversation with him:

Doctor: *You had a very serious car crash. You are lucky that you didn't kill yourself or anyone else. What are you going to do about your drinking problem?*

Patient: *I only had a couple of beers, that's all. I don't have a problem.*

D: *Your alcohol level was 190.*

P: *Look, everyone goes out with their friends and drinks a little. Don't make such a big deal about it. Just sew me up so I can get out of here. I have to get up early and go to school.*

D: *Sir, I've been an ER doctor for many years. 190 is more than a few drinks. I know when someone is an alcoholic and has a drinking problem. You'll be ready to go as soon as I finish suturing this laceration, but you must stop drinking and driving! Next time you may end up dead! (All the while, doctor is wagging his/her finger at the patient.)*

Q: What problems are inherent in this type of provider-patient communication?

This interaction demonstrates some common problems and traps encountered when attempting to counsel a patient.[10] In this dialogue, the physician is using his authority and expert status to shame the patient into compliance with his prescription for behavior change. The heavy-handedness and one-sidedness of this approach may actually increase the patient's resistance to change.

The physician's first interactions are important, as they will set the tone for the remaining encounter. In beginning the interaction by telling the patient he has a serious problem, the physician fell into the *confrontation-denial trap.* The patient responded predictably by denying a problem and any necessity for change. The doctor ended up arguing one side more and more aggressively, while the patient, feeling trapped, defended his behavior more and more adamantly. For example, D: "Well John, you should stop drinking." P: "Yes, but I'll lose my friends. . . ."

It is also important to avoid the *labeling trap.* "You are an alcoholic" or "your drinking problem . . ." and so on. This may lead to a power or control struggle between the doctor and patient. The physician may then appear judgmental, ending with more resistance on part of the patient.

This leads us to another trap to avoid, the *expert trap*. Here the physician appears to have all the answers and the patient is placed in the passive role, negating the importance of eliciting the patient's own motivation for change.

Additional traps to avoid include the *blaming trap*, which implies that the problem is someone's or something's fault. Time and effort is displaced on an outside focus, and the patient becomes defensive. Instead, the focus should be placed on the patient's own concerns and what *he* might wish to do about them.

Early in the interaction, the physician should attempt to avoid the *question-answer trap* in which the interviewer elicits only short, one-or two-word answers on the part of the patient. While this may be productive during an initial medical history, it should be avoided once the provider begins to raise the issues around change. If not, the patient assumes a passive role and is not afforded the opportunity to make self motivational comments.

Finally, one of the most difficult challenges for the ED physician is to avoid the *premature focus trap*. The physician has a limited time for each patient interaction and will need to focus on the issues expediently, while the patient may have another agenda involving larger issues and problems. To avoid a struggle, one must first acknowledge the patient's concerns. Sometimes this is just something simple like providing a drink of water, offering a phone for contact with a significant other, or alleviating anxiety about finding a way home.

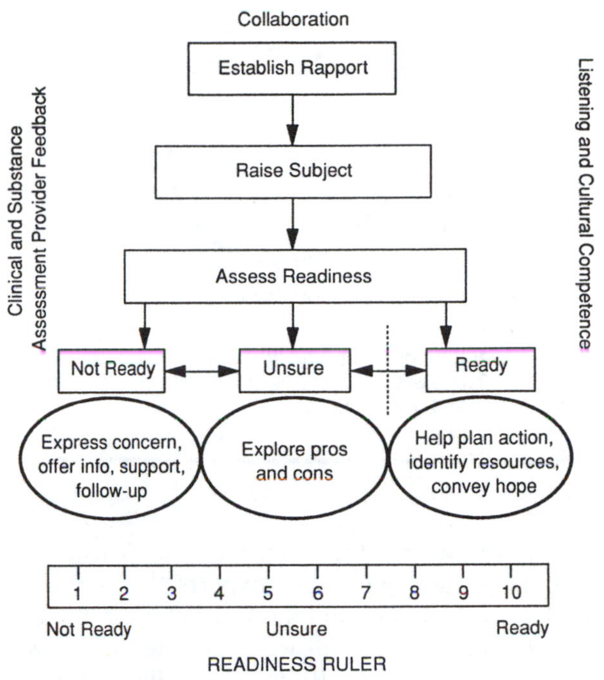

Q: What alternative approach might avoid these traps and offer a better prognosis for behavior change?

The Brief Negotiation Interview (BNI) is a strategy to assist patients to recognize and change behaviors that may be significant risks to health (Figure 31-1). Most often patients are ambivalent and reluctant to change.[10] The goals of the interaction are to help the patient resolve some ambivalence by exploring conflicting motivations and to provide possible strategies for change, depending on the patient's readiness to change. Knowing that resources are available, or how to access them is often enough to "get unstuck."

Figure 31-1 Brief Negotiation Interview

Information should be patient-centered, permitting freedom of choice, and not advice giving.[11,12] The physician cannot persuade the patient to change, as in "if you don't...this may happen," a style which will surely elicit the "yes, but..." response. Studies of noncompliance reveal that most patients do not fully follow doctors' orders. Half of all patients do not take their prescribed drugs correctly,[13] and lifestyle changes (diet, alcohol intake, and smoking) are even less likely to follow customary physician interventions.

Paulo Freire, an educator, attributes the failure of traditional models of education to what he calls a "banking" theory of knowledge; teachers deposit knowledge into passive recipients, just like money into bank accounts. He encourages instead a model in which learning goes both ways, in which the learner can also impart knowledge to the teacher.[14] In the BNI, for example, the patient possesses a unique store of knowledge that is essential for behavioral change to occur—his own life history—which is just as important for achieving the goal of lifestyle change as the physician's expertise.[9] The physician-

Figure 31-2 Stages of Change Model

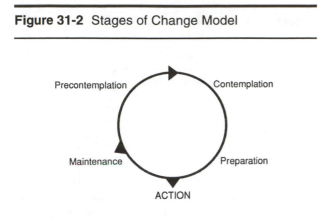

SOURCE: Adapted from *The Transtheoretical Approach: Crossing Traditional Boundaries of Therapy*, James Prochaska and Carlo DiClemente, 1984. Pacific Grove, CA: Brooks/Cole. Figure 3-3, p. 30.

patient encounter then becomes, as Tuckett describes, "a meeting between experts."[1]

Figure 31-1 presents the basic steps in the brief negotiation interview process, adapted from work originally outlined by Rollnick and Bell, who used motivational interviewing with excessive drinkers.[15] The goal of the BNI is to increase intrinsic motivation so that change arises from within rather than being imposed from without. Overall principles include (1) assisting the patient to recognize and actively initiate behavioral change; (2) leaving the responsibility of change to the individual; and (3) creating a positive atmosphere conducive to change.

Q: What is known on a theoretical level about how people come to change high-risk behaviors?

A model of how people change has been developed by psychologists James Prochaska and Carlo DiClemente.[16] They have described a series of stages through which people pass in the course of changing behavior (Figure 31-2). The circle implies that it is normal for patients to go through the process several times. The first point of entry is the "precontemplation" stage. Here the person is not even aware that a problem exists, or that change is necessary. More often, someone else, such as a significant other, or health care provider, knows of the person's problem. At this stage, the person needs information and feed-

back to raise the possibility of a problem necessitating change. The "contemplation" stage occurs once one is aware that a problem exists and is characterized by ambivalence. At this stage, the person may go back and forth with reasons for and against change. This is where the brief negotiation interview may be most useful to tip the scale towards change. The "preparation" stage is where a provider can assist the person to find a strategy for change that is appropriate for that individual, offering a range of accessible, effective strategies. The "action" stage is where the person participates in specific actions in order to initiate change. Once a change is made, however, there is no guarantee that it will persist. During the "maintenance" stage one attempts to sustain the change without relapse.

Prochaska, DiClemente, and Velicer found that among smokers, 35% were in the precontemplation stage, 50% in the contemplation stage, and only 15% in the action stage.[17] Rollnick et al. found that among hospitalized excessive drinkers, 29% were in the precontemplation stage, 45% in the contemplation stage, and 26% were in the action stage.[18]

Q: How might a Brief Negotiation interview (BNI) be conducted in the context of the ED?

Table 31-1 illustrates the tasks of the BNI, describes appropriate goals for the practitioner, and lists some open ended questions that can be used to elicit information and move the interaction forward. In the situation described in the case study, the attending physician was actually listening outside the curtain while the resident was giving advice. He was not happy with the outcome, and decided to intervene to correct the damage. This is the way the BNI was structured:

Case Continuation

Doctor: You had a very serious car crash. Do you remember what happened?

Patient: Not much. I remember leaving my friends at the bar. The rest is all a blur.

D: You mentioned you had a previous crash this year. What happened?

P: Oh, nothing really. I hit an embankment. It was a very slippery night.

Table 31-1 The BNI

Tasks		Goals	Questions
Establish rapport		—to understand patient's concerns and circumstances; —to explain provider's role; —to avoid a judgemental stance.	Sit down on chair at bedside and ask open-ended questions that show concern for patient as a person, i.e., how are you feeling today? Are you comfortable? If I could see the situation through your eyes, what would I see? Help me to understand.
Raise subject		—to get patient agreement to talk about alcohol and drug use.	Would you mind spending 5 minutes talking about your use of ___? How do you see it affecting your health?
Assess readiness		—to evaluate readiness to accept a referral	How do you feel about your use of ___? How ready are you to change your use of ___? (Use ruler).
Provide feedback		—to raise patient awareness of the medical aspects of alcohol and drug use and consequences of further use; —to let patient know provider's concerns.	How much do you know about what caused the reason for your ED visit? What do you make of all this?
Readiness Ruler:	Not Ready	—to offer further contact if the patient desires; —to offer to present your feedback and concerns if the patient wants; —to offer card with referral options	Is there anything you would want to know about ___? Would you mind if I tell you about my concerns for your health? What would it take to get you to consider thinking about a change? If you ever decide to stop, what would you do?
	Unsure	—to facilitate the patient's ability to name the problem by discussing pros and cons of use; —to understand ambivalence and how to work with it.	What are the good things you like about ___ or what it does for you? What are the not so good things/things you don't like about ___? What concerns do you have about your use of ___?
	Ready	—to help patients name solutions for themselves, choose a course of action and decide how to achieve it; —to encourage patient choice.	1. Emphasize a) there are many options; b) you know what has worked for you in the past and for other people; c) you are the best judge of what suits you and can work for you. 2. List options. 3. Ask, "What will work for you?" 4. Offer back-up support and referral.

Figure 31-3 Principles of Reflective Listening

REFLECTIVE LISTENING

ATTITUDE: Provider acceptance of
                        patient's experience

TECHNIQUES: Empathy and Rapport
                        Validation and Respect
                        Summary and Clarification

BASIS OF CHANGE: Patient ambivalence

BENEFITS TO   Accurate Assessment
PROVIDER: Appropriate Referrals
                        Role Satisfaction

Table 31-2 General Principles for Negotiating
Behavior Change

- Respect for autonomy of patients and their choices
- Readiness to change must be taken into account
- Ambivalence is common; it needs to be understood
- Targets need to be selected by the patient, not the expert
- The expert is the provider of the information and support
- The patient is the active decision maker

Source: Rollnick, 1994

D: *That must have been frightening. Would you mind spending a few minutes talking about your drinking?*

P: *Look, I go out with my friends a lot. I have a few drinks. Who doesn't. What's the big deal?*

D: *I'm concerned about your drinking, and especially when you drive. How ready are you to change your drinking behavior?*

P: *I don't have a problem with my drinking.*

D: *That may be the case, but help me to understand what drinking does for you? What do you like about it?*

P: *I work hard. It helps me relax. I hang out with my friends, listen to music.*

D: *Are there any things not so good about your drinking?*

P: *Right now my only problem is getting up for school. Sometimes I can't think straight in the morning because I have such a bad hangover.*

D: *And that doesn't seem right to you.*

P: *I need to be alert for school as I have very little time to study outside class. Lately I'm not thinking as clearly.*

D: *And you think this may have something to do with your drinking?*

P: *Yes, and my girlfriend is always nagging me about it.*

D: *So, on the one hand it helps you relax and hang out with your friends, and on the other it impairs your thinking in the morning, and upsets your girl-*

friend. Anything else that is less good about the drinking?

P: *What happened tonight was not too good about the drinking.*

D: *What about it?*

P: *I wasn't as alert as I should have been.*

D: *Like in school.*

P: *Worse.*

D: *Where does this leave you?*

This alternative interaction illustrates the principles of *reflective listening* (Figure 31-3) and the use of open-ended questions in an effort to encourage the patient to talk.[10] It also offers several possibilities for exploring the connection between drinking and driving with the patient. There is no attempt to assign blame or label a problem in the initial encounter. Table 31-2 outlines some general principles to keep in mind during the BNI. Table 31-3 illustrates some dangerous assumptions about behavior change that the provider should avoid.

An important concept in the BNI is the use of reflective listening. It is a way of checking what the person meant by a statement. Because it is a nonjudgmental technique, it is less likely to build resistance or block further conversation and instead encourages further thought and reflection on the part of the patient. Reflective listening takes into account what the speaker meant, what the speaker said, what the listener heard, and finally what the listener thought the speaker meant. Intonation in reflective-listening statements should usually turn down at the end of the remark in order to encourage the patient to

Table 31-3 Dangerous Assumptions Regarding Behavior Change

- This person ought to change.
- This person is ready to change.
- This person's health is a prime motivating factor for him/her.
- If he/she does not decide to change his/her behavior, the consultation has failed.
- Patients are either motivated to change, or not.
- Now is the right time to consider change.
- A tough approach is always best.
- I'm the expert—he/she must follow my advice.

SOURCE: Rollnick, 1994

Table 31-4 Facilitating the Naming Process

Develop Discrepancies: Explore Pros and Cons

- Facilitate patient awareness of consequences.
- Demonstrate discrepancy between present behavior and the patient's own expressed goals.
- Empower the patient to name the problem; use the patient/client and his consequences as a source of arguments for change.

SOURCE: Adapted with permission from May PA, Miller JH, Wallerstein N. Motivation and community prevention of substance abuse. *Experimental and Clinical Psychopharmacology* 1993, Vol. 1, No. 1–4, pp. 68–79. Copyright © 1993 by The American Psychological Association.

respond. An upward intonation should be avoided, because it can suggest a challenge or threat.

Q: What is this "readiness to change" approach?

Measuring readiness to change ("The Readiness Ruler", Figure 31-1) is an important part of the BNI. Rollnick has developed this linear model based on Prochaska and DiClemente's wheel of change and has applied it to drinking, smoking, diet, exercise, drug use, and compliance with therapeutic regimens. At the left end of *The Readiness Ruler*, patients self-identify as NOT READY to consider change. Those on the right side are READY to change, and those in the middle are ambivalent (UNSURE). Patients may move forward and backward along this continuum. Attempting to move someone along before they are ready will only lead to an inappropriate strategy resulting in resistance. Helping patients to move toward readiness is an acceptable outcome of the BNI, even if the patient does not commit to change at the present time.

Q: What should be included in a discharge plan for referral and safety?

Once the patient's degree of readiness to change is assessed, the physician can choose from a menu of

strategies[18] (Tables 31-1, 31-4, 31-5, 31-6).[19] The case study illustrates the use of the concept of readiness:

Case Continuation

D: *Where does this leave you?*

P: *What do you think I should do, doctor?*

D: *Well, you told me what you liked and disliked about your drinking. Based on that, do you feel like you're ready to change your drinking behavior?*

Table 31-5 Choosing Solutions That Will Work

Support Self-Efficacy, Patient Choice and Responsibility

- Belief in the possibility of change is an important motivator.
- The patient is responsible for choosing and carrying out a plan for personal change that works for him.
- There is hope in the range of alternative approaches available.
- Solicit a menu of options from the patient; add to it as needed.

SOURCE: Adapted with permission from May PA, Miller JH, Wallerstein N. Motivation and community prevention of substance abuse. *Experimental and Clinical Psychopharmacology* 1993, Vol. 1, No. 1–4, pp. 68–79. Copyright © 1993 by The American Psychological Association.

Table 31-6 Handling Ambivalence

Roll with Resistance

- Use momentum to good advantage.
- Shift perceptions.
- Expect resistance.
- Invite—don't impose—new perspectives.
- Empower patients to name the solution.

SOURCE: Adapted with permission from May PA, Miller JH, Wallerstein N. Motivation and community prevention of substance abuse. *Experimental and Clinical Psychopharmacology* 1993, Vol. 1, No. 1–4, pp. 68–79. Copyright © 1993 by The American Psychological Association.

P: It seems like it might be better to cut back.

D: What about your drinking and driving?

P: That's a mistake. I can find someone else to drive, or take the bus.

D: Would you like to speak with someone about trying to cut back on your drinking?

P: No, I can do it on my own.

D: Some people can cut back on their own, but sometimes that proves to be very difficult. If you find that you need help, I can give you the names and phone numbers of some people here you can contact.

Table 31-7 [18]summarizes important guidelines for helping patients with decision making. If the patient is *ready* to change as in the above example, the physician assists him to name the solution or option that is best for him, and a course of action. Referral and support are offered accordingly. If the patient is *not ready*, the physician can express concern and offer appropriate information, as in this case about drinking and driving and about possibilities for speaking with someone in the future. Sometimes in the ED, the physician is mandated to report behaviors or compelled by professional and or ethical standards to give written and verbal discharge instructions regarding high-risk behavior. This may mean simply stating: "Do not drink and drive."

If the patient is *unsure*, the physician assists the patient to express the pros and cons of change as in the above example and understands their ambivalence. Concern and follow-up are offered. The physi-

Table 31-7 Guidelines for Helping Patients with Decision Making

- Do not rush patients into decision making.
- Present options for the future rather than a single course of action.
- Describe what other patients have done in a similar situation.
- Emphasize that "you are the best judge of what will be best for you.
- Provide information in a neutral, nonpersonal manner.
- Failure to reach a decision to change is not a failed consultation.
- Resolutions to change often break down. Make sure that patients understand this and do not avoid future contact if things go wrong.
- Commitment to change is likely to fluctuate. Expect this to happen and empathize with the patient's predicament.

SOURCE: Rollnick, Heather, and Bell, 1992. Negotiating behavior change in medical settings: The development of brief motivational interviewing. *Journal of Mental Health* 1:25–37.

cian hopes the patient moves ever so slightly to the right on the readiness scale and may at a future time be all the more ready to change.

CONCLUSION

Many physicians are reluctant to accept responsibility for negotiating behavior change. This is especially a problem in the high-pressure setting of a busy ED. However, patients presenting to EDs have high rates of injury and chronic disease risk and often lack other sources of routine health care. It is therefore imperative that the ED physician be educated to identify these problems and intervene effectively.[20] Often physicians are unaware that even a brief intervention may trigger a positive change in behavior or encourage patients to seek further treatment.[21] It is possible during a 10-minute Brief Negotiation Interview to assess a patient's readiness to change and empower a patient to find his or her own solutions. Early referral and treatment may have a dramatic effect and avert a lifetime of consequences. The BNI works best when the ED offers a system for easy access to treatment and has appropriate referral resources. So, as a physician, HOW READY ARE YOU TO CHANGE YOUR BEHAVIOR?

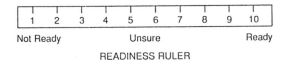

READINESS RULER

NOTES

1. Tuckett D, Boulton M, Olson C, Williams A. *Meetings between experts.* New York: Tavistock, 1985.
2. Orleans CT. Understanding and promoting smoking cessation: Overview and guidelines for physician intervention. *Ann Rev Med* 1985; 36: 51–61.
3. Russell M, Wilson C, Baker C, Taylor C. Effect of general practitioners' advice against smoking. *BMJ* 1979; 2:231–5.
4. Wallace P, Cutler S, Haines A. Randomized controlled trial of general practitioner intervention in patients with excessive alcohol consumption. *BMJ* 1988; 297:663–8.
5. Walsh D, Hingson RW, Merrigan DM, et al. The impact of a physician's warning on recovery after alcoholism treatment. *JAMA* 1992; 267:663–7.
6. Stott NCH, Pill RM. "Advise yes, dictate no"—Patients' views on health promotion in the consultation. *Fam Pract* 1990; 7:125–31.
7. Kaplan S, Greenfield S, Ware J. Assessing the effectiveness of patient centered interactions on the outcome of chronic diseases. *Med Care* 1989; 27:110–27.
8. Ockene J, Kristeller J, Goldberg R, Amick T, Pekow P, Hosmer D, Quirk M, Kalan K. Increasing the efficacy of physician-delivered smoking interventions. A randomized clinical trial. *J Gen Inter Med* 1991; 6:1–8.
9. Roter DL, Hall JA. *Doctors Talking with Patients/Patients Talking with Doctors.* Westport, CT: Auburn House, 1993.
10. Miller WR, Rollnick S. *Motivational Interviewing: Preparing People to Change Addictive Behavior.* New York: Guilford Press, 1991.
11. Roter DL, Hall JA, Katz NR. Physician-patient communication: A descriptive summary of the literature. *Pat Ed Counseling* 1988; 12:99–119.
12. Stewart M, Roter D. *Communicating with Medical Patients.* London: Sage, 1989.
13. Haynes RB, Taylor DW, Sackett DL (eds.). *Compliance in Health Care,* 2nd ed. Baltimore: John Hopkins University Press, 1981.
14. Freire, P. *Pedagogy of the Oppressed.* New York: Seabury Press, 1970.
15. Rollnick S, Bell A. Brief motivational interviewing for use by the nonspecialist. In Miller W, Rollnick S. *Motivational Interviewing: Preparing People to Change Addictive Behaviors.* New York: Guilford Press, 1991.
16. Prochaska J, DiClemente C. Toward a comprehensive model of change. In Miller WR, Heather N (eds.). *Treating Addictive Behaviors: Processes of Change.* New York: Plenum Press, 1986.
17. Prochaska J, DiClemente C, Velicer W. Comparative analysis of self-help programs for four stages of smoking cessation. In Glyn T (Chair). *Four National Cancer Institute funded self-help smoking cessation trials.* Symposium conducted at the Annual Association for the Advancement of Behavior Therapy Convention, New York, 1988.
18. Rollnick S, Heather N, Bell A. Negotiating behaviour change in medical settings: The development of brief motivational interviewing. *J Mental Health* 1992; 1:25–37.
19. May PA, Miller JH, Wallerstein N. Motivation and community prevention of substance abuse. *Exp Clin Psychopharm* 1993; 1:68–79.
20. Bien T, Miller WR. Brief interventions for alcohol problems: A review. *Addiction* 1993; 88: 315–36.
21. Bernstein E. Speaking sober in the emergency department. *Acad Emerg Med* 1995; 2:762–4.

Unit V

Preparations for the Twenty-First Century

32

Managed Care: New Challenges and Opportunities for Emergency Medicine

RICHARD M. MCDOWELL

CONTENTS

CHAPTER SUMMARY

Emergency medicine provides the safety net that catches many patients who would otherwise fall through the cracks of the health care system. It is on the frontline, treating patients regardless of the type of problem, time of day, or ability to pay, providing an interface between specialty care for inpatients, resources for follow-up care, and primary care for outpatients. As a result of this unique perspective, the voice of emergency must be heard in the design and implementation of an improved health care system.

Emergency medicine is part of the solution to many problems in the health care system today, but ED visits have been characterized by some as part of the problem. Criticism has been focused on two tar-

gets: so-called "inappropriate" ED visits, and high ED visit charges. This has led insurance companies to propose solutions which seek to decrease ED visits by either turning patients away from the ED or by denying payment for care which is rendered. These solutions are poor public policy based on oversimplified evaluations of the complex problems of emergency departments and their patients.

Certainly, efforts must be made to reduce ED overcrowding by providing reasonable access to primary care. But in the absence of national health policy that provides such care, the ED physician has an obligation to provide medical diagnosis and treatment to patients who present in need. A more thorough analysis of ED care can provide solutions that address high ED charges and high utilization with effective public policy that is not harmful to patients and does not create impossible ethical dilemmas for the emergency medicine practitioner.

Several managed care strategies that deny emergency department care are clinically ineffective, ethically inappropriate, legally unrealistic, and threaten the entire safety net. They ignore the reality that adequate primary care is not available to patients in many areas. There are moral, legal and logistical problems with turning patients away from an ED, which may be their only realistic route to care. Emergency medicine, which represents only 1 to 2% of the total health care bill, is a major source of high-quality care that prevents problems from worsening and driving up the cost of health care delivery. It is vital that the system not only fully support emergency departments but also fully integrate them into an expanded and accessible primary care network.

INTRODUCTION

The process illustrated in these case presentations is called "preauthorization," "prior approval," or "gatekeeping." Several scenarios have been selected to illustrate actual cases which occur in many EDs where managed care organizations exist. Emergency departments have different policies and procedures to guide this preauthorization process and also differ in location, staffing, and volume, just as patients themselves differ in educational level and resources, but these managed care preauthorization scenarios do occur daily throughout the entire spectrum of hospitals and patients.

Although the actual details of the encounter vary from hospital to hospital, several aspects are typical. The patient enters the triage and registration area of the hospital ED and, at some point during the process, is identified as an enrollee of a managed care organization (MCO). Hospital ED personnel have been instructed to call the MCO to "authorize" or "approve" the visit—that is, to give "permission to be seen" or to "refuse the visit." A telephone call is made to a representative of the MCO, who may be a nurse or primary care physician (PCP)—the "gatekeeper" whose role is to judge whether ED visits are appropriate or inappropriate. This gatekeeper may or may not know the patient. If the visit is "not allowed" by the MCO gatekeeper, the patient is so informed by ED personnel. At this point, the patient will be told that the MCO will not "allow" or pay for the ED visit, and the patient may be given additional information, including an alternative site and time for an exam by the PCP. The patient may or may not be satisfied with this information. The patient may or may not be seen again by the triage nurse or by the emergency physician. Finally, documentation of the details of this entire process varies considerably from hospital to hospital.

Case #1

A 24-year-old female arrives in the ED with her 6-month-old daughter at 2000 hours on a weekday evening, and the baby is seen by the triage nurse on arrival. The nurse documents a triage exam in a note that includes normal vital signs except for a temperature of 101°F. The note says that the child has had symptoms of

a URI for 2 days, including a runny nose and congestion, and presents to the ED because of the fever that began several hours ago. The triage exam documents nasal congestion, clear lungs, and a baby in no apparent distress.

The mother is then shown to the registration area where she shows a clerk an insurance card which shows that she participates in a MCO which "requires" preauthorization. The clerk completes the information for the medical record, calls the gatekeeper, and receives a return call from the primary care physician 30 minutes later. The clerk reads the information from the triage note to the PCP over the telephone and is told that the patient's visit is "not approved" and the mother should come to the PCPs office in the morning.

The registration clerk tells the mother that the visit has not been approved and she is to take the baby to the PCP in the morning. She says she understands and leaves the ED. The clerk informs the triage nurse that the patient has left and voids the ED chart.

Case #2

A 55-year-old male comes to the ED at 1500 hours with symptoms that he describes as heartburn that began 3 hours ago and that he attributes to a large, greasy lunch. He has no prior history but left work to come to the hospital because of the persistence of the symptoms, which were initially severe but now improved.

The triage nurse is busy with a queue of patients, and the security guard directs the patient to the registration clerk, who proceeds with a preauthorization process, which is similar to the one described in case #1. The PCP answers the phone and tells the clerk to have the patient come to his office now to be seen. There is no triage note and the patient leaves before an ED chart is generated.

Case #3

An 11-year-old female is brought to the ED at 1800 hours by her parents for a sore throat, which began 3 days ago. The triage nurse notes a normal exam except for a temperature of 102° and swollen tonsils, which are difficult to visualize because of the patient's gagging. The patient is registered and the PCP is contacted by the triage nurse, who explains the situation. The patient is instructed to see the PCP the next day in the office. The parents both work and one of them will have to miss work to take the child to the doctor. The triage nurse informs them that their insurance will not pay for the visit but they may have the child seen in the ED if they choose. They elect to leave and seek treatment the next day. The nurse documents this conversation on the triage note and attaches it to the ED chart, which is tabulated by the QA audit as a patient who leaves the ED without treatment.

Q: What are the potential negative outcomes if these three patients do not receive timely care?

In all three cases, there is a risk of sudden death if serious conditions are not appropriately diagnosed. The baby may have occult bacteremia and develop meningitis, the symptoms of the 55-year-old male may represent an evolving M.I., and the child may have a peritonsillar abscess.

Q: Why does the emergency department call for preauthorization, and what does preauthorization really mean?

Managed care organizations want telephone triage of their enrollees in order to direct some of them away from care in the emergency department and into a less costly setting for health care delivery. This preauthorization is for payment of the ED visit, not for permission for ED care. The agreement to seek preauthorization is part of the contract between the insurance company and the enrollee and is not part of the relationship between the ED and the patient. ED personnel call, however, because the patient requests it or, or because hospital clerical staff have been told that it is their responsibility to make the call as part of the registration process. In many instances, the hospital has signed a preauthorization agreement with the MCO in order to decrease instances of nonpayment for emergency services. Unfortunately, the ED which participates in preauthorization is confronted with a monumental risk management problem.

Q: What is the liability exposure of the ED if these patients have bad outcomes—if the baby has occult bacteremia and subsequently develops meningitis, or the man has new onset coronary insufficiency and an M.I. or arrhythmia en route to the office, or the child has a peritonsillar abscess that is not treated because neither parent can get excused from work?

Patients may perceive denial of payment by the insurance company as a refusal to treat by the ED, which has apparently turned them away. There may be serious problems with the managed care gatekeeper's suggestion for an office visit follow-up, including time delay in diagnosis and treatment, lack of transportation, and inability to reschedule work or child care obligations. If a bad outcome results, the hospital ED has significant malpractice risk exposure.

Q: If there is litigation, is the documentation of this encounter adequate?

The managed-care decision maker who received the call can claim that information given by hospital personnel was inadequate; the visit would have been authorized if the situation had been described accurately. If the telephone call was made by a clerk with no medical expertise, or if the call was made by an appropriate person, such as the ED triage nurse, but there is no formal documentation of the details of the conversation, a strong case can be made for liability. Even a written note can be suspect, since it is only one party's impression of the encounter. Taped recordings may be accurate, but there are ethical and legal problems involved in taping of telephone conversations, and storage of such records presents formidable difficulties.

Furthermore, the managed care organization will claim, correctly, that no one refused to authorize care for the patient. What was refused was authorization for *payment* for the visit. The hospital ED now is in the position of having turned the patient away without care because the patient is now, in effect, uninsured. Ironically, the patient with no insurance and no income who presented to the same ED would, in most cases, have received full treatment.

Q: Does this encounter satisfy the federal regulations regarding emergency treatment and transfer (EMTALA/COBRA)?

In addition to the civil liability inherent in this encounter, there is federal legislation that specifically governs activities in hospital emergency departments known as the Emergency Medical Treatment and Labor Act, EMTALA, also known as COBRA or OBRA.[1] This federal law closely regulates the triage, treatment, and transfer of patients who present to hospital EDs and specifically prohibits the use of insurance status to influence care. Significant penalties of up to $50,000 and loss of Medicare license can be assessed to physicians and hospitals found in violation. Under EMTALA, emergency departments that participate in preauthorization activities by calling managed care organizations for approval of ED visits are at significant risk.

Calling for preauthorization for care in the ED is a clinical and ethical problem that is complicated by reimbursement issues. But as a risk-management issue alone, it poses an enormous liability. Many emergency physicians feel that the best way to manage this liability is to refuse to participate in this ED preauthorization activity in any form.[2] Managed care organizations do not have the same liability as EDs in this scenario and will push hospitals to sign contracts that require ED preauthorization calls in an attempt to keep patients out. Exposure to litigation lies with the hospital ED and physician but not with the managed care organization, which does not claim to practice medicine or refuse care in the ED. In addition, the MCO has some protection from state malpractice and insurance regulations under the Employee Retirement Income Security Act (ERISA).[3] These gatekeeper systems in managed care can create a conflict in physician-patient relationships. In medical malpractice lawsuits, cost-containment is not considered as a factor by judges and juries.[4]

Q: Are there any risk-management strategies that can be used in this scenario to improve the preauthorization protocol in order to minimize physician and hospital exposure?

Hospital EDs try to manage the risk in various ways. If the preauthorization call results in nonapproval, the patient might be given a form which says that the ED is willing to treat, but the patient will be billed and has financial responsibility for the visit. This solution is problematic, since the patient is still being treated differently as a result of insurance status. Perhaps all patients should be informed that their insurance company may not cover their bill.

Also, EMTALA regulations prohibit coercing a patient to transfer to another facility based on the fact that the patient would be billed unless transferred.[5] Could ED preauthorization activities be similarly construed? Some hospital EDs have the patient personally make the call and speak with the gatekeeper, since it is a contractual insurance matter between the patient and their insurer. But none of these stopgaps completely solve the problem, and the concept of preauthorization is simply a bad technique for cutting health care costs. Costs can be controlled and problems between insurance companies and emergency departments can be solved in a different and better way.

BROADER DISCUSSION

Q: What problems have given rise to the concept of preauthorization?

Insurance companies have focused on two aspects of emergency care: high charges and so-called "inappropriate" visits. Preauthorization, or prior approval or gatekeeping, for ED visits is the proposed solution, because patients can then be redirected from the ED into a primary care office. ED charges are certainly high in comparison to a visit in a primary care office, partly because of the practice of cost shifting, in which hospital charges are based on overall payer mix and thus do not always reflect actual costs. Insurance companies view many ED visits as "inappropriate," since some patients receive a diagnosis that retrospectively is considered nonurgent. These are valid concerns, but preauthorization for ED visits is not the answer.

Q: What other problems make the concept of refusing ED care attractive?

Overcrowding in EDs has become a significant problem, especially in large urban hospitals that deliver a disproportionate share of uncompensated care. Many emergency health care providers agree with managed care organizations that we need to build a stronger primary care network. Two articles in *JAMA* in 1991 discussed the problem of patients in large public hospital EDs queuing for care and then leaving without treatment, despite the fact that many of them needed immediate medical attention.[6,7] Many of the patients who had urgent problems either left or had to wait for a long time to be seen. Many who left but did not have urgent problems could not afford clinic care or did not have access to another site for care.

Overcrowding causes patients to leave EDs without being seen by an M.D. in all types of hospitals, although the number is greater in EDs with long waiting times and with a higher percentage of uninsured.[8] Overcrowding affects all patients who are treated there, not just those who are truly nonurgent and have no alternative to receiving episodic care. The American College of Emergency Physicians has recommended five strategies for addressing ED overcrowding, including adequate primary care services and insurance coverage for all citizens.[9]

In an effort to address these issues, a few EDs have taken the concept of preauthorization for care and have tried to change it into a more acceptable model. The requirement for a telephone call to a third party who is not in the ED, who cannot reliably identify the acuity of the patient, and who has limited liability is a significant problem. In an attempt to replace this telephone triage conversation, some EDs have developed their own triage guidelines to iden-

tify patients who could be refused care in the ED and referred elsewhere.[10–13] However, these guidelines for refusal of care have not been validated in other studies and institutions.[14,15] Such guidelines would have to achieve consensus about the definition of an emergency, and such consensus is difficult to achieve.

Q: Why is preauthorization or refusal of ED care unworkable and unacceptable?

The problem is that the concept of an "inappropriate" ED visit is fundamentally flawed. It is easy to invoke, but: (1) what is the definition of an emergency? and (2) where will this care be delivered if the patient is turned away from the ED? Definitions of emergent situations must be comprehensive enough to include not just medical but emotional and social aspects of health. These definitions must also be not just medically tenable, but legally justifiable.

Q: What constitutes an emergency?

An emergency is in the eye of the beholder.[16] Patients and physicians evaluate the necessity for emergency department care based on the reason for the visit. Insurance companies, however, define emergencies based only on retrospective review of medical records, using a discharge diagnosis based on a complete history, physical, testing results, and subsequent consultations. Retrospective review allows MCOs to refuse reimbursement for a large number of ED visits and saves them money, but it is unfair to their enrollees. Patients are put in the position of having to make their own diagnoses correctly before an ED visit or be responsible for the bill. What patients need is a prospective tool to help identify emergencies. The American College of Emergency Medicine uses a definition of an emergency that is useful prospectively and comprises what a "prudent layperson" would judge to be an emergency.[17] This ACEP definition has been used in several state legislative acts and medical society positions, and three states—Arkansas, Maryland, and Virginia—have formally accepted the prudent layperson definition as state law.[18]

Review of the literature suggests that there is considerable disagreement about the number of ED visits that might be categorized as nonurgent. A widely quoted study by the U.S. General Accounting Office in 1993 labeled 43% of 1990 ED visits in their broad sample as nonurgent, using a "threat to life or limb" definition.[19] Derlet at University of California, Davis, Medical Center prospectively triaged 18% of patients away from the ED as nonurgent,[12,13] but rates are quite different in other studies.[14,15] Internists and emergency physicians retrospectively reviewed ED charts and arrived at different numbers for nonurgent visits—64% and 10%, respectively; the patients themselves thought that only 16% of their problems were less than either very or fairly urgent. In a number of other studies published between 1964 and 1994, the number of ED visits characterized as "nonurgent," "inappropriate," or "not emergency" varied from 6% to 82%, depending on the definition of emergency and the method of evaluation (retrospective versus prospective).[20]

Q: If we triage "inappropriate" ED patients away, where will they go?

Preauthorization for ED visits in managed care plans was designed for several reasons, including high ED charges and nonurgent visits. It may be inappropriate, however, to call these nonurgent ED visits "inappropriate." There may be opportunities to cut costs for these ED visits, but the preauthorization concept itself is unacceptable and unworkable and should be rejected.

In a 1991 *JAMA* editorial, Dr. Arthur Kellermann points out that the problem is not inappropriate, nonurgent ED visits, but the unmet need for primary care.[21] The Graduate Medical Education Advisory Committee predicted in 1980 that increases in accessibility of ambulatory care would cause fewer nonurgent visits to EDs. We are still without national health care insurance, however, and the number of uninsured has continued to grow and currently stands at 41 million, most of whom are uninsured workers and their families.[22] Growth in ED visits has paralleled the growth in population, from 82 million visits in 1980 to 99 million in 1990, an increase of 19%. Dr. Kellermann concludes that use of hospital EDs for

nonurgent care cannot be dismissed as inappropriate, if patients do not have access to primary care elsewhere.

Patients who are triaged away from EDs may not receive any care. Follow-up information on pediatric patients from low-income, inner-city families turned away from an ED by the preauthorization process was unobtainable in a significant segment, either because they failed to keep their PCP appointment or had no telephone.[23] The 1993 GAO report on emergency departments found that patients covered by Medicaid and Medicare and uninsured patients accounted for the largest growth segment, resulting in disproportionate increases in unreimbursed ED patient care costs.[19] In addition, urban EDs had a large percentage of uninsured patients and more visits related to AIDS, alcohol, drugs, and violence. From 1985 to 1990, visits to physician offices increased 11%, while ED visits increased by more than 19%, with growth due mainly to visits by the uninsured, the elderly, and the more seriously ill patients. Several barriers to access to non-ED care were identified. These included lack of a primary care provider, no willing primary care provider because of lack of insurance or inadequate reimbursement schedules, and transportation problems.

By late 1993, 36 states were using managed care plans as part of their Medicaid programs, and it is estimated that all states will ultimately participate. The American College of Emergency Physicians has published a number of serious problems with the use of managed care health care.[24] Medicaid recipients in urban areas have limited access to outpatient care other than hospital EDs. The Medicaid Access Study Group studied alternatives to visits to the ED for Medicaid recipients for nonemergency problems in 10 cities.[25] Timely access to non-ED outpatient care is limited by financial considerations, as well as heavy patient booking, limited office hours, and not enough primary care providers in some neighborhoods. They concluded that many of the poor will have nowhere to go if outpatient care in the ED is restricted before acceptable alternatives are put into place.

Studies from large urban public hospital emergency departments identify major nonfinancial obstacles that discourage access to care outside of EDs, emphasizing that universal coverage alone will not guarantee continuity of medical care. In one study, over 60% of patients reported no regular source of care and identified barriers such as no transportation, exposure to violence, need for care after hours, dependency on others, no telephone, and lack of education.[26] In a similar ED, 16% of patients identified the ED as their regular source of care; 28% had no regular source of care and received 42% of their care in an ED; 56% identified another regular source of care, but 24% to 36% of all their recent M.D. visits were in an ED.[27] In some large urban areas, health care delivery to the poor relies heavily on public hospital emergency departments. Unless primary care sites are available to meet these needs, policies which restrict access to these EDs may adversely affect the health of these patients. Reducing the number of uninsured and underinsured patients will help but will not be the solution to this problem; demand for nonurgent care in the ED will not necessarily decline when everyone is covered by health insurance.

Q: Will ED preauthorization work to decrease ED visits?

The effectiveness of preauthorization strategies has also been questioned. Although some EDs have reported decreased visits with increased managed care penetration, it is unclear whether this is related to ED preauthorization or to effective increases in the availability of primary care. Glotzer et al, from an urban public pediatric ED reported that the majority of primary care physicians and ED staff were unhappy with ED gatekeeping policies for clinical, ethical and legal reasons.[28] They were reluctant to deny care to a child brought to the ED, and, as a result, these policies had no impact on ED utilization. These authors point out that other alternatives must be as available and at least comparable in cost. One test of whether managed care actually makes primary care available to patients who are denied access to the ED is whether those patients can in fact be persuaded to use other resources.

Warren et al., in an article entitled "Cost Containment and Quality of Life: An Experiment in Compassion for Physicians" reviewed ED visits before and after PCPs were "liberated" from gatekeeping during night hours.[29] They found that there was no increase in ED utilization or cost, but that the PCPs were very pleased to get more sleep at night.

Studies of utilization patterns among certain subsets of ED patients reveal that health insurance status and access to primary care are not the only determinants.[30] Greater availability of prenatal ultrasound, screening mammography, and childhood immunizations have not by themselves increased utilization rates for those services. Just because a system makes important services more available and affordable does not guarantee the desired utilization of those services by the public.

Q: Can emergency departments be part of the solution rather than part of the problem?

Because emergency departments have been characterized as expensive and having "inappropriate" visits, they are generally viewed as part of the health care problem. As a result, poorly designed "fixes" such as preauthorization or denial of ED care have been suggested. The proper approach is to look at EDs as part of the solution to some of the problems in the health care system.

Because of variability and unpredictability in both the volume and the timing of life-threatening emergencies, there are periods of time and situations where resources and staff are actually underutilized. Principles of economy of scale can make inclusion of nonurgent patients economically practical in these circumstances, especially if physician extenders are utilized for "nonacute" patients. If nonemergency visits could be billed at a more flexible and variable rate, inclusion of nonurgent patients could actually be cost-saving and reduce the fixed costs of maintaining an ED. For example, an ED with a "fast track," or urgent-care component, might contract with a managed-care Medicaid program to provide low-cost services aimed at getting patients referred into primary care. Such a contract would be attractive to an ED because it would cover patients who present for care, and it would be attractive to a managed-care organization, because prevention and primary care referrals reduce the long-term costs of providing care for these patients.

Emergency departments provide the safety net for the health care system and will continue to function in this critical role regardless of preauthorization or other policy changes. However, policies that characterize EDs as part of the problem jeopardize this safety net and will risk unintended adverse long-term consequences for the health of many citizens. In a 1994 *JAMA* editorial, Kellermann says we should not penalize patients for not following rules when these rules do not take into account any nonfinancial problems such as lack of transportation. A system of health care that meets the patients' needs must instead be fashioned, and current problems of restricted access must be resolved.[31] Patients, hospitals, and emergency care providers are currently being punished by a system which does not acknowledge the reality of people's lives, or the realities of health care delivery, or the scope of the problem. Policy which integrates ED treatment more fully into an expanded and more accessible system of outpatient care will improve the health care system, and ensure that patients are not turned away from the ED (or any other source of care) without receiving diagnosis and treatment. The ED can be a valuable link in case finding and referral of preventable conditions, and could thus, in the long run, reduce medical care and social expenditures.

Cost does not have to be a deterrent to such policy. Hospital ED charges are high because they include dollar margins for buffering of large amounts of uncompensated care. Charges per patient would decrease if universal coverage were available, and there were no need to compensate for the patients who are uninsured and underinsured.

Current practices of preauthorization, in situations where the patient must legally be seen whether or not authorization is obtained, are counterproductive since they encourage cost shifting and thus increase the charges per patient. Retrospective chart reviews are clearly inadequate for evaluating whether or not there was a true emergency. Better solutions are needed.

Establishing adjacent fast tracks or urgent clinic sites which are open until midnight and on weekends and are immediately available to patients who present to the ED for episodic care reduces per patient charges and costs. Roles for nurse practitioners and physician assistants should be explored as a further means of lowering cost and raising efficiency in the care of nonurgent patients.

Cost and charge issues are not the only avenues to pursue in making emergency medicine part of the solution. Emergency physicians are working to organize multiple EDs and design a computer medical record database for large groups of Medicaid recipients, in order to link them all together with a primary care office network.[32] This effort links EDs and primary care networks in an effective partnership, working together to take good care of patients. Another possibility is that home telephone advice for patients, delivered before they present to the ED for care, might be examined as a part of an insurance company benefit, but it must be structured very carefully to direct patients to appropriate sites for care, rather than to provide second-rate and superficial diagnosis and treatment. Telephone advice should be protocol driven with medical quality assurance/quality improvement methods in place, in order to limit the serious legal liabilities which could arise from careless design or implementation.

In the recent national health care discussions, emergency physicians engaged in the debate over specialty care versus primary care. However, emergency medicine provides both types of care, 24 hours a day for anyone in need. Emergency medicine provides episodic and unscheduled care, which includes true emergency care, a specialty of its own, as well as primary care for a large number of patients who lack realistic alternatives. We are on the frontline of health care delivery and are the real gatekeepers for both specialty and primary care, in the hospital and in the community. The problems that are currently occurring under managed care are not monolithic, and with a little effort, reasonable solutions can be achieved that will benefit patient and provider alike. Maryland, for example, has recently legislated that patients should not be required to seek authorization for an emergency department visit.[33] In the next few years, as managed-care organizations grow and consolidate throughout all parts of the country, emergency medicine practitioners will have many opportunities to demonstrate leadership and provide proactive solutions to cost containment needs, while continuing to improve access and quality of care for our patients.

NOTES

1. Public Law 99-272, signed into law in 1986.
2. Hill H. Preauthorization for Care. In Henry G, (ed.). *Emergency Medicine Risk Management: A Comprehensive Review.* Dallas: American College of Emergency Physicians, 1991.
3. Grady B. Trouble at the gate. *Texas Med* 1994; 36–8.

4. Lydon D, Hamilton FN, Ross CS. Knocking at the gate: Gatekeeper system creates liability concerns for ED physicians. *Emerg Legal Brief* 1994; 5:73–8.

5. Cordover M. What's new with OBRA: Part II. *Emerg Depart Law* 1995; 7:15.

6. Baker DW, Stevens CD, Brook RH. Patients who leave a public hospital emergency department without being seen by a physician. *JAMA* 1991; 266:1085–90.

7. Bindman AB, Grumbach K, Keane D, et al. Consequences of queuing for care at a public hospital emergency department. *JAMA* 1991; 266:1091–6.

8. Stock LM, Bradley GE, Lewis RJ, et al. Patients who leave emergency departments without being seen by a physician: Magnitude of the problem in Los Angeles County. *Ann Emerg Med* 1994; 23:294–8.

9. ACEP. Measures to deal with emergency department overcrowding. *Ann Emerg Med* 1990; 19:944–5.

10. Derlet RW, Kinser D, Ray L, et al. Prospective identification and triage of nonemergency patients out of an emergency department: A 5-year study. *Ann Emerg Med* 1995; 25:215–23.

11. Derlet RW, Nishio DA. Refusing care to patients who present to an emergency department. *Ann Emerg Med* 1990; 19:262–7.

12. Derlet RW, Nishio DA, Cole LM, et al. Triage of patients out of the emergency department: Three-year experience. *Am J Emerg Med* 1992; 10:195–9.

13. Derlet RW, Kinser D. The emergency department and triage of nonurgent patients. *Ann Emerg Med* 1994; 23:377–9.

14. Lowe RA, Bindman AB, Ulrich SK, et al: Refusing care to emergency department patients: Evaluation of published triage guidelines. *Ann Emerg Med* 1994; 23:286–93.

15. Birnbaum A, Gallagher EJ, Utkewicz M, et al. Failure to validate a predictive model for refusal of care to emergency department patients. *Acad Emerg Med* 1994; 1:213–7.

16. McCabe JB. What is an emergency, and who wants to know? *Ann Emerg Med* 1994; 23:872–3.

17. ACEP *State Stat*, January 1995.

18. ACEP. Landmark state legislation passes. *ACEP Newsletter* 1995; 14:1.

19. US General Accounting Office: Emergency Departments unevenly affected by growth and change in patient use. Washington DC: GAO, 1993.

20. Foldes SS, Fischer LR, Kaminsky K. What is an emergency? The judgments of two physicians. *Ann Emerg Med* 1994; 23:833–40.

21. Kellermann AL. Too sick to wait. *JAMA* 1991; 266:1123–5.

22. Current Population Survey, 1994. Washington DC: Bureau of the Census.

23. Shaw KN, Selbst SM, Gill FM. Indigent children who are denied care in the emergency department. *Ann Emerg Med* 1990; 19:59–62.

24. Maclean CB. Medicaid managed care and emergency care. *Ann Emerg Med* 1993; 22:116–8.

25. Kellermann AL. Access of medicaid recipients to outpatient care. *NEJM* 1194; 20:1426–30.

26. Rask KJ, Williams MV, Parker RM, et al. Obstacles predicting lack of a regular provider and delays in seeking care for patients at an urban public hospital. *JAMA* 1994; 24:1931–3.

27. Baker, DW, Stevens CD, Brook RH. Regular source of ambulatory care and medical care utilization by patients presenting to a public hospital emergency department. *JAMA* 1994; 271:1909–12.

28. Glotzer D, Sager A, Socolar D, et al. Prior approval in the pediatric emergency room. *Pediatrics* 1991; 88:674–80.

29. Warren BH, Bell PL, Isikoff S, et al. Cost containment and quality of life. *Arch Intern Med* 1991; 151:741–4.

30. Hand R, Koshy M, Dorn L, et al. Health insurance status and the use of emergency and other outpatient services by adults with sickle cell disease. *Ann Emerg Med* 1995; 25:224–9.

31. Kellermann AL: Nonurgent emergency department visits. *JAMA* 1994; 271:1953–4.

32. Robert Doe, M.D. Personal communication.

33. ACEP *State Stat*, April 1995.

33

Health Promotion and Disease Prevention in the Emergency Department

RICHARD M. GOLDBERG
EDWARD BERNSTEIN
DEIDRE ANGLIN
MIRIAM COTLER
RICK HAYNE
ROOSEVELT TRAVNITZ

CHAPTER SUMMARY

Although health care expenditures in the United States have more than tripled from the $250 billion spent in 1980, there has been a progressive deterioration in the delivery of care to the nation's uninsured and underinsured. Existing Medicaid programs and the services of public institutions have been sharply curtailed in recent years as government agencies at all levels attempt to deal with severe budget deficits.[1,2] As a result, a substantial segment of the population has become medically disenfranchised. Approximately 40% of the population lacks adequate financial protection from medical expenses. Nearly half of the elderly are not covered for long-term needs.[3,4] Emergency departments (EDs) have become, de facto, major providers of primary care. Additionally, many patients now seen in EDs have needs for public and preventive health services not previously felt to be within the scope of the specialty of emergency medicine, either practically or philosophically.[5–9] Recent studies and editorials have suggested that the province of emergency medicine may indeed be expanded to accommodate these needs,[7–17] but little has been written regarding a format for such a process.

We have attempted to address this question by considering what additional health services could be provided by EDs to their medically indigent and underserved populations (defined as all patients with Medicaid and self-pay insurance status as well as all patients over the age of 65). Using criteria of (1) low cost of administration, (2) ease of implementation, (3) potential impact, and (4) relevance of service to population served, we identified five areas as being suitable for development within a general protocol: vaccinations, screening services, expanded social services, educational materials, and provision of medications. In this chapter, we present a discussion of elements of the protocol as well as a general plan for its implementation.

VACCINATIONS

The impact of vaccinations as a public health measure has been profound. With the exception of safe water, no other modality, including antibiotics, has had such a major effect on mortality reduction.[18] Moreover, vaccines are economical, with highly favorable benefit-cost ratios having been demonstrated.[19] Yet there is evidence that current strategies for providing access to immunizations are insufficient. Up to 50% of children less than age 5, regardless of insurance status, are not adequately immunized.[20,21] This fact is not without practical consequences. The measles epidemic of 1989–1991, resulting in more than 55,000 cases and 11,000 hospitalizations, was due to underimmunization.[22,23] The Centers for Disease Control and Prevention (CDC) have established a national goal of achieving 90%

immunization coverage among 2-year-olds by 1996.[24] In addition, the CDC recommends that people over the age of 65, as well as other high-risk individuals, be immunized with pneumococcal and influenza vaccines. Coverage goals are 80% immunization for this population.[25,26]

There are numerous references in the recent medical literature to the ED as a potential site for the routine administration of vaccinations.[10–12,17,21,27] Additionally, the CDC, in collaboration with a 35-member working group representing a broad array of public and private interests, recently published *Standards for Pediatric Immunization*. Among their guidelines is the recommendation that ". . . each encounter with a health care provider, *including an ED visit* . . . is an opportunity to screen immunization status and, if indicated, administer needed vaccines."[22]

SCREENING SERVICES

Domestic Violence

Each year in the United States, at least 1.5 million women seek medical care for injuries resulting from domestic violence, with the ED often being the initial point of assessment.[28–30] Studies have shown that between 22% and 35% of women who seek care for any reason in the ED are victims of domestic violence.[31] Those who are not identified or appropriately referred have more health problems and make more frequent visits to health care providers.[32] Moreover, failure of health care providers to respond to a victim seeking help increases her feelings of hopelessness and despair and perpetuates her sense of isolation and entrapment in the abusive relationship.[33]

It has been recommended that questions about domestic violence be part of routine screening examinations and, when indicated, appropriate assessment, documentation, safety plans and referrals be made.[30,34]

Substance Abuse

Smoking. Tobacco-related illness and death have been identified as the largest public health epidemic of our time.[35] Several studies support the value of brief clinical interventions for tobacco use. These interventions include routine assessment of tobacco use in all patients, cessation counseling, prescribing pharmacological aids, distribution of educational materials, and the provision of follow-up support.[36–38] The ED can serve as an important point of access to these interventions.

Alcohol and drug abuse. One in every ten deaths in the United States is related to alcohol, and 20% of the total national health expenditure for hospital care is spent on alcohol-related illness.[39] Additionally, the economic cost of drug abuse to society has been estimated to be over $58 billion.[40] As with tobacco, there is evidence that brief interventions by physicians and referral for alcohol and drug treatment have the potential for positive impact.[41–43] The use of routine screening questions in the ED for the detection of alcoholism and drug abuse has been recommended.[10,16]

Infectious Diseases, Sexually Transmitted Diseases (STDS), Tuberculosis (TB), and Human Immunodeficiency Virus (HIV)

Recent data document the need for increased vigilance in the detection of STDs. The CDC in 1991 reported more than 620,000 cases of gonorrhea and 128,000 cases of syphilis.[44] Likewise, there is an upward trend in the number of cases of TB, with more than 26,000 cases being reported in 1992.[45,46] Furthermore, in 1992, there were more than 47,000 new cases of AIDS.[47] Studies on the seroprevalence of HIV in ED populations indicate a range of 0.4 to 14.6%.[48–51]

It is well beyond the ability of the average ED to pursue fully the diagnosis of these diseases in all individuals potentially at risk. However, at least some if not all of the following measures may be considered: (1) Screening questions for symptoms of STD; (2) treatment of STD contacts when possible; (3) screening questions for AIDS, with provision for routine or anonymous testing; (4) screening questions for tuberculosis with application of skin tests and chest x-rays for individuals at high risk; (5) provision of educational materials regarding the above diseases when appropriate.

Cervical Cancer

Hogness et al. reported on 706 women in an urban county hospital-based ED who had Pap smears added to their pelvic examinations. They concluded that there was a high prevalence of cervical dysplasia and advised routine Pap screening in urban EDs as a component of a cervical cancer control program.[13]

Breast Cancer

Breast cancer is now the second leading cause of cancer deaths in women.[52] Studies have confirmed the effectiveness of clinical breast examination and screening mammography in reducing breast cancer mortality.[53–55] The National Cancer Institute now recommends monthly breast self-examination and regular clinical breast examination for all women, and annual mammography for women between the ages of 50 and 75.[56] EDs can aid in surveillance efforts by identifying women in need of these services, providing educational materials and facilitating appropriate referrals.

Hypertension

Studies indicate that substantial numbers of patients presenting to the ED have undetected hypertension.[57–59] Most EDs should be able to implement a detection, counseling and referral program.

SOCIAL SERVICES

Social services rendered in the ED appear to follow a trimodal distribution, with children requiring services dealing with abuse and neglect, young adult patients requiring assistance with drug abuse and crisis intervention, and elderly patients requiring financial and placement services.[60,61] Several studies have demonstrated the cost-effectiveness of having social workers staff the ED on a full-time basis: (1) they are able to divert some admissions previously necessitated by social and marginal medical reasons; (2) they are able to arrange for assistance benefits, medication programs, home care services, and shelter placement; (3) they provide counseling services for victims of rape and domestic violence, as well as assessment and referral for patients with a variety of emotional problems; and (4) they reduce substan-

tially the time demands on ED staff who would otherwise be attempting to provide many of these services.[60–64]

EDUCATIONAL PAMPHLETS

Educational materials in the form of pamphlets can be obtained and distributed at very little cost on a variety of topics relating to public health and preventive services.

DISTRIBUTION OF FREE MEDICATIONS

The Senate Special Committee on Aging recently reported that 84% of poor or near-poor elderly Americans do not qualify for Medicaid prescription drug coverage and must pay for their medications. These patients, numbering approximately 10 million, are eligible for a variety of free drug programs.

Awareness of these programs is low, however, and many patients have experienced long waiting times before receiving their medications. The Pharmaceutical Manufacturers' Association has responded to this report by compiling a directory of 59 available programs from 44 companies and has established a toll-free number for information on access.[64] Information on these programs can be provided by ED staff. Additionally, a number of medications can be dispensed in limited amounts from EDs at relatively little cost.

PLAN OF IMPLEMENTATION

Although portions of the protocol may be implemented with existing personnel in some EDs, it is likely that full implementation will require a team of designated personnel, to include the ED physician (EP), a needs assessment nurse (NAN), and a medical social worker (MSW). The latter two positions would be staffed 7 days per week, with coverage provided at the very least during peak hours of patient flow. All patients within the target population would be surveyed with a Needs Assessment Form (NAF) on arrival in the ED (Figures 33-1, 33-2). Forms would be reviewed by the NAN, who would then direct implementation of the protocol in the following manner (Figure 33-3).

Figure 33-1 Protocol Flow Sheet

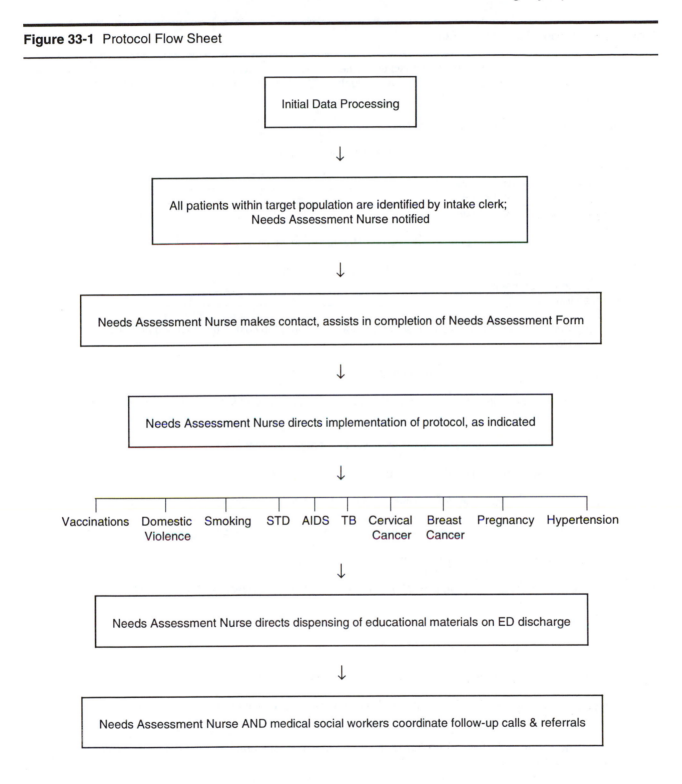

Figure 33-2 Needs Assessment Form

We feel it is very important that you receive basic public health care. Your answers to these questions will enable us to provide you some basic services. Your answers are voluntary. This form is confidential and does not become a part of your medical record.

1. Has your child had the following vaccinations:

Vaccinations	Don't know	No	Yes	If yes, when
Hepatitis B				_____
DPT (Diphtheria, Pertussis, Tetanus)				_____
Haemophilus influenzae Type B				_____
MMR (Measles, Mumps, Rubella)				_____

2. If you are more than 65 years of age, have you had the following vaccinations:

Vaccinations	Don't know	No	Yes	If yes, when
Pneumococcal pneumonia				_____
Influenza virus				_____

3. If you are more than age 65, have you ever not been able to afford the cost of medications prescribed for you?
   Yes_____   No_____

4. (a) Have you ever been injured or threatened by someone in your home?   Yes_____   No_____

   (b) Have you ever been injured or threatened by an intimate partner outside your home (i.e., boyfriend)?
       Yes_____   No_____

5. Do you smoke at all or are you exposed to smokers in your home or work place?   Yes_____   No_____

6. Have you ever had an alcohol or drug abuse problem: Yes_____   No_____

7. Have you been drinking or using drugs within the past 24 hours?   Yes_____   No_____

8. Have you recently noticed any sores or abnormal discharge from your penis or vagina?   Yes_____   No_____

9. Are you at any risk for acquiring AIDS infection?   Yes_____   No_____

10. Have you experienced fevers, cough, or weight loss for more than three weeks?   Yes_____   No_____

11. For women:

   A. Have you had a Pap Smear within the past year?   Yes_____   No_____

   B. Do you examine your breasts for lumps regularly?   Yes_____   No_____

   C. If you are over age 40, have you had a breast examination by a doctor within the past year?
       Yes_____   No_____

   D. If you are between the ages of 50 and 75, have you had a mammogram within the past two years?
       Yes_____   No_____

   E. Are you pregnant?   Yes_____   No_____   Unsure_____

Figure 33-3 Assessment and Services Protocol

I. VACCINATIONS

The needs assessment nurse (NAN) will assess vaccination status. For patients in need of vaccinations:

A.   Appropriate information pamphlets will be distributed and informed consent will be obtained.

B.   Vaccines will be administered according to the schedule given below. Patients for whom immunization status is unknown or indeterminate will receive immunizations appropriate for age.

C.   A vaccination will not be administered to patients appearing acutely ill or who have fever greater than 101°F.

D.   A vaccination will not be administered if there is a history of allergy or severe reaction to the vaccine.

II. SCREENING

Domestic violence: For patients identified as being victims of domestic violence:

A.   The emergency department physician (EP) will assess for specific injuries, documenting them in the medical record, drawing body maps, and obtaining photographs when indicated;

B.   The medical social worker (MSW) and EP will assess the patient with regard to:
(1) Emotional state (suicide/homicide risk); (2)Relationship with perpetrator; (3) Involvement of children; (4) Assessment of lethality; (5) Short- and long-term risk for violence; and (6) Short- and long-term plans for safety, including referral to shelter.

C.   NAN will notify police if legally mandated or requested by patient.

D.   The MSW will dispense appropriate educational materials.

Smoking: For patients identified as being either active smokers or having passive exposure to smoke, the NAN and EP will:

A.   Assess readiness to stop;

B.   Offer educational materials, prescription for nicotine patches, or enrollment in cessation programs as indicated by assessment.

Alcohol & drugs: For patients responding either "yes" to question 1 or to both questions 1 and 2:

A.   The EP will conduct focused examination as indicated;

B.   The MSW will assess, distribute educational materials and make referrals as indicated.

STD: For patients with suspected STD:

A.   The EP will conduct focused examination and treat as indicated;

B.   The NAN will conduct follow-up interview to provide educational materials, and arrange for treatment of contacts, as well as notification of public health department.

AIDS: For patients at risk for AIDS:

A.   The EP will conduct a focused examination, with laboratory evaluation and referral as indicated;

B.   The NAN will distribute educational materials.

Tuberculosis: For patients with possible tuberculosis:

A.   The EP will conduct a focused examination, including skin tests and x-rays as indicated;

B.   The NAN will coordinate the follow-up in terms of educational materials, reading of skin tests and liaison with the public health department.

Cervical Cancer: If patient is overdue for cervical Pap smear:

A.   The EP or NAN will obtain Pap smear;

B.   The NAN will dispense educational material and ensure appropriate follow-up with test results.

Breast Cancer:

A.   The NAN will instruct all women unfamiliar with the technique of breast self-examination;

B.   All women over age 40 who have not had a clinical breast examination or mammogram within the past year will receive appropriate referral;

C.   Educational material on breast cancer will be dispensed to all women.

Continued

Figure 33-3 Assessment and Services Protocol *(continued)*

Pregnancy: If patient may be pregnant or is pregnant and not currently receiving prenatal care:
A. The EP will order a pregnancy test, also conducting a focused examination if indicated by presenting complaint;
B. The EP will dispense a prescription for vitamins with iron and folic acid;
C. The NAN will dispense educational material and refer to a prenatal clinic.

Hypertension:
A. The NAN will identify patients as being hypertensive if, on two separate readings, 30 minutes apart, patients less than age 50 have systolic blood pressure greater than or equal to 140 mmHg. systolic or 90 mmHg. diastolic; for patients 50 years of age or more, systolic blood pressure of 160 mmHg. or greater and diastolic blood pressure of 95 mmHg. or greater;
B. The EP will conduct a focused examination with treatment and referral as indicated.
C. The NAN will dispense educational material.

III. SOCIAL SERVICES
The MSW will be available to implement specific aspects of the protocol as indicated above. Additionally, assessments by the MSW may also be requested for patients needing financial assistance, assistance benefits, shelter, emotional counseling/crisis intervention, evaluation for child or elder neglect, rape counseling, or home care.

_____ Financial assistance
_____ Assistance benefits
_____ Shelter
_____ Emotional counseling/crisis intervention
_____ Domestic violence
_____ Substance abuse
_____ Child/elder neglect
_____ Home care
_____ Rape counseling

IV. EDUCATIONAL MATERIALS
Educational materials on the following topics will be distributed, as indicated above:

Vaccinations	Domestic Violence
Smoking	Substance Abuse
STD	AIDS
Tuberculosis	Cervical Cancer
Breast Cancer	Pregnancy
Hypertension	

V. MEDICATIONS
1. The following medications will be available for dispensing at the direction of the EP:
First generation cephalosporin
Prenatal vitamins with iron and folic acid
Erythromycin preparation
Phenytoin
Oral steroid agent
Topical steroid agent
Nonsteroidal antiinflammatory agent
Antihypertensive
Oral narcotic analgesic
Beta agonist inhaler
Antihistamine

2. The NAN will assist elderly patients in gaining access to free medication programs.

Vaccinations

Administration of vaccines would follow standard guidelines with regard to timing, informed consent and associated educational materials. As per current recommendations, patients with mild febrile illness (less than 101° orally) and patients with unknown vaccination status would be administered vaccines according to schedule.[22]

Screening Services

Domestic violence. Patients identified as being victims of domestic violence would be assessed by the NAN, MSW, and EP with regard to the following considerations: (1) emotional state, including suicidal and homicidal risk; (2) specific injuries; (3) relationship of perpetrator; (4) involvement of children; (5) assessment of lethality; (6) short-term and long-term risk for violence; (7) immediate plans for safety, including overnight stay in ED if indicated; and (8) long-term plans for leaving the abusive environment, including referral to a shelter. As indicated, all injuries would be described (including photographs, body maps, etc.), treated, police would be notified if legally mandated or requested by the patient, educational materials would be distributed and appropriate referrals would be made.

Smoking. Patients identified as either being active smokers or having passive exposure to smoke would be identified, counseled by the NAN and EP, and an assessment for readiness to change would be made. Interventions ranging from dispensing educational materials to expanded discussion of benefits and costs to enrollment in cessation programs would then be offered.

Alcohol and drugs. Patients would be screened using the following questions: (1) Have you ever had an alcohol or a drug abuse problem? (2) Have you been using alcohol or drugs of potential abuse within the past 24 hours? Patients answering affirmatively to question number 1 or both questions 1 and 2 would have an assessment by the MSW, with distribution of educational materials and referral for treatment as indicated.

Infectious diseases. Patients would be asked screening questions regarding STDs, risk of AIDS, and TB. Patients with possible STDs would receive a focused examination by the EP and follow-up by the NAN in terms of educational materials, contact of public health agencies and provision for treatment of contacts. Patients at risk for AIDS would receive a focused EP examination and appropriate laboratory evaluation, including provision for anonymous testing if requested. Educational materials would be distributed by the NAN. Patients at risk for TB would receive a focused EP examination, skin tests and x-rays as indicated, and follow-up coordinated by the NAN in terms of educational materials, readings of skin tests, appropriate referral and liaison with the public health department.

Screening services for women. Women within the target population would be asked screening questions regarding Pap smear and mammogram, ability to perform breast self-examinations, and possibility of pregnancy. Women overdue for Pap smears would have them performed in the ED, either by the EP or NAN. Women unfamiliar with the technique of self-examination of the breast would be offered instruction in a private examination room by the NAN. All women over age 40 would be referred for annual clinical breast examination, and all women between the ages of 50 and 75 would be referred for mammography if no such examination has been performed within the past year. Appropriate educational materials on cervical and breast cancer would be dispensed.

Pregnancy tests would be performed on women suspected of being pregnant. All women with positive tests as well as all women known to be pregnant but not receiving prenatal care would be given appropriate educational materials, a prescription for vitamins, iron and folic acid, and a referral to a prenatal clinic for follow-up.

Hypertension. Adult patients (age 18 or older) within the target population would have blood pressure measurement by the NAN and would be considered hypertensive if, on two separate readings, 30 minutes apart, they exceeded the American Heart Association criteria of (1) for age <50, a systolic blood pressure of ≥ 140 mmHg or diastolic blood pressure of ≥ 90 mmHg, or (2) for ≥ 50 years, a systolic blood pressure of ≥ 160 mmHg or diastolic pressure of ≥ 95 mmHg.[65] All hypertensive patients would be assessed and treated by the EP as indicated. Those patients with no prior history of hypertension would receive appropriate referral and educational materials.

Social Services

Based on the NAF as well as any other information obtained during the ED visit, the MSW would offer patients a variety of services including financial assistance, assistance with benefits, shelter referral, emotional counseling and crisis intervention, rape counseling, assessments regarding domestic violence, child or elder neglect, substance abuse, and assistance obtaining home care services.

Educational Materials

As indicated, educational materials would be dispensed to patients on such topics as domestic violence, smoking cessation, alcohol and other substance abuse, seat belts, drinking and driving, bicycle and motorcycle safety, TB, STDs, AIDS, cancer prevention, prenatal care, hypertension, and risk factors for coronary artery disease and stroke.

Dispensing of and Provision for Medications

Patients within the target population would have any of the following medications dispensed from the ED in sufficient amounts to constitute a course of treatment: a first-generation cephalosporin, an erythromycin preparation, a nonsteroidal antiinflammatory agent, prenatal vitamins with iron and folic acid, an antihypertensive agent, an oral narcotic agent, phenytoin, an oral steroid agent, a beta-agonist inhaler, a steroid topical preparation, and an antihistamine. Additionally, elderly patients identified by the NAN as being unable to afford the cost of their prescribed medications would be supplied with information on applicable medication assistance programs.

COST CONSIDERATIONS

The cost of implementing the protocol will depend primarily on the level of staffing assigned to it. Harrington recently reported that the cost of providing MSW coverage for 15 hours on a daily basis (2.8 FTE) in a Massachusetts ED was approximately $160,000, including benefits.[62] The cost of providing a registered nurse to fill the role of NAN for 12 hours on a daily basis (2.5 FTE) would be approximately $100,000, including benefits, in Southern California.[66] The cost of dispensing medications listed in the protocol is difficult to estimate. If, however, five courses of antibiotics and one course of every other medication listed were dispensed on a daily basis, the approximate cost to the hospital would be $43,000.[67] The cost of vaccines and educational materials is assumed to be negligible in most areas of the country. Overall administrative costs are also assumed to be negligible though this may not be the case if data-gathering is required or if more comprehensive services are offered.

Balanced against these expenses are to be considered a number of potential savings. Recent studies have shown that MSW services provided in the ED can result in a reduction in hospitalization for marginal medical reasons, an increase in compensible ancillary services rendered, and an increase in compensible consultation charges generated.[60-63] It has been estimated that the combination of expenses saved and revenues received may approximate or even exceed MSW salaries.[62]

In the absence of actual cost-benefit studies, the extent to which the cost of a NAN or free medication program would be offset by a long-term reduction in the amount of uncompensated care delivered is unknown. However, the potential for long-term savings is considerable. The facility cost, for instance, of an ED visit in Southern California may range from $40 to $1,310 depending on the level of service rendered. Likewise, the cost of a medical bed may range from $700 to $1,500, a telemetry bed from $1,050 to $3,000, and an intensive care bed from $2,350 to $6,000 per day.[68]

Available data indicate that elderly patients and patients with lower socioeconomic status are more likely to use the ED as their primary care resource. When hospitalized, these patients have been shown to stay up to 27% longer and incur charges up to 13% higher than other patients.[69-71] Such data do suggest that attempts by ED personnel to deal more comprehensively with the public health and preventive services needs of this patient population could help mitigate the costs of future ED visits and hospitalizations.

As a final cost consideration, the scope and success of the protocol within a given community may well depend on two factors. The first is the adequacy of reimbursement for at least some of the services rendered. The second is the ability of the ED to develop adequate linkages to primary care, home care, and social service resources. Without such linkages, patients will continue to cycle back to the ED, with ever-increasing cost to the system.[5,72,73]

CONCLUSION

In 1991, Pane et al, presented their findings on the extent to which medically indigent patients rely on the ED as their source of primary care. They state, among their conclusions, that until such time as major health care reform is achieved, "the overloaded emergency medical care system will continue to serve as the safety net for many of our country's health care and social ills that are being addressed inadequately in other sectors."[5]

There is now ample documentation of the degree to which the health care needs of this large segment of our population are inadequately addressed: Fifty percent of children less than the age of 5 are underimmunized;[19] homeless children have higher rates of dental decay, anemia, and decreased visual acuity;[74,75] lack of insurance is the strongest predictor of women between the ages of 45 to 64 not getting a Pap smear or breast examination;[76] homeless adults have increased rates of TB and pneumonia from pneumococcus influenza and haemophalus influenzae;[77] a substantial percentage of welfare women of childbearing age have iron-deficiency anemia;[24] and minorities suffer inequities in health care such that the death rates for heart disease, hypertension, and diabetes are higher for blacks than for whites and the life-expectancy for blacks is 6 years shorter.[78] Likewise, Hispanic women suffer a higher incidence of cancer of the cervix for reasons believed due to inadequate access to care.[79,80]

A new and major concern is the fact that the number of homeless people is increasing each year.[81]

Furthermore, they are undergoing a dramatic demographic shift with growing numbers of young adults and families with children among their ranks.[82,83]

As part of the reaction to this crisis in the delivery of health care to the medically indigent, a number of recent studies and editorials have appeared suggesting that EPs can include within their scope of practice the provision of certain public health and primary care services.[7-17] The protocol presented is an attempt to develop a formal process by which this may be done. A number of prominent health concerns, including nutrition and obesity, family planning, environmental health, physical fitness, oral health, and injury prevention are not addressed. Despite these limitations, the protocol is meant to be broadly generic and adaptable in its elements to a variety of practice settings, patient populations and cost restraints. Ultimately, however, the protocol assumes that the ED is well integrated within a comprehensive system of health care delivery. This implies adequate provisions for reimbursement of services rendered and adequate resources within the community for referrals and linkages to be made.

NOTES

1. *Statistical Abstract of the United States: 1994,* 114th ed. Washington, DC: U.S. Bureau of the Census; 1994.
2. Ginzberg E: Improving health care for the poor: Lessons from the 1980s. *JAMA* 1994; 271:464–7.
3. Enthoven A, Kronick R. A consumer-choice health plan for the 1990s: Universal health insurance in a system designed to promote quality and economy. *NEJM* 1989; 320:29–37, 94–101.
4. Ginzberg E. Medical care for the poor: No magic bullets. *JAMA* 1988; 259:3309–11.
5. Pane GA, Farner MC, Salness KA. Health care access problems of medically-indigent emergency department walk-in patients. *Ann Emerg Med* 1991; 20:730–3.
6. Davis JE. National initiative for care of the medically needy. *JAMA* 1988; 259:3171–3.
7. Baker DW, Stevens CD, Brook RH. Patients who leave a public hospital emergency department without being seen by a physician: Causes and consequences. *JAMA* 1991; 266:1091–6.
8. U.S. General Accounting Office. *Emergency Departments: Unevenly Affected by Growth and Change in Patient Use.* Washington, DC: U.S. Printing Office, 1993.

9. Lowe RA, Young GP, Reinke B, White JD, Auerbach PS. Indigent health care in emergency medicine: An academic perspective. *Ann Emerg Med* 1991; 20:790–4.

10. Bernstein E, Goldfrank LR, Kellermann AL, Hargarten SW, Jui J, Fish SS, et al. A public health approach to emergency medicine: Preparing for the twenty-first century. *Acad Emerg Med* 1994; 1:277–86.

11. Rodriguez RM, Hoffman JR. Public health and the emergency department (editorial). *Emerg Med News* 1994; XVI:2,18–20.

12. Rodriguez RM, Baraff LJ. Emergency department immunization of the elderly with pneumococcal and influenza vaccines. *Ann Emerg Med* 1993; 22:1729–32.

13. Hogness CG, Engelstead LP, Linch NM, Schorr KA. Cervical cancer screening in an urban emergency department. *Ann Emerg Med* 1992; 21:933–9.

14. Ernst AA, Romolo R, Nick T. Emergency department screening for syphilis in pregnant women without prenatal care. *Ann Emerg Med* 1993; 22:781–5.

15. Hibbs JR, Ceglowski WS, Goldberg M, Kauffman F. Emergency department-based surveillance for syphilis during an outbreak in Philadelphia. *Ann Emerg Med* 1993; 22:1286–90.

16. Green M, Setchell J, Hanes P, Stiff G, Touquet R, Priest R. Management of alcohol-abusing patients in accident and emergency departments. *J Royal Soc Med* 1993; 83:393–5.

17. Polis MA, Davey VJ, Collins ED, Smith JP, Rosenthal RE, Kaslow RA. The emergency department as part of a successful strategy for increasing adult immunization. *Ann Emerg Med* 1988; 17:1016–18.

18. Plotkin SL, Plotkin SA, Rodewald LE, Szilagye PG, Humiston SG, Raubertas RF. A short history of vaccination. In Plotkin SA, Mortimer EA Jr. (eds.). *Vaccines.* Philadelphia: Saunders, 1988, pp. 1–7.

19. Hinman AR: Public health considerations. In Plotkin SA, Mortimer EA Jr. (eds.). *Vaccines.* Philadelphia: Saunders, 1988, pp. 587–611.

20. Humiston SG, Rodewald LE, Szilagyi RG, Raubertas RF, Rochmann KJ, et al. Decision rules for predicting vaccination status of pre-school age emergency department patients. *J Peds* 1993; 123:887–92.

21. Lindegren ML, Atkinson WL, Farizo KM, Stehr-Green PA. Measles vaccination in pediatric emergency departments during a measles outbreak. *JAMA* 1993; 270:2185–9.

22. Ad Hoc Working Group for the Development of Standards for Pediatric Immunization Practices. Standards for pediatric immunization practices. *JAMA* 1993; 269:1817–22.

23. The National Vaccine Advisory Committee. The Measles Epidemic: The Problems, Barriers, and Recommendations. *JAMA* 1991; 266:1547–52.

24. U.S. Department of Health and Human Services. *Healthy People 2000. National Health Promotion and Disease Prevention Objectives.* Washington, DC: Public Health Service; 1990. U.S. Department of Health and Human Services Publication PHS 91-50213.

25. Centers for Disease Control. Pneumococcal polysaccharide vaccine. *MMWR* 1989; 38:64–76.

26. Centers for Disease Control. Prevention and control of influenza. *MMWR* 1991; 40:1–15.

27. Bell LM, Lopez NI, Pinto-Martin J, Casey R, Gill FM. Potential impact of linking an emergency department and hospital-affiliated clinics to immunize pre-school-aged children. *Pediatrics* 1994; 93:99–103.

28. Flitcraft A. Physicians and domestic violence: Challenges for prevention. *Health Affairs* 1993; 12:154–61.

29. McLeer SV, Anwar R. Education is not enough: A system of failure in protecting battered women. *Ann Emerg Med* 1989; 18:651–3.

30. American Medical Association Diagnostic and Treatment Guidelines on Domestic Violence: *Arch Fam Med* 1992; 1:39–47.

31. Warshaw C. Domestic violence: Challenges to medical practice. *J Women's Health* 1993; 2:73–80.

32. Campbell JC, Pliska MJ, Taylor W, Sheridan D. Battered women's experiences in the emergency department. *J Emergency Nursing* 1994; 20:280–8.

33. Randall T. Domestic violence intervention calls for more than treating injuries. *JAMA* 1992; 264:939–40.

34. Council on Scientific Affairs, American Medical Association. Violence against women: Relevance for medical practitioners. *JAMA* 1992; 267:3184–9.

35. Whitlock EP. Routine smoking cessation intervention in healthcare systems (epitome). *West J Med* 1994; 161:64.

36. Duncan C, Stein MJ, Cummings SR. Staff involvement and special follow-up time increase physicians' counseling about smoking cessation: A controlled trial. *Am J Public Health* 1991; 81:899–901.

37. Rollnick S, Kinnersley P, Stott N. Methods of helping patients with behaviour change. *BMJ* 1993; 307:188–190.

38. Hollis JV, Lichtenstein EL, Vogt TM, Stevens VJ, Biglan A. Nurse-assisted counseling for smokers in primary care. *Ann Intern Med* 1993; 118:521–5.

39. Cyr MG, Wartman SA. The effectiveness of routine screening questions in the detection of alcoholism. *JAMA* 1988; 259:51–4.

40. NIDA. *Drug Abuse Treatment: An Economic Approach to Addressing the Drug Problem in America.* Washington, DC: ADAMHA, 1991.

41. Miller WR. The effectiveness of treatment for substance abuse: Reasons for optimism. *J Subst Abuse Treat* 1992; 9:93–102.

42. Walsh D, Hingson RW, Merrigan DM, Levenson SM, Coffman GA. The impact of a physician's warning on recovery after alcoholism treatment. *JAMA* 1992; 267:663–7.

43. Mayfield D, McLeod G, Hall P. The CAGE questionnaire: Validation of a new alcoholism screening instrument. *Am J Psychiatry* 1974; 131:10,1121–3.

44. Centers for Disease Control. Summary of Notifiable Diseases, United States, 1991. *MMWR* 1992; 40:1–55.

45. Centers for Disease Control. Tuberculosis morbidity, 1992. *MMWR* 1993; 42:363.

46. Cantwell MF, Snider DE, Cauthen GM, Onorato IM. Epidemiology of tuberculosis in the United States, 1985 through 1992. *JAMA* 1994; 262:535–9.

47. Haverkos HW. Reported cases of AIDS: An update. *NEJM* 1993; 329:511.

48. Baker JL, Kelen GD, Sivertson KT, Quinn TC. Unsuspected human immunodeficiency virus in critically ill emergency patients. *JAMA* 1987; 257:2609.

49. Kelen GD, Fritz S, Qaqish B, et al. Unrecognized human immunodeficiency virus infection in emergency department patients. *NEJM* 1988; 318:1645.

50. Kelen GD, DiGiovianna T, Bisson L, Kalainov D, Sivertson KT, et al. Human immunodeficiency virus infection in emergency patients: Epidemiology, clinical presentations, and risk of health care workers. The Johns Hopkins experience. *JAMA* 1989; 262:516.

51. Schoenbaum EE, Webber EP. The under-perception of HIV infection in an inner city emergency room. *Am J Public Health* 1993; 328:327–35.

52. American Cancer Society. Cancer facts and figures—1989. New York:The Society,1990.

53. Shapiro S, Benet W, Strax L, Roesser R. Selection, followup and analysis in the health insurance plan study: A randomized trial with breast cancer screening. National Cancer Institute Monographs 1985; 67:65–74.

54. Tabar L, Gad A, Holmberg LH, Ljungquist V, Eklund G, et al. Reduction in mortality from breast cancer after mass screening with mammography. *Lancet* 1985; 1:829–32.

55. Verveek ALM, Hendricks JHCL, Holland R, Mravunac M, Sturmans F, et al. Reduction of breast cancer mortality through mass screening with modern mammography: First results of the Nijmegan Project, 1975–1981. *Lancet* 1984; 1:1222–4.

56. National Cancer Institute. *Working Guidelines for Early Cancer Detection.* Bethesda, MD: U.S. Department of Health and Human Services, 1987.

57. Kaszuba AL, Matanovski G, Gibson G. Evaluation of the emergency department as a site for hypertension screening. *JACEP* 1977; 7:51–5.

58. Slater RN, DaCruz DJ, Jarrett LN. Detection of hypertension in accident and emergency departments. *Arch Emerg Med* 1987; 4:7–9.

59. Hamaker JB, Baker BK, Weinberger M, Neill PJ. The emergency room and the hypertensive patient. *Med Care* 1984; 22:755–9.

60. Wrenn K, Rice N. Social-work services in an emergency department: An integral part of the health care safety net. *Acad Emerg Med* 1994; 1:247–53.

61. Brookoff D, Minniti-Hill M. Emergency department-based home care. *Ann Emerg Med* 1994; 23:1101–6.

62. Harrington DV. The ER social worker: Cost-effective, crisis-oriented discharge planning and more. *Discharge Planning Update* 1991; 11:8–11.

63. Ponto JM, Berg W. Social work services in the emergency department: A cost-benefit analysis of an extended coverage program. *Health Soc Work* 1992; 17:66–73.

64. More Awareness of Free Drug Programs for Indigent Patients is Needed, Says Senate Committee on Aging (News). *Am J Hosp Pharm* 1992; 49:2646.

65. 1984 Report of the Joint National Committee on Detection, Evaluation and Treatment of Hypertension. *Arch Intern Med* 1984; 144:1045.

66. Personal communication, Rick Hayne R.N., Nurse Manager, Department of Emergency Medicine, Saint Joseph Medical Center, Burbank, California.

67. Personal communication, Dale Wheeler, Pharm.D., Pharmacy Department, Saint Joseph Medical Center, Burbank, California.

68. Personal communication, Business Services Office, Saint Joseph Medical Center, Burbank, California.

69. Stern RS, Weissman JS, Epstein AM. The emergency department as a pathway to admission for poor and high-cost patients. *JAMA* 1991; 266:2238–43.

70. Munoz E, Laughlin A, Regan DM, Teicher I, Margolis IB, et al. The financial effects of emergency department-generated admissions under prospective payment systems. *JAMA* 1985; 254:1763–71.

71. Munoz E, Soldano R, Laughlin A, Margolis IB, Wise L. Source of admission and cost: Public hospitals face financial risk. *Am J Public Health* 1986; 76:696–7.

72. Bernstein E. National Conference to Link Primary Care, HIV, Alcohol and Drug Abuse Treatments. *Acad Emerg Med* 1992; 4:8–10.

73. Allison EJ, DeHart KL. The ultimate safety net (editorial). *Ann Emerg Med* 1991; 20:820–1.

74. Fierman AH, Creyer BP, Acker PJ, Legano L. Status of immunization and iron nutrition in New York City homeless children. *Clin Ped* 1993; 32:151–5.

75. Miller DS, Lin EHB. Children in sheltered homeless families: Reported health status. *Pediatrics* 1988; 81:668–73.

76. Braveman P, Oliva G, Miller MG, Schaaf VM, Reiter R. Women without health insurance: Links between access, poverty, ethnicity and health. *West J Med* 1988; 149:708–11.

77. O'Connell JJ. Nontuberculosis respiratory infections among the homeless. *Seminars in Respiratory Infections.* 1991; 6:247–53.

78. Council on Ethical and Judicial Affairs. Black-white disparities in health care. *JAMA* 1992; 263:2344–6.

79. Munoz E. Care for the Hispanic poor: A growing segment of American society. *JAMA* 1988; 260:2711–2.

80. Ginzberg E. Access to health care for Hispanics. *JAMA* 1991; 265:238–41.

81. Burt MR, Cohen BE. America's homeless: Numbers, characteristics and programs that serve them. Washington DC: The Urban Institute Press; 1989. Irvin Institute Report 89-3.

82. Wright JD, Weber E. *Homelessness and Health.* New York: McGraw-Hill, 1987.

83. Institute of Medicine. *Homelessness, Health and Human Needs.* Washington, DC: National Academy Press, 1988.

Index

Access, 10–11, 141
Activities of Daily Living (ADL) Scale, 191–192, 193
Addiction Severity Index (ASI), 67
Adolescent Social Action Program (ASAP):
    case studies, 265–266
    Hospital/Detention Center (H/DC) experience, 266
    role of ED providers in, 268
Advocacy, 13, 72–73, 165, 255
African Americans:
    asthma and, 152–157
    barriers to health care of, 10–11, 274
    domestic violence and, 96
    drugs and pregnancy and, 272
    sexually transmitted diseases and, 37
    smoking and, 71
    tuberculosis and, 25
    and violence
        case studies, 84–85
        causes of, 85–87
        eradicating, 90–91
        firearms, 84, 87–89
        gang activity, 84
        overview, 83–84
        role of ED and, 89
        symptoms of, 89–90
        treatment for, 90
Agency for Toxic Substances and Disease Registry
    (ATSDR), 223, 236
AIDS (Acquired Immunodeficiency Syndrome):
    case studies, 45–49
    communicating a diagnosis in an ED setting, 45–50
    cost and, 10
    discrimination and, 10
    education and, 10
    ethical dilemmas and, 10
    HIV exposure and, 9

    insurance and, 10
    as an issue common to public health and emergency
        medicine, 4, 9–10
    late diagnosis of HIV disease in women, 47
    prisoners and, 203
    risk factors for, 46
    testing, 46–47
    tuberculosis and, 24, 28
    women and, 11
Air bags, 7
Airborne exposures:
    Agency for Toxic Substances and Disease Registry
        (ATSDR), 223
    carbon monoxide, 220–221
    case studies, 219–222
    Chemical Transportation Emergency Center
        (CHEMTREC), 224
    HAZMAT teams, 224
    Material Safety Data Sheets (MSDS), 222
    Radiation Emergency Assistance Center/Training
        Site (REAC/TS), 224
    Regional Poison Control Centers, 223
    sentinel event notification system for occupational
        risks (SENSOR), 223
    sentinel health events, 222–223
Alcohol:
    Adolescent Social Action Program (ASAP), 264–269
    blood alcohol concentration (BAC), 54–55
    breath analyzer, 55
    case studies, 51–57
    as a critical public health/emergency medicine prob-
        lem, 8
    dual diagnosis and, 66–68
    and increase in violence in the ED, 130
    and legislative change, 57–59
    injuries and, 7, 52–53, 243